Can Physicians Manage the Quality and Costs of Health Care?

The Story of The Permanente Medical Group

Can Physicians Manage the Quality and Costs of Health Care?

The Story of The Permanente Medical Group

John G. Smillie, M.D.

Foreword by
Bruce J. Sams, Jr., M.D.
Executive Director (Retired)
The Permanente Medical Group, Inc.

McGraw-Hill, Inc.
New York St. Louis San Francisco Auckland Bogotá
Caracas Lisbon London Madrid Mexico Milan
Montreal New Delhi Paris San Juan São Paulo
Singapore Sydney Tokyo Toronto

Library of Congress Cataloging-in-Publication Data

Smillie, John G.
    Can physicians manage the quality and cost of health care? : the
story of The Permanente Medical Group / John G. Smillie ; foreword
by Bruce J. Sams, Jr.
        p. cm.
    Includes bibliographical references and index.
    ISBN 0-07-060886-5 :
    1. Permanente Medical Group (Oakland, Calif.) — History.   2. Kaiser-
Permanente Medical Care Program — History.   3. Health maintenance
organizations — California — History.   I. Title.
    [DNLM: 1. Permanente Medical Group (Oakland, Calif.)   2. Kaiser-
Permanente Medical Care Program.   3. Health Maintenance
Organizations — history — California.   W 275 AC2 S58c]
RA413.3.3.P37S55   1991
362.1′0425 — dc20
DNLM/DLC
for Library of Congress   91-17423
                                                                    CIP

1 2 3 4 5 6 7 8 9 0   DOC/DOC   9 7 6 5 4 3 2 1

ISBN 0-07-060886-5

*The editors for this book were Theodore C. Nardin and Barbara Toniolo, the
editing supervisor was Caroline Levine, and the production supervisor was
Donald F. Schmidt. It was set in Baskerville by McGraw-Hill's Professional
Books Group composition unit.*

In memory of
Sidney R. Garfield, M.D.
(1906-1984)
the Founder

Contents

Foreword

This history sprang from Dr. Smillie's resolve that our younger generation of Permanente physicians know of their heritage, and the lessons to be learned from it. As he began to put the book together, however, he and many of us felt that the story of Kaiser Permanente would be interesting and useful to a wide group of people outside our own ranks—especially those grappling with the problems of organizing, delivering, and financing health care.

Dr. Smillie has, therefore, written a comprehensive and scholarly history of the conception, birth, and formative years of a truly innovative model for health care delivery. Here the principles of Kaiser Permanente—which include prepayment, group practice, physician responsibility, and mutually exclusive contracting between Health Plan and Medical Group—are described and analyzed. The story is enriched and enlivened by the human side of this adventure, in which strong personalities searched for ways to reconcile their own goals with those of the overall program.

It has been my privilege to be Executive Director of The Permanente Medical Group, Inc., in the Northern California Region for the past 15 years, the era subsequent to the one described in this book. I can report that the principles of prepayment, group practice, and physician responsibility for quality and cost have been proven over and over again to be sound. Our policy of contracting exclusively with each other has bound us together as mutually supportive and mutually dependent partners. The formula is working.

For physicians the story told here is especially pertinent. It provides insights into the advantages (and challenges) of closer interaction with business, lawyers, financiers, and others who have their own interests in the health care world. The days in which physicians rendered services to patients for a fee paid totally out of the patient's pocket are long gone. Patients, except for the wealthy few, could never afford today's highly technical medicine without third-party financial help. Physicians, no matter how motivated or skilled, could not deliver this care without complex organizations to support them.

Physicians must, therefore, accept a new responsibility in addition to their traditional one of providing personal care to individual patients. They now must develop and support organizations which will facilitate the practice of high-quality medicine while providing the financing and structure necessary to make patient care available in the first place. Physicians who do not accept this new responsibility will simply be left out of the planning — and are likely to be dissatisfied with the results. This book provides proof that physicians can mold their own destiny.

At a time when more traditional health care delivery systems appear to be failing, it is comforting to realize that we are not inextricably entrapped in these systems.

Kaiser Permanente was developed in a spirit of pioneering and innovation. Dr. Smillie would be well pleased if, in addition to educating and entertaining its readers, this inspiring book kindles in them a fresh interest in new approaches to today's and tomorrow's health care delivery challenges.

Bruce J. Sams, Jr., M.D.

Acknowledgments

I am indebted to all my colleagues of The Permanente Medical Group for their commitment to a medical practice that serves people with good quality care in a socially responsible manner. This history of The Permanente Medical Group is intended to reward them with the knowledge that they made a difference. Dr. Morris Collen cautioned me to be certain that the book is factual and well documented. Dr. Cecil Cutting read the manuscript in draft and made numerous valuable suggestions. He also helped select the photographs. Dr. Bruce Sams, Jr., Executive Director of the Medical Group, is primarily responsible for leading and pushing me to complete the work. Dr. Richmond Prescott has been of enormous assistance in working out many editorial changes and management details. Avram Yedidia and Jack Chapman of the Kaiser Foundation Health Plan related interesting, colorful, and often amusing anecdotes. Scott Fleming, of the Central Office staff of Kaiser Foundation Health Plan corrected some misconceptions. The Board of Directors of The Permanente Medical Group has been gracious and generous with financial assistance. Group Health Foundation and the Kaiser Family Foundation have also supported this effort financially. My daughter Christina Smillie, M.D., a skilled and experienced editor of medical literature and formerly a staff physician in Community Health Care Plan in Bridgeport, Connecticut, made invaluable suggestions and corrections from the viewpoint of a young physician learning how a prepaid group practice Health Maintenance Organization works. To many others who asked questions that should be answered and who showed an interest in reading this book, I am profoundly grateful.

John G. Smillie, M.D.

Can Physicians Manage the Quality and Costs of Health Care?

The Story of The Permanente Medical Group

1

The Desert Song—
1933–1938

It was not planned. It just happened. And yet once it happened—once prepaid group medical practice proved itself in the Mojave Desert of southern California during the Great Depression—a chain of events was set in motion that would profoundly affect the delivery of medical care in America.

In July 1933, a young doctor by the name of Sidney Roy Garfield encountered an opportunity in the desert. He did not know it at the time, but this opportunity contained within itself the formative elements of a new kind of medical practice. This interaction of desert opportunity, Sidney Garfield's pragmatic intelligence, and the social ambitions energizing the large-scale public works projects with which America sought to offset the Depression coalesced in the creation of a medical care delivery system destined to grow in numbers and importance over the next half century.

In 1933 Sidney Garfield, MD, was completing his training in general surgery at the Los Angeles County Hospital. Like so many of his generation, Garfield was facing an uncertain future despite long years of study and the even longer struggle of his parents, who had first directed him toward medicine. Bertha and Isaac had emigrated from Russia as a young couple, each of them aged 18, acquired a new name, Garfield, and the chance for a better life. Isaac Garfield began his professional career as a clothes peddler on the streets of New York City. He prospered, and in time he was able to open his own men's clothing store in

Elizabeth, New Jersey, where Sidney Roy Garfield was born on April 17, 1906. The Garfield family — Isaac, Bertha, an older daughter Sally, and Sidney — formed a tight patriarchal household, emphasizing hard work, education, and music. Young Sidney, a lively boy with red hair inherited from his mother and clear gray eyes, was kept busy helping around the family store, washing windows, sweeping the sidewalk, delivering trunks. In his spare time, he took violin lessons and his sister Sally studied the piano. He started public school at the precocious age of 4, having been passed off by his parents as a 5 year old. Sidney did exceptionally well in mathematics and science and wanted to be an engineer. As a boy during World War I, he designed bridges, tunnels, and military works in his spare time. Directed by his parents toward medicine, he acquiesced, but he would never be a traditional physician. Significantly, large-scale engineering works — aqueducts, dams, shipyards — shaped his experience as a young physician.

When it came time for Sally Garfield to marry, her parents selected Harry Blackman, a mechanical engineer working in a local shipyard. Harry played the saxophone and had his own band. As much as they admired Harry for his good job at the shipyard and for his musical abilities, Isaac and Bertha Garfield decided that their son-in-law should become a dentist. Sidney was already in his first year of premed at Rutgers. Sidney the doctor, Harry the dentist: Isaac and Bertha wanted the best for the next generation. Like thousands of other Americans searching for expanded opportunities, they cast their glance across the country to the rapidly developing city of Los Angeles and moved there in 1923. With $40,000 realized from the liquidation of his New Jersey properties, Isaac Garfield bought an apartment house, a grocery store, and a music store on Central Avenue in south Los Angeles. Sally ran the grocery store while her husband Harry and her brother Sidney enrolled at the University of Southern California (USC).

Sidney Garfield missed the academic stimulation of Rutgers. After a year at USC, he decided to apply to medical school at the end of his sophomore year. Reading the report of a visiting German commission on the five best medical schools in the United States, he applied to all five of them at the age of 18. Four turned him down; the fifth, the University of Iowa, accepted him. Having begun school at age 4 and having bypassed the last 2 years of college, Sidney Garfield was on the way to becoming a very young physician. At Iowa, Sidney Garfield joined a fraternity, played junior varsity basketball, drove a greenish-blue Buick roadster with a folding windshield and a rumble seat, and took his MD degree in 1928. The son of a one-time clothes peddler now solidly middle class, Garfield first displayed during his medical school years a life-long taste for fine tailoring. His hair was even curlier and redder than in his childhood. His face was lean and angular, and his gray eyes were frequently concealed behind a seemingly deliberate narrowing, as if Garfield were a spectator of his own life.

After a year as an intern at the Michael Reese Hospital in Chicago, he returned to Los Angeles in 1929 to continue his postgraduate training at the County Hospital. There he was offered a 3-year residency in surgery, which he completed in 1933. He was 27 years old, a physician and a surgeon, and he wanted to establish himself as a reputable surgeon in fee-for-service practice in Los Angeles. Holding a respected position in life, after all, was one of the main arguments his parents had used to persuade him to change his course from what they considered the uncertain path of engineering to what they believed was the more secure path of medicine. It was, however, the worst year of the Depression, and opportunities for solo practice were scarce.

While serving as a surgical resident at Los Angeles County Hospital, Sidney Garfield experienced another possibility—group practice. At County he formed a close friendship with two residents in internal medicine: Raymond M. Kay, a short, round-faced, good-natured graduate of the Stanford Medical School, and Kay's roommate, Justin Wallace Neighbor, a University of Michigan Medical School graduate. The three friends played tennis and dated the same group of student nurses together.

Garfield, Kay, and Neighbor shared with each other the fascinating clinical experiences of Los Angeles County Hospital. They referred cases back and forth to each other and, over a period of time, developed a collegiality that would last for a lifetime and that was, in fact, a basic element in their later partnership. As a large public hospital in a major metropolis, Los Angeles County Hospital offered these young residents a medical education in a mutually supportive social context that was in many ways its own form of group practice. Playing together, learning from each other, they acquired their medical skills in a socially responsive hospital setting where patients were treated without consideration of payment. The young physicians absorbed a sense of medicine as a form of social practice that was part and parcel, not only of Los Angeles County, but of America itself during the Depression years. Under the assault of economic hardship, the social dimension of American experience was asserting itself against an already established philosophy of individualism. These young doctors were learning not only from each other and from the teams of physicians at Los Angeles County, but also from the philosophy of social responsibility that animated a great public hospital at a time of economic stress.

While solo fee-for-service practice remained the career expectation for these physicians in training, they also glimpsed the possibility that there could be another way of practicing medicine: as members of a group. Another resident, Harry Kirby, brilliant and respected by his colleagues, was already proclaiming a preference for a life of medicine in a more organized social setting than fee-for-service would allow. While never penetrating the inner core of the friendship shared by Garfield, Kay, and Neighbor, Kirby challenged them professionally with an example of an accomplished young physician searching out a more cooperative way of practicing medicine.

Of the three friends, only Raymond Kay was able to establish a part-time fee-for-service practice in Los Angeles. Kay, however, was faced with poor collections from patients in financial distress, as so many were during the Depression. Kay knew that some physicians covered this shortfall by doing more than was really necessary for those patients able to pay. Equally disturbing, Kay felt that he did not have enough patients to maintain the clinical sharpness that had peaked at the end of his residency. Finding that he functioned best in a large public hospital setting, where the variety of cases presented ample challenge to his skills and where the opportunity existed to work with other experienced physicians, Kay chose to limit his fee-for-service practice to half-time and returned to County Hospital as a staff physician and teacher of interns and residents. Kay also began to ponder the imbalance in a system that would see capable young doctors out of residency treating colds and other trivia in private practice while Los Angeles County Hospital was deluged with serious cases.

Meanwhile, Wallace Neighbor also found himself disinclined to enter fee-for-service practice, although in Neighbor's case the alternative was on the other end of the social ladder from Los Angeles County Hospital. Neighbor obtained a salaried job as house physician at Arrowhead Springs, a fashionable resort hotel outside Los Angeles, favored by the Hollywood crowd. It was not the sort of practice Neighbor intended as his lifetime career, but this was the Depression and Arrowhead Springs offered an opportunity for a diversified practice, and the tennis was excellent. Going their different ways, Kay, Neighbor, and Garfield—friends in medicine, each of them deeply affected by their experiences at Los Angeles County—would within a few years be reunited in group medical practice.

Sidney Garfield, meanwhile, unable to open a solo surgical practice in the disastrous economic climate of the Depression, was looking for a salaried job. Another Los Angeles County graduate, Gene Morris, who had trained under Garfield as an intern, was in general practice in the little town of Indio on the edge of the Mojave Desert 140 miles east of Los Angeles. Hearing that Garfield was looking for a salaried job, Morris notified him that the Metropolitan Water District of Los Angeles, then in the process of building an aqueduct from the Colorado River to Los Angeles, was looking for a physician to staff a small medical unit in Indio.

In October 1923, the year the Garfields arrived in Los Angeles, the city engineer of the growing metropolis, William Mulholland, led a group of engineers on a survey of the Colorado River. Although Los Angeles had completed an aqueduct from the Owens River in the Sierra in 1913, Mulholland and his colleagues knew that Los Angeles—and all of southern California, in fact—would need even more water if its growth rate were to continue. In July 1924 the City of Los Angeles filed a claim with the Bureau of Reclamation for 1.1 million acre-feet per year of water from the Colorado River, nearly four times as much as it was then drawing from the Owens River. Empowered by a $2 million bond issue, Los Angeles and 11 other cities formed the Metropolitan Water District of Southern California and surveyed 25,000 square miles of mountains and desert for the best possible aqueduct route. In 1931 the voters of the district authorized a $220 million bond issue to finance the dams, reservoirs, and aqueducts that would give it access to the Colorado. In December 1932 the advance guard of what became a labor army 11,000 strong took to the field. For 8 long years, 3 shifts a day worked 7 days a week blasting, gouging, scraping, drilling, welding, and laying cement. By 1941 they had constructed a 242-mile-long aqueduct.

It was a heroic enterprise, involving more than 20 construction companies and subcontractors; but when Sidney Garfield applied for the job in Indio, the Metropolitan Water District offered him a mere $125 a month to work in its clinic. Even in those desperate times, Garfield felt the salary inadequate for a trained surgeon. Three hundred dollars, he believed, would have been more appropriate. Declining the position, Garfield drove back to Indio and discussed the matter with Gene Morris. With 5000 workers in the field, the two young physicians decided, there were more opportunities for medical practice than those offered by the Metropolitan Water District. In the course of the conversation, Garfield and Morris conceived a plan. Garfield would borrow money to build a small hospital near Desert Center, 60 miles east of Indio. Morris would continue to practice in Indio and contribute between $300 and $400 a month toward start-up costs. Once the Desert

Center Hospital was built, the partners would offer fee-for-service industrial medical care for on-the-job compensable injuries and illnesses. The hospital would also offer fee-for-service nonindustrial medicine on an individual basis.

Sidney Garfield borrowed $2500 from his father. It might have been his own money that he borrowed, his friend Wally Neighbor later speculated in an interview. Garfield and his father worked closely together on money matters. "Even when he began to make money," Neighbor reminisced, "his father would dole out the money to him. His father was a very shrewd investor."[1] It is hard to believe that Sidney Garfield, even as a just-graduated surgical resident, was ever completely without funds. He continued to manage the family apartment buildings during the early days of his medical practice.

In any event, empowered by the $2500, Garfield approached various insurance companies and contractors to ascertain their interest in the project. The insurance agents told Garfield that if he built the hospital, they would support it. One contractor, Ely Dixon, was so enthusiastic about the hospital that he offered Garfield a plot of land for its location. A builder in Indio agreed to construct the 12-bed hospital at Desert Center for the $2500 down payment and to carry the balance over the following 5 years or the duration of the aqueduct project, whichever came first. Western Surgical Supply Company, anxious to sell its wares in a difficult Depression market, equipped the hospital on a monthly payment basis, with no down payment, providing such necessities as an autoclave and X-ray equipment. General Electric provided air conditioning, then an innovative technology, for 10 percent down, the rest in monthly payments. Garfield also bought a washing machine on time and shaded the hospital windows against the fierce desert glare with the newly invented venetian blinds. He personally selected a soothing color scheme and equipped the diminutive wards with flower containers and personal radios. The design and building of Contractors General Hospital, as it came to be called, launched Garfield on a lifetime of concern for hospital design. In later years, the designing of hospitals became his second career.

All in all, Garfield and Morris assumed a $50,000 debt to get Contractors General Hospital into operation. "It was not like any industrial hospital or first-aid camp that anyone had ever seen in the history of large construction," Wally Neighbor later recalled. "The usual first-aid shack was just what the name implies, an old shack; but this hospital was air conditioned, it had a surgery, rooms, and good-looking nurses. Sidney had a way of influencing nurses to come and work for him."

Garfield also hired a married couple to cook, clean, do the laundry, perform maintenance, and drive the ambulance. The entire hospital crew was on call 24 hours a day. Once a month the married couple got the weekend off, which left Garfield and Betty Runyon, one of the two nurses, to do the cooking and run the washing machine. Once a month, Gene Morris would come down from Indio and relieve Garfield for the weekend. On his weekend off, Garfield frequently visited Wally Neighbor at Arrowhead Springs. "It wasn't as if he went out in the desert and became a monk," Wally Neighbor later reminisced. "He was in and out constantly."[2]

Garfield and Morris had gambled on being able to treat a high volume of insured, on-the-job injuries. There was no problem, initially, with having patients turn up. They came with cuts, bruises, infected fingers, broken bones, boils, and chronic sores on hands and feet caused by the damp soil in the tunnels. They came with back injuries, pneumonia, heart attacks, hernias, burns, snake and spider bites. When prostitutes established themselves in tent cities outside the camps, they came with syphilis and gonorrhea. Venereal disease, however, was considered a nonindustrial illness and was not covered by insurance.

A growing percentage of the patients arriving at the hospital were there for off-the-job illnesses or injuries. Earning 50 cents an hour, few had the money to pay for their care. Since there was no county hospital to receive such nonpaying patients, Garfield felt obliged to admit them, hoping that income from the indemnified industrial injuries would carry him through. The insurance companies, however, quibbled over his fees for simple on-the-job injuries and suggested that the hospital was overservicing its patients. Payments were discounted, and seriously injured patients, once their condition stabilized, were transferred at the request of the insurance companies to more favored hospitals and doctors in metropolitan Los Angeles.

"The insurance companies had the money," Garfield said of this period, "but they were anxious to keep it. We got a patient and we would treat him with tender loving care and we would bill the insurance company, and more often than not, they would come back and discount our bills, saying that we treated the patient too many times." The one sure thing he learned in the desert, Garfield claimed, was that in medical care whoever pays the bills usually controls the services.[3]

Within 7 months of its opening, with 20 different employers scattered along hundreds of miles and with insurance companies reluctant to pay (and with their payments slow in coming), Contractors General Hospital was on the verge of bankruptcy. It became nearly impossible to meet the payroll. The two nurses were working without pay. It was also difficult to keep up payments to the surgical supply house and to the contractor who built the hospital. Gene Morris asked to dissolve the partnership, forcing Garfield to buy him out over a series of monthly payments. Damaged as an entrepreneur, Garfield was also affronted in his professional pride. As long as the insurance carriers maintained supreme control over his patients, he could have no autonomy, and his doctor-patient relationships were severely compromised. Indeed, the lesson was clear: the one who pays the bills controls the service.

When word got out that Sidney Garfield was contemplating closing the hospital down, the contractors and the insurance companies found themselves faced with the prospect of becoming, once again, the sole source of emergency care near the work sites. The largest insurance company involved in the project was the San Francisco–based Industrial Indemnity Exchange, established in 1921 by a group of contractors, among them W. A. Bechtel and Henry J. Kaiser. By 1934 Kaiser, Bechtel, and John Phillips owned the Industrial Indemnity Exchange outright. Kaiser installed his right-hand man, A. B. Ordway, as executive vice president. The chief planner and strategist for the company was Harold Hatch, a brilliant engineer afflicted by a spinal deformity that had stunted his growth and hunched his back. Hatch appeared in the desert in 1934 on an inspection tour of construction sites. Meeting Garfield at the Contractors General Hospital in Desert Center, the brilliant engineer turned insurance agent and the equally brilliant surgeon turned medical entrepreneur became good friends over the course of a number of visits. As an insurance agent, Hatch was interested in standardizing and containing costs. As an employers' representative, he did not want to lose medical coverage for the construction workers. Dramatically, Hatch suggested a new method for financing medical care at the Contractors General Hospital: prepayment. As it was, 25 percent of the workers' compensation insurance premium was already being allocated for medical and hospital expenses. The Industrial Indemnity Exchange, Hatch suggested, would be willing to pay half that premium, 12.5 percent, to Garfield to care for its indemnified workers. The remaining 12.5 percent would be used to pay the costs of patients needing to be transferred to Los Angeles. This 12.5 percent payment amounted to $1.50 per worker per month or a nickel a day. Hatch then persuaded the employers to offer a voluntary payroll deduction of an additional nickel a day for complete nonindustrial coverage. Both Hatch and Garfield felt that it was essential that enrollment and prepaid coverage be voluntary. With 5000 construction workers covered by this plan if all joined, some $500 a day would then be generated for the support of Garfield's hospital. The proposal was implemented, and very quickly Contractors General Hospital was back in business. After this, Garfield remembered, "we were able to meet our bills, pay off our creditors, meet our payroll, and begin to get some impressive results."[4]

2

Beneath the simple surface of Harold Hatch's recommendation of prepayment for comprehensive group-practice medical coverage and Sidney Garfield's willingness to implement Hatch's recommendation lay an important piece of unfinished business in American medicine. While present from the start in American history, prepaid group medical practice offering comprehensive coverage nevertheless remained only a latent possibility, a minor chord, in the solo practice sovereignty that by the end of the nineteenth century dominated American medicine. As early as 1790 the Boston Dispensary offered group-practice prepaid coverage to its membership. Similar clinics were founded in New York, Philadelphia, and elsewhere. During the presidency of John Adams, Secretary of the Treasury Alexander Hamilton established a health-care program for sick and disabled members of the American merchant marine. Empowered by Congress in 1798, the Marine Hospital Service offered comprehensive medical coverage to American merchant mariners and sailors working on the inland waterways. Hospitals were ultimately established in Boston, Pittsburgh, on Lake Champlain in Vermont, and in San Francisco, where a marine hospital opened in 1851 at the height of the Gold Rush. Also in the west, in 1868 the Central Pacific (later Southern Pacific) Railroad offered comprehensive medical care for sick and injured employees. The railroad hired physicians and built a hospital in Sacramento. The Southern Pacific thus pioneered comprehensive industrial medicine in the United States. It must be pointed out, however, that the merchant marine program did not involve a voluntary enrollment or assessment. It and the Southern Pacific program were, in fact, prototypes of industrial medicine as opposed to more comprehensive programs.

A number of isolated lumbering and mining companies in the west also offered similar programs, although few of them were as extensive as or of the quality of the health-care system established by the Southern Pacific. Southern Pacific staff surgeons, for instance, were the first to perform appendectomies west of the Mississippi and were also responsible for developing a number of other innovative surgical techniques. The railroad also emphasized preventive care. Officers and employees of the railroad were encouraged to have periodic checkups so that ailments could be detected and treated before they caused serious damage to health. On the other hand, the mining and lumber company programs were voluntary. Workers paid a percentage of their own wages, dropping their contribution for the company physician into a box or jar on payday, a primitive form of payroll deduction. Physicians were compensated on the basis of services performed. These twin principles of free choice and capitation (from the Latin word for "head count") represented a significant development in the evolving concept of prepaid comprehensive medical care.

With the exception of the railroads and mining and lumbering companies, however, American industry did not follow suit in establishing industrial health plans. There were a few exceptions, of course, such as the Consolidated Edison Company of New York, which in 1891 established a company-sponsored mutual aid society to administer a prepaid medical care program for its workers. In the early 1900s, the Endicott-Johnson Company, a shoe manufacturer in Johnson City, New York, and the Standard Oil Company of Baton Rouge, Louisiana, also established health-care programs for their employees.

European immigrants, meanwhile, were also sponsoring the practice of the so-called lodge or contract medicine in certain large American cities. Modeled on the medical benefit societies that were popular in both Europe and England at the time (some million members in England alone), these organizations or lodges collected dues and with the money placed physicians under contract to offer prepaid medical care to their membership. In New York's lower east side there were between 1500 and 2000 benevolent associations, most of them contracting for the services of a lodge doctor. The French community of San Francisco, for example, established *La Société Française de Bienfaisance Mutuelle* during the Gold Rush. For a monthly fee of 1 dollar, members of the French community and others, mostly European immigrants, enjoyed a comprehensive program of medical services in the society's 20-bed hospital at the corner of Bush and Taylor. By 1869 the program was enrolling nearly 4000 members in an expanded facility at Fifth and Bryant. In 1896 an even grander hospital was constructed on the square block bordered by Geary, Anza, Fifth, and Sixth Avenues. The fact that such early lodge or benevolent society programs were prepaid and voluntary and tended toward comprehensive coverage represented a significant advance in the evolving concept, as did the fact that the French program in San Francisco owned its own hospital.

As the late nineteenth century became the twentieth, most major industrial countries in Europe were in the process of evolving some form of national social insurance, including medical benefits. In the United States, by contrast, such legislation took another 30 years to surface. Social Security, which did not then include health insurance, was not enacted until 1935. On the other hand, in 1908 the United States enacted a workers' compensation law for federal employees. Beginning around 1910 at the height of the progressive era, many states began to enact workers' compensation laws requiring employers and employees to contribute to the cost of health-care insurance for job-related injuries. In most instances, the fees were kept in a state-controlled fund that paid physicians on a fee-for-service basis for treating job-related injuries. Some states allowed employers to establish a form of self-insurance, which could consist of contract physicians available to injured workers. In certain cases, this coverage was expanded, for a fee, to include non-job-related illnesses or injuries.

In 1929 the Department of Water and Power of the City of Los Angeles contracted with Drs. Donald Ross and H. Clifford Loos of the Ross-Loos Medical Group in Los Angeles for prepaid medical coverage for its 12,000 employees and 25,000 dependents. Each subscriber to the plan paid $2 per month for medical coverage exclusive of hospitalization, which was billed separately. Involving as it did prepayment, comprehensive care, and group practice, the Ross-Loos program is of historical importance. It also provoked the ire of the Los Angeles County Medical Society, which withdrew its opposition when the program voluntarily limited its membership. The rising cost of hospitalization also provoked in 1929 the so-called Blue Cross approach, first developed by Baylor University in Dallas, Texas, and formally endorsed by the American Hospital Association in 1933.

The fact that the Los Angeles Department of Water and Power contracted with a privately owned group-practice medical clinic in 1929 underscores a significant convergence of two innovative principles: prepayment for comprehensive coverage and the group practice of medicine. Many of the prepayment programs that emerged in the nineteenth and early twentieth centuries involved some form of group medical practice. According to Princeton University medical historian and sociologist Paul Starr, author of the Pulitzer Prize–winning *The Social Transformation of American Medicine* (1982), the Mayo Clinic, founded by a physician father and his two physician sons in the 1880s in Rochester, Minnesota, is the prototype of the privately owned, progressive group-practice medical clinic. By 1914, the Mayo Clinic included 17 doctors on its staff; by 1929, when the Mayo Clinic was housed in its own 15-story building, that figure had grown to 386 physicians and dentists, backed by 895 support staff. So impressed was Charles F. Menninger, a Topeka, Kansas, general practitioner, by his visit to the Mayo Clinic in 1908, that he joined with his three physician sons to form a similar institution, the Menninger Clinic in Topeka. While the Menninger Clinic was a single-specialty organization oriented toward psychiatric practice, it did follow the guidelines of group medical practice established at Mayo. According to Starr, the experience of American physicians in the armed forces during World War I sensitized many of them to the benefits of medical practice in a group situation. In any event, various forms of group medical partnerships and/or clinics were established in the years immediately following World War I, such as the Ross-Loos Medical Group in Los Angeles, whose 1929 contract with the Department of Water and Power provides such a prophetic paradigm of the course that prepaid group medical practice would eventually take in the United States.

Both prepayment and group medical practice alike, however, ran counter to the model of solo fee-for-service practice that the American medical community had determined to be the best model for medical practice in the United States. Paul Starr has chronicled the process whereby American physicians gained sovereignty over the practice of medicine in the nineteenth and early twentieth centuries by eliminating or controlling all agencies and factors that could possibly intercept the direct, primary, and unqualified relationship between physician and patient. Whether it be government agencies, insurance companies, lodges, mutual aid associations, or benevolent societies, the American medical establishment was quick to limit the influence of any and all factors outside of this physician-patient relationship. The medical establishment also gained control of hospitals, medical schools, and state licensing boards. Group practice, as Paul Starr points out, "changed the relationships of physicians to each other. Unlike lodge practice, it gathered physicians into a single organization, often with business managers and technical assistance, in a new and more elaborate division of labor. Typically, some doctors brought capital as well as labor to the enterprise and became its owners, while other doctors were their employees. And so group practice, though under the control of members of the profession, introduced a type of hierarchical, profit-making organization into medical practice."[5] Even the Mayo Clinic, Starr notes, despite the preeminent level of medicine it practiced, was severely criticized by established physicians.

Physicians in multispecialty group practice, however, were quick to point out its advantages. Physicians in different specialities were available to each other for ready referrals. Sharing medical records created, automatically, a continuous de facto process of peer review. Group-practice physicians were continuously educating one another in the day-to-day practice of medicine. The sharing of hospital and clinic space; the consolidation of laboratory, X-ray, and other ancillary disciplines into one location; together with the unification of records keeping, billing, and other administrative procedures, all made for great efficiency and cost effectiveness.

Despite these and other benefits, group practice, running as it did counter to the established model, remained a minor development in the early twentieth century. By 1932, a year before Sidney Garfield went out to the Mojave Desert, fewer than 2000 American physicians were in any form of group practice in the United States. While the American Medical Association never attacked group practice outright, it was always eager to point to its disadvantages, especially the fact that group practice invariably put physicians into an employer-employee relationship with each other. Specialists resented the fact that group practice cut down on the number of outside referrals. The medical establishment was also deeply suspicious of the corporate aspects of group practice, with its emphasis upon capital investment, hierarchical controls, and corporate profit. While it was ethical and sound public policy for physicians to profit from their skills, the medical establishment did not want a competitive capitalist economy to invade American medicine and restructure it along corporate lines. This is why, among other reasons, the medical establishment made sure that large hospitals, which emerged in the late nineteenth and early twentieth centuries as places to practice medicine, remained organized as nonprofit enterprises, whether publicly or privately controlled.

Local medical societies were invariably suspicious, therefore, of any form of group medical practice in their area, particularly if any form of prepayment was involved since prepayment involved the interposition of another organization—the lodge, the benevolent society, the employer, the union, the insurance company—between the physician and the patient. Thus, in established medical thought, prepayment constituted a threat to the integrity of the physician-patient relationship and should be opposed wherever it appeared. In 1929 when Dr. Michael A. Shadid established the Farmers' Union Cooperative Hospital Association, a rural medical cooperative in Elk City, Oklahoma, he was repeatedly harassed by the county medical society despite the fact that the association was enthusiastically received by the farmers of the community.

The competitive economic advantages of prepaid group medical practice were totally evident in the program established by Ross-Loos physicians to the Los Angeles Department of Water and Power employees and their dependents. In 1931, for a total payment of $216,410, subscribers to this plan received an estimated $499,378 worth of medical services, if calculated on a fee-for-service basis. No wonder the Los Angeles County Medical Society sought to restrict Ross-Loos's growth. Such competitive advantages of prepaid group-practice programs haunted solo-practice physicians whose careers and livelihoods were so fundamentally structured according to the fee-for-service model.

3

Fortunately, Sidney Garfield faced no medical society opposition in the Mojave Desert. Since there were no competing doctors, he represented no economic threat. Nor was he hampered by regulations designed to curb prepaid practice. All he needed was his license to practice medicine in California, which he already had. For Garfield, prepayment was a godsend. The $500 generated each day from the Industrial Indemnity prepayment and the nickel voluntarily contributed as a payroll deduction each day by each worker for off-the-job coverage allowed him to practice medicine at Contractors General Hospital in Desert Center to the best of his ability. Without the insurance companies watching his every move, second-guessing and quibbling with his every decision, Garfield regained autonomy in medical matters. He had the confidence to extend as much care as he thought necessary. It was now the doctors, not the insurance companies, who made the decisions that certain patients needed to be transferred to Los Angeles. Experience soon demonstrated that the insurance companies no longer needed to retain the 12.5 percent of the premium they had earmarked for Los Angeles hospitals and doctors. As a result, Industrial Indemnity Exchange increased the contribution to Garfield from 12.5 to 17.5 percent.

Occasionally, there were misunderstandings, some of them humorous. A worker came to the hospital at the end of the month and asked Garfield, "How about giving me a dollar's worth of aspirin for the five cents a day I paid you?" Garfield, on his part, continued to work as hard as ever, helping out in the kitchen, doing the laundry when necessary. On one occasion, when the call came into the hospital that a worker had broken his leg, it was Garfield who drove the ambulance out to the desert site, the orderly sitting in the right-hand seat. Garfield and the orderly carefully placed the injured man on a stretcher and drove him back to the hospital. When Garfield began to scrub, however, in preparation for setting the bone, the patient bolted up from the operating table, saying, "That ambulance driver isn't going to touch my leg!" It took a little while for the staff to convince the patient that the boyish young man who had carried him on the stretcher was also the physician in charge of the hospital.

Prepayment reversed the economics of medicine. Instead of being paid for the treatment of injuries or illness, Garfield and his colleagues were now being paid to care for the overall health of the subscribing membership. Two of the most common injuries Garfield encountered were nail punctures through rubber-soled boots and head injuries caused by falling rocks or collisions with shoring in the tunnels. Legend later had it, incorrectly, that Garfield himself went around to construction sites, hammer in hand, and pounded down the dangerous nails. What he did do, however, was to go out and persuade the contractors to have their men pound down the nails. He would also inspect tunnels for dangerous shoring. "Prior to the prepayment deal with the insurance companies," he later admitted, "we were anxious to have the injured come into our hospitals. We were sort of ashamed of that. After we got on prepayment, we started safety engineering."[6] There were other medical benefits as well. Workers who had previously avoided coming in for care until they were so sick that they had no other choice now came in when they first felt sick. This, in turn, strengthened the preventive aspects of Garfield's program, allowing him to treat patients at an earlier stage when he could possibly affect the outcome of an illness.

By this time, Garfield's hospital was responsible for construction sites strung out over 125 miles extending from Desert Center to the location of the proposed Parker Dam on the Colorado River. It was from the reservoir, now named Lake Havasu, created by the proposed Parker Dam that the Los Angeles Aqueduct would draw its water. Garfield initially dealt with the problem of his scattered sites by assigning first-aid men to distant camps, but when Parker Dam entered the construction phase, Garfield decided to build a second hospital at that site. A possibility existed that the medical care plan could be expanded to include not only the aqueduct workers but also the dam builders as well. The Six Companies, a consortium of contractors that included the Henry J.

Kaiser Company, had been awarded the contract to build Parker Dam because of the consortium's proven record in the recently completed Hoover Dam project. Joseph Reis, a Kaiser Company executive representing the Six Companies, negotiated with Garfield regarding the proposed medical care program. During the construction of the Hoover Dam, the Six Companies had supported through the Industrial Indemnity Exchange a medical care program similar to the program Garfield was providing for the Metropolitan Water District. That program, however, involved no voluntary payroll deductions in prepayment for off-the-job illness or injury. Garfield offered Reis a comprehensive program at the 17.5 percent rate for industrial injury care, augmented by the nickel a day voluntary contribution for nonindustrial care, exactly the package that was supporting the Metropolitan Water District aqueduct program. Reis, however, refused to offer more than a 12.5 percent rate of compensation and bluntly told Garfield that either he accept that rate or the Six Companies would move their own medical crew down from Hoover Dam and provide their own medical coverage program. Since the Henry J. Kaiser Company was a major owner of Industrial Indemnity, Reis was in effect bidding against his own employer in that Industrial Indemnity was already paying Garfield the 17.5 percent rate.

Garfield had to take Reis's ultimatum seriously. For some time now, he had been promising the construction sites that he would soon be establishing a second hospital at Parker Dam. Wanting both the contract and the second hospital, Garfield yielded to Reis's aggressive bargaining and agreed to 12.5 percent of the workers' compensation premium. When A. B. Ordway of the Industrial Indemnity Exchange heard of this, he summoned Garfield to his office in San Francisco.

"I got a call from him to come to San Francisco right away," Garfield later remembered, "and I rode up all night on the train wondering what he wanted. I got there and he had his whole crew, including Harold Hatch and his attorneys, all in this big room. He looked at me and said, 'How can you make such a fool out of me in my organization by giving Reis a lower rate than you're giving us? Everybody knows about this, and they will all blame us for an inefficient operation.' I listened to him for a while, and then I told him that the only reason I agreed to the lower figure was to give better service over all because we had to have that job to provide service to the far end of the line. Finally I said, 'If you feel that strongly about it, Mr. Ordway, just reduce your payment to 12.5 percent and I'll try to make a go of it.' Ordway stopped talking for a minute, and then he said, 'Come outside. I want to talk to you.' He took me next door into another room, and he said, 'Don't you ever offer to give me back money like that! You need that money to do the job you're doing. Now you get out of here and don't you ever do anything like that again.' Ordway did the whole thing just to impress his people. He didn't want me to reduce the rate. Actually, what happened with Parker Dam—after six months—was that they voluntarily raised their rate to 17.5 percent."[6]

Sidney Garfield built and staffed the Parker Dam Hospital. At the request of the Six Companies, he also built and staffed a third hospital at the construction site of Imperial Dam, 150 miles south of Parker. Constructed by the Six Companies, Imperial Dam was not part of the Los Angeles Aqueduct project; it was intended, rather, to store and provide water for the irrigation of the Imperial Valley in southeastern California. Ordway cautioned Garfield not to build an overly elaborate hospital at the Imperial Dam site. "He told me just to build the bare necessities," Garfield recalled. "I didn't believe in that. I wanted the third hospital to be as good as the others, and I really built a nicer place there. I had learned how to plan and to build better, so I wound up building a nicer place in Imperial than I did in the other two sites. Mr. Ordway got rather upset at me for spending so much money."[7]

The three hospital locations—Desert Center, Parker Dam, and Imperial Dam—formed a geographic triangle. Garfield staffed each hospital with at least one physician, who worked for him as an employee. His first recruit was Dr. Harry Kirby, who was leaving the Army Reserves after spending 6 months in the snows of Montana in charge of a Civilian Conservation Corps Company. Kirby had trained with Garfield at Los Angeles County Hospital and had even then impressed Garfield by his medical skills and his thoughtful approach to questions of medical organization and delivery. Garfield located other doctors at certain key first-aid stations between the hospitals. As the only fully qualified surgeon, Garfield traveled the 85 to 150 miles between the three hospitals to provide specialized surgical care.

Throughout these desert years, 1933–1938, Sidney Garfield kept in contact with his friends from Los Angeles County Hospital. When Pat Allen, a nurse from County, contracted polio in the 1934 Los Angeles polio epidemic, Garfield brought her out to Desert Center to recuperate. During this time, Garfield visited Los Angeles on the average of a weekend a month. Ray Kay and Wally Neighbor would occasionally make it out to the desert, or more frequently Garfield would visit them at Arrowhead Springs or Los Angeles. The three physicians would frequently talk of their differing medical experiences. Both Kay and Neighbor were impressed with Garfield's success with prepaid care.

As well they might have been. After building and equipping three small hospitals, after employing physicians, nurses, and support staff to provide medical care for 5000 workers spread across a great desert, Sidney Garfield had retained earnings from the 5-year period of $250,000. It was an astonishing sum in 1938 when the average *annual* American income, excluding those on relief, was $1350. Sidney Garfield had every intention of using his earnings to finance a solo fee-for-service practice in Los Angeles. But it did not happen that way. A telephone call intervened.

2
Grand Coulee— 1938–1941

As the only surgeon serving the three Mojave Desert hospitals, Sidney Garfield spent a lot of time on the road. It was his habit to call in to Desert Center from gas stations for his messages. On a hot morning in July 1938, Garfield turned his Buick into a gas station between Desert Center and the Imperial Dam. Calling the hospital at Desert Center, he asked for his messages. A. B. Ordway, president of the Industrial Indemnity Exchange, had telephoned. Garfield returned the call.

"Sid," Ordway asked over the long-distance line, "do you know Edgar Kaiser?"

"I've never met him," Garfield answered.

"Kaiser just got the award for Coulee Dam in Washington," Ordway replied. "He heard about the job you did for us down here, and he wants you to do the medical job up there. Can you come up to Portland to talk to him?"

This was not an offer Garfield wanted to hear. With a quarter of a million dollars in the bank, he had more than ample means to establish himself in a fee-for-service surgical practice in Los Angeles. The desert years, after all, had been an interruption. It was time to get back into a more conventional practice.

"I don't want to take on another temporary job," Garfield told Ordway. "I want to get into private practice and put my roots down some place."

"I'd rather not get into that," Ordway responded. "Please just go up to Oregon as a favor to me and talk to Edgar Kaiser—just go up and talk to him and advise him what to do." Ordway explained that he had

19

practically promised Edgar Kaiser that Garfield would go up to Portland for the interview.

"I'll go up," Garfield acquiesced. A. B. Ordway, after all, had played a major role in making the aqueduct program possible. But there was no doubt in Garfield's mind that he would turn down any proposal that Kaiser would make. Just before he rang off, Ordway cautioned Garfield that Edgar Kaiser was a forceful persuader.[1]

The Grand Coulee Dam along the Columbia River in central Washington State was the third major dam project to involve the Henry J. Kaiser companies. In 1931 Henry Kaiser joined a consortium of construction companies, the Six Companies, that was awarded the contract by the Bureau of Reclamation to build the Hoover Dam on the Colorado River. At 726 feet high, set on a 650-foot-thick base, the Hoover Dam was completed by the Six Companies in 1936, two years and two months ahead of schedule. At the time it was the largest dam ever built. The Six Companies next won the contract to build the Bonneville Dam on the Columbia River, the boundary between Oregon and Washington. Two dynamic young men, Henry J. Kaiser's son Edgar, 25, who had started as a shovel supervisor on the Hoover Dam project, and Clay Bedford, 30, emerged during the Bonneville project as key leaders in the field. Edgar Kaiser saw to finance and administration; Clay Bedford supervised engineering and construction. Bonneville Dam was completed in 1938, a year ahead of schedule.

Henry Kaiser then moved the same team 467 miles up the Columbia River to the Grand Coulee in Washington, where a reorganized Six Companies had won the contract to complete a Bureau of Reclamation dam three and a half times wider than the Hoover. The Mason-Walsh-Atkinson-Kier group had previously won the contract for excavation and foundation work. Consolidated Builders, Inc., with the Kaiser companies represented by Edgar Kaiser and Clay Bedford as managing contractors, was to build the dam itself. Four-fifths of a mile long, the Grand Coulee Dam required twice as much concrete as Hoover Dam. Hammerhead cranes moved continuously across a steel trestle built above the dam, pouring concrete. In one day 20,684 cubic yards of concrete were poured, a record that still stands. Employed on the project were some 6500 workers, divided into three crews, each pitted against the other in competition. Grand Coulee Dam was completed a year and a half ahead of schedule.

Upon assuming responsibility for the project, Edgar Kaiser discovered that he had a problem with medical services at the dam site. Mason City—a company town of 15,000 construction workers, contractors, government inspectors, and dependents—had one hospital. The previ-

ous contractors had hired physicians for the hospital. They were expected to treat construction workers on a prepaid basis for salaries
ranging from $200 to $300 per month. The rest of their income was
expected to come from fee-for-service. A two-tier system soon developed. Patients capable of paying were given the red carpet treatment.
Construction workers were asked to stand in line, literally at the rear of
the hospital. Sensing that the Kaiser management was already responsive in the matter of health care, union leaders threatened to start their
own program if medical services were not improved. There was even
talk of a strike. At this point, Edgar Kaiser telephoned A. B. Ordway,
who telephoned Sidney Garfield, reaching him in the Mojave Desert.

Garfield flew up to Portland and checked into the Multnomah Hotel,
where Edgar Kaiser had rooms and a temporary office. "I called,"
Garfield later recounted, "and was told Mr. Kaiser was busy. They
would call me. I waited and waited, getting more irritated." Kept waiting for a number of hours, Garfield became progressively more restless
and angry. He began to check with the local airline for flights back to
Los Angeles. Finally, after 6 hours of waiting, Garfield was called.

"As I walked up the stairs to the Kaiser rooms," Garfield remembers,
"I rehearsed what I would say: 'Mr. Kaiser, I'm not interested in this
job. Thank you. Good-bye.'"

Garfield knocked at the door, and Sue Kaiser, Edgar Kaiser's wife,
opened it. "Oh, Dr. Garfield," she said, "I'm so happy to see you. We
think Becky has the measles."

"The kid did have the measles," Garfield recounted, "and I was able to
reassure her. When I went to see Edgar, I wasn't as mad as I had been."

In the conversation that followed, Edgar Kaiser explained the situation. Angered by the shabby treatment they had received from the previous contractors, the unions wanted to set up their own medical coverage program. "This was a challenge to Edgar," remembered Garfield.
"He didn't want the unions involved in the medical care. Ordway had
persuaded him that the way we handled people and our health plan was
so good that Edgar could sell our service to the people."

The next day Edgar and Sue Kaiser were motoring up to Grand Coulee from Portland, a drive of 200 miles. Edgar Kaiser invited Sidney
Garfield to come along. During the drive, Kaiser quizzed Garfield as to
how his Los Angeles Aqueduct program had worked. Kaiser in turn described the Coulee project to Garfield. It was a single work site. A working hospital already existed. Wives and children of employees were living on the location. Kaiser then asked Garfield a crucial question, Could
prepaid coverage be provided to dependents as well as to employees?

"I didn't want to do that," Garfield later admitted. "I didn't know how we would take care of them or what to charge on prepayment. I said we would have to start out in fee-for-service for dependents and feel our way along and then see what we could do."[2]

Edgar Kaiser was reluctant to agree. He did not want a two-tier system to develop between his employees and their dependents, the employees receiving comprehensive prepaid care, the dependents receiving only what they could pay for, which was next to nothing. Edgar Kaiser's reluctance, expressed on the drive north to Grand Coulee, was a practical response to union pressures for full coverage. It was the unions and the Kaiser companies, voicing themselves through Edgar Kaiser, and not Sidney Garfield, who were at this point envisioning what was soon to be implemented: a comprehensive prepaid group practice covering employees and dependents. It would take another year, however, for this complete program to be put into effect.

Arriving at the dam site at Grand Coulee, Garfield instantly understood its advantages over the Los Angeles Aqueduct project, whose workers were spread over hundreds of square miles of desert. At Grand Coulee a stable community of 15,000 lived in the company town of Mason City. As rundown as the 35-bed Mason City Hospital was, it also offered an opportunity for a truly integrated group medical practice – unlike the desert, where Garfield's doctors were rarely in one place together. Touring the site, Garfield became convinced that Grand Coulee offered an opportunity to test what had been learned on the California desert. It also offered him the opportunity to assemble a hand-picked team of medical peers. Garfield decided to defer fee-for-service practice in Los Angeles for another 2 or 3 years and accept Edgar Kaiser's offer.

Garfield organized his program on two fronts, refurbishing the Mason City Hospital and recruiting qualified physicians. The hospital was cleaned and painted, and three operating rooms were reequipped. At Desert Center in the Mojave, Garfield had established one of the earliest air-conditioned hospitals in the country. In the torrid summer of 1938, he decided to do the same thing at Grand Coulee. In fact, Garfield promised the unions that the hospital would be air-conditioned before he went to the board of directors of the Kaiser companies to ask for funds. The boards turned down his request. Funds from the Kaiser Company were for hospital care, Garfield was told, not luxuries. Since he had already promised the unions the air conditioning, Garfield went to Spokane and purchased $8000 worth of air-conditioning equipment, which he negotiated down to a $6000 payment. Shortly after the air conditioning was installed, Garfield later reminisced, "Edgar called me in and he was very disturbed. He said, 'I thought we turned down your air conditioning, and I see you bought it.' I said, 'I bought it with my own money.' But he said, 'We can't have you do that. Don't ever do that again.' He then returned to me the $6000 I had paid."[3] All in all, Garfield spent between $75,000 and $100,000 (reports differ on the amount) refurbishing the Mason City Hospital into an air-conditioned, state-of-the-art treatment center. Meanwhile, he was making every effort to recruit a medical staff.

Since he would be dividing his time between Grand Coulee and the Los Angeles County Hospital, where he had accepted an appointment to supervise surgical residents, Garfield needed a strong medical director for the Grand Coulee operation. He turned to his friend Wally Neighbor, a native of Washington State, who was then in his fifth year of practice at the Arrowhead Springs Resort in southern California.

"I was delighted," Wally Neighbor remembered. "I was tired of taking care of the movie colony and the neurotics, although I had some beautiful experiences there that I wouldn't trade for anything, but it was not the most exciting kind of medical care."[4]

Neighbor went up with Garfield to Grand Coulee for a 3-day stay. Conditions at the local rooming house were so primitive that Garfield insisted that Neighbor take the one available bed while he slept on a set of box springs resting directly on the floor. Despite the primitive conditions, so different from the resort luxury of Arrowhead Springs, Neighbor accepted Garfield's offer to coordinate medical care, eventually for 15,000 workers and their dependents. Garfield also approached another friend from Los Angeles County days, Ray Kay, but Kay had already committed himself to teaching for the USC School of Medicine at Los Angeles County Hospital.

Wally Neighbor was a Washingtonian, and initially Garfield thought that he could recruit other physicians from Washington as well from county and university-affiliated hospitals. Going over to Seattle, Garfield interviewed residents at the county hospital. It was a disappointing experience. "I asked to meet with residents in the specialties I wanted," Garfield remembered. "The administrators set up the meeting. The residents met with me but they turned me down cold. The reason given was the bad reputation of the medical care at Coulee....So I next went to Portland, Oregon. No takers there."[5]

Garfield next turned his attention to San Francisco General Hospital, which was partially staffed by Stanford Medical School residents. The administrator of San Francisco General recommended a 28-year-old resident in surgery by the name of Cecil Cutting. A native Californian, Cutting had graduated from Stanford and the Stanford Medical School. Then in the final stages of his residency, Cutting had tentatively accepted an offer to join a prominent San Francisco orthopedist.

"I had my future all staked out," Cutting recollected. "One day I was relaxing playing pool. I got a call from a doctor from Los Angeles who wanted to talk to me about a job up in Washington. I wasn't particularly interested." Garfield said that he would call back in a few days after Cutting had time to think it over.

In the course of this first telephone conversation, Garfield told Cutting that he was also interested in obstetrics and gynecology residents. Cutting told his friend and fellow Stanford classmate, Ray Gillette, the chief resident in ob/gyn at San Francisco County General Hospital, about the conversation. A native Washingtonian, Gillette expressed interest in Garfield's proposal. He told Cutting that he would seriously consider Garfield's proposal if Cutting himself would seriously consider it. When Garfield called Cutting back a few days later, Cutting asked him to come up to the Stanford Medical School in San Francisco to talk the matter over with Dr. Loren Chandler, the Dean.

"I considered myself kind of a fair-haired boy," Cutting remembers, "or at least Dr. Chandler was the kind of fellow that made all the students feel special."

Sidney Garfield arrived at the Lane Hospital of the Stanford Medical School in San Francisco in a bedraggled condition from the 3-hour flight in a single engine airplane from Los Angeles. He had a terrible headache. Cutting fetched him some aspirin. Thus fortified, Sidney Garfield entered Dean Chandler's office to explain to him the concept of prepaid group practice which he was trying to sell to some of his residents.

Chandler bristled. He told Garfield that he would not permit Cutting to go up to Grand Coulee because—as Garfield remembered—"it was an unethical way to practice medicine and Dr. Cutting would lose his status with the medical societies and it would be a mark against him for life. I asked him how else you could take care of workers without a health plan. They hadn't any money. He said, 'Well, you have to figure it out like everybody else figures it.' He would not permit Cece to go up there and work on a health plan that might affect his whole future life."

Undaunted, Garfield continued the argument. He guaranteed Chandler that Cutting would not be barred from the medical society if he went to work at Grand Coulee. Chandler replied that he would buy Garfield a steak dinner if Cutting took the job and was also admitted into a medical society. Leaving the interview, Garfield stood with Cutting in the hallway outside the dean's office and told him that he thought the matter was hopeless, that Dean Chandler would never permit Cutting to join the Grand Coulee venture. Nevertheless, Garfield took the time to outline to Cutting the challenges and opportunities of what he was offering.

"Let me think about it," Cutting said, "and I'll be in touch with you." A week later, he called Garfield and said that he would like to visit the Grand Coulee hospital.

"Dr. Garfield went on home, expecting probably I wouldn't join," Cutting recalls. "But I got to thinking about it....It seemed to me that I would always be a small boy going in with another doctor, the senior doctor in San Francisco. To go as chief surgeon to a new hospital—active, lots of work in a big, industrial project—would at least give me a lot more experience the first few years. I was young and eager, active, anxious to work, so I called Dr. Garfield and told him that in spite of Dr. Chandler's recommendation, I'd go up and take a look at it." The more Cutting thought of the offer, the more intriguing it became. It was not the concept of prepayment, however, but the chance for surgical experience, that led Cutting to go up to Grand Coulee and to take a second look.[6]

Returning to San Francisco, Cutting talked the matter over with his wife Millie, a nurse whom he had married during his internship year. Since Cutting himself was making only $30 a month as a resident, Millie Cutting was carrying two jobs, working downtown during the day in a pediatrician's office and at night for an ophthalmologist. When Cutting outlined Garfield's offer, his wife said that she would do whatever he wanted. Shortly after, the couple packed their belongings into their Dodge and headed north to Washington.

Thanks to his initial contact with Cutting, Garfield was also able to recruit from Stanford, Ray Gillette, an obstetrics and gynecology specialist, and Richard Moore, a resident in surgery and orthopedics. Garfield also recruited a classmate from the University of Iowa School of Medicine, Gene Wiley, a general practitioner with training in surgery, and Chuck Olson, an internist. A number of nurses from San Francisco General also signed up, including Winifred Wetherill, who met and married Wally Neighbor in Grand Coulee, and Jerry Searcy, a nurse-anesthetist. All in all, SR Garfield MD and Associates, as the group was called, initially included an internist, an obstetrician-gynecologist, two surgeons (including the mostly absent Garfield), and two general practitioners. The first thing the six doctors did upon getting settled in Grand Coulee was to study for their Washington State licenses. They went over in a group to Olympia and took their examinations together. Everyone passed. Also on the staff was an osteopath practicing as a physiotherapist. "Our wives all loved him," Wally Neighbor later remarked, "for rubbing their necks and removing their tensions and whatnot."[7]

The early months of SR Garfield MD and Associates were not idyllic. The location was remote and conditions primitive. Aside from Mason City, there was Government Town, where staffers from the Bureau of Reclamation lived, and Grand Coulee itself, which was mostly a red light district. Cecil and Millie Cutting resided in the company hotel. They were flat broke. The young couple had exhausted their resources getting to Washington. Neither of them thought of asking for an advance. "My wife couldn't take the heat very well," Cutting remembered, "and she would lay on the bed with a wet sheet over her; and we didn't have enough money to eat, really. She would go over to the cafeteria and see how far she could stretch a few pennies to eat; and of course I ate well at the hospital, and it had air conditioning and everything. She finally learned to come over and sit in the waiting room on the very hottest days. Since then, Dr. Garfield has laughed at us and said, 'Why didn't you ask me for money?' We didn't know enough to do that!"[8]

At the end of this first discomforting month, Cutting received his first paycheck for $350. He and Millie moved into a remodeled schoolhouse, the largest home in the community, and it soon became the social center for the physicians and the Kaiser executives.

After the first few months, Sidney Garfield did not spend much time at Grand Coulee. Basing himself in Los Angeles, where he continued at the County Hospital, Garfield flew up to Grand Coulee every sixth weekend to relieve Cutting. Cutting and the other physicians were on duty 24 hours a day. Every sixth weekend they were off. Since construction crews were working around the clock, full 24 hour-a-day coverage was absolutely necessary. "Many a night we'd get out on the job at two o'clock in the morning or so," Cutting later recalled. "A fellow had fallen off the dam and smashed up, so we had to get him in."[9]

Although an absentee landlord, Garfield could also be a hard taskmaster. On one occasion he called the doctors together in the hospital dining room and told them that the patients were waiting too long. Certain doctors were taking breaks while the patients were waiting. Everyone had to buckle down and take care of the patients. Cecil Cutting took offense. "I talked to him afterwards, saying that I was running all the time. I couldn't work any harder. If that was not satisfactory, then I'd better give it up right now. He assured me that he wasn't talking about me and asked me to stay on. I came that close to leaving. Not because I didn't like it, but because I didn't like the lecture."[10]

The Grand Coulee plan was similar to that of the desert. SR Garfield MD and Associates was paid a percentage of the workers' compensation premium for industrial coverage. A voluntary payroll deduction of 50 cents per week per employee insured coverage for nonindustrial injuries or illness. Initially skeptical, the workers and their union leadership soon became satisfied, even appreciative, of the care they were receiving under this health plan. Their wives and children, however, continued to be treated on a fee-for-service basis because Garfield, as he himself admitted, continued to resist expansion of the program because he remained unable to devise a satisfactory computation of prepaid rates for dependent coverage. Because of the fee barrier, dependents deferred seeking the medical attention they needed. The doctors noted that dependents were coming into the hospital with complications of pneumonia, mastoid infections, ruptured appendixes, and other serious problems that were only rarely encountered in the construction workers. Not surprisingly, once the program had established itself, the union leadership began to put pressure on the Kaiser Company and on Garfield to provide prepaid coverage for dependents. The unions even threatened to go on strike unless such a program was devised. Thus pressured, Garfield met with Edgar Kaiser, and the two of them, almost arbitrarily, settled upon a rate of 50 cents per week per adult, 25 cents per week per child. With this agreed upon, prepaid health plan coverage was extended to dependents. To handle the new members, pediatrician George Agnew was added to the staff. The rate worked, and the expanded program, now covering 15,000 workers and their dependents, thrived. With prepaid comprehensive coverage extended to workers and dependents, with multispecialty group medicine being practiced at the hospital, a major innovation in the delivery of medical services had occurred, almost by accident.

As in the case of the Mojave Desert project, prepaid comprehensive coverage at Grand Coulee resulted in a high level of preventive medicine. The physicians at Coulee noticed a change in the types of conditions for which dependents sought medical care. They saw simple acute appendicitis, instead of peritonitis; earaches instead of mastoiditis; upper respiratory infections and less pneumonia; early lumps in the breast instead of metastatic carcinoma. Of course, in 1939–1940, they did not have penicillin or other antibacterial chemotherapy for pneumonia or ear infections, but hospital care, fluids, and other symptomatic care seemed to prevent most serious complications. Garfield was especially pleased by the ability of his program to ward off fatal pneumonia. "We no longer saw terminal pneumonias," he later remembered of the prepaid program for dependents after it was 6 months in operation. "We saw the early pneumonias, and we were able to treat them early to prevent complications and in many cases, we felt, prevent them from dying."[11] With the medical skills of group practice, the Coulee physicians were also capable of handling just about any case that came their way, including serious cancer surgeries. Only one patient, a suspected brain tumor, had to be referred to Spokane.

Paradoxically, the group's fee-for-service income increased when comprehensive coverage for dependents went into effect. It had been expected to decrease, but the wives of workers, commenting about their experiences with the employee health plan to others who were not covered, stimulated a new level of medical care consciousness in the community. "We gave good care and we gave one class of service. The fellows with concrete blisters on their feet or sand in their eyes," Cecil Cutting claimed, "were just as important to us as the fellows with appendicitis or chest pain."[12] The prepaid membership came from construction workers and their dependents and government workers associated with the project. Townspeople from Coulee Center came in on a fee-for-service basis, including a few entrepreneurs who used a red light to advertise their services.

Grand Coulee was by and large a happy time for the physicians of SR Garfield MD and Associates, and in later years the memory of Grand Coulee, where they had first sustained a prepaid comprehensive group practice covering both workers and dependents, was considered the second founding, after the desert, of the Kaiser Permanente Medical Plan. It was easy to remember these years, moreover, because they were so pleasant. The group was, most fundamentally, young men and women who had taken their training together and bonded as friends during these formative years. Cecil Cutting, Ray Gillette, and Richard Moore had all been residents together in the Stanford program at San Francisco General Hospital where Winifred Wetherill and Jerry Searcy had been on the nursing staff. Mildred Cutting, Isabel Moore, and Hazel Gillette were classmates in the Stanford Nursing School. Gene Wiley had gone through the University of Iowa School of Medicine with Sidney Garfield, and Wally Neighbor and Garfield had been close friends since their residencies at Los Angeles County Hospital. Relationships became further bonded when Wally Neighbor married Winifred Wetherill and Charles Olson married Evelyn Sanger from the nursing staff. The Neighbors had their first son born to them at Grand Coulee and the Gillettes had their second child.

The medical group made friends with the Kaiser staff: with Edgar and Sue Kaiser, Clay and Kit Bedford, Joe Reis of Industrial Indemnity, Mike Miller, the estimating engineer for the Kaiser company, Hal Babbitt, who ran the hotel and acted as personnel officer, and Todd Waddell, who ran the safety department and the insurance programs. Friendships were also formed with Bureau of Reclamation staff living in a government settlement across the Columbia River. The Reclamation people even had lawns, on which one could stretch out for a picnic.

The Cuttings had their converted schoolhouse moved into the center circle of Mason City, where it functioned informally as the focus of social activity during off hours. Progressive parties would begin there, then move on to the Kaisers or the Bedfords, with increasing merriment. Often after midnight, when the temperature had at long last cooled down, the group would meet for badminton in the company gymnasium. The Kaisers, the Bedfords, the Cuttings, and the Neighbors were intense badminton devotees. Wally Neighbor and Charles Olson loved the outdoor life: fishing, swimming, duck and pheasant hunting, together with the ice skating, skiing, and tobogganing available in the winter. At Christmastime, there would be caroling and Dickensian tableaus in the great dining room, which the company would decorate so that, as Wally Neighbor remembered, "It looked like the finest nightclub you could imagine. They would import and bring in great huge mirrors, beautiful drapes. You've never seen anything so beautiful."[13] Here also was held a gala New Year's Eve celebration. When it came time to get away, Spokane was only a hundred miles distant and even Seattle was possible on a long weekend. "The doctors would all take turns going into the city," Garfield remembered, "and when they did it was quite a holiday. But being all together in quite a social group, all liking each other—we picked people who liked each other—we really didn't feel too cut off. We felt like we were enjoying ourselves."[14]

The most fundamental satisfaction of these years was the practice of medicine in a prepaid, hospital-based group practice. "We knew we liked the way the practice of medicine was being carried out," remembers Cecil Cutting. "The prepayment made so much sense. We didn't have to worry about putting claims to the insurance company for every visit and billing the people for every service that we gave them. It was sort of a continuation of the same sort of practice that you had as a house officer in medical school. We were all enthusiastic about that—

the advantages of working together with a group of specialists, and prepayment method budgeting and forecasting of our expenses, meeting
our payroll and so on."[15]

The hours were long and the work intense. Physicians worked 6 days
a week with only two or three Sundays off a month. Since three shifts
were working on the dam around the clock, up to 50 workers could
show up for a midnight sick call. "You were there to do the job and you
did it," was how Wally Neighbor remembered these years. "There was
no complaining."[16] Even Sidney Garfield, the group proprietor, did his
full share of work on the weekends he came up from Los Angeles.
"Once at Grand Coulee," nurse anesthetist Jerry Searcy remembers,
"Sid was walking around the hospital without his white coat, looking
very youthful with his bright red hair and casual clothes. A patient saw
him and shouted, 'Boy! Would you take care of this?' pointing to his
bedpan. Sid wasn't at all offended. He laughed and emptied the bedpan. Of course the patient had no idea who Sid was. When Sid performed surgery at Grand Coulee, he used to sing 'My heart belongs to
daddy.' He loved to sing."[17]

As hard-pressed as they were, the young doctors and nurses had the
satisfaction, as Neighbor remembered it, of experimenting in prepaid
medicine with no interference from the outside. "In Coulee," Neighbor
remembered, "there was no county medical society involved. If there
was, we didn't know about it. So here we were, experimenting with what
was in those days unethical...or that's what they later said we were."[18]
According to Garfield, the group applied to the American Medical Association for permission to start its own medical society chapter. A
Grant County Medical Society was informally organized, its existence
acknowledged by a letter from the Washington Medical Association.
Thus the Grant County Medical Society was organized entirely on a
group-practice prepaid basis. Technically, Sidney Garfield had won his
bet with Dean Chandler of the Stanford Medical School. Chandler's
protégé Cecil Cutting was now a member in good standing of a medical
society. "I wrote back to Chandler that he'd lost his bet," said Garfield,
"but he never did pay off that steak dinner."[19]

While most of the married nurses tended to their families, Mildred
Cutting—who had spent her first month at Grand Coulee broke, hun-
gry, and exhausted from the heat—recovered sufficiently to start a well-
baby clinic in the local community church. Working on a volunteer basis, Mildred Cutting organized the clinic and solicited funds for it door
to door, including the houses of ill repute on the hill. "The madams
were very friendly," says Cecil Cutting. "The community church pro-

vided the space, and the houses of ill repute the money—a very compatible community."[20]

All times, especially good times, come to an end. In its fourth year this tightly knit medical family, SR Garfield MD and Associates, faced the prospect of dissolution as the Grand Coulee Dam neared completion. In the evenings, the physicians would often get together for discussions of their future. They would speculate about establishing a prepaid group practice in a permanent community such as the San Francisco Bay Area or Los Angeles. "We had a plan which could stand on its own feet," remembered Sidney Garfield, "pay its own way, build and pay for its own facilities, pay decent remuneration to the doctors. We even felt that in a permanent operation we could provide funds for training, teaching and research."[21]

It was an idealistic dream. Three big hurdles loomed. Opposition from the American Medical Association and its state and county medical society affiliates was a certainty. Would people in a permanent community have any notion of prepaid group practice? In isolated communities such as Grand Coulee and the Mojave Desert, prepaid care was easily understood and accepted by enrollees. It was the only care available. In a permanent urban community, people would have established patterns of getting medical and hospital care. How could they be introduced to the advantages of prepaid group practice programs? To advertise was, in the ethos of that era, unethical and unthinkable.

The third hurdle was capital. The physicians and the Kaiser businesspeople knew that it would take substantial funds to establish a prepaid health plan in a permanent community while being forced to resist established medical opposition and educate consumers to a new way of delivering health care. The Kaiser Company was not in the medical business. A medical care program was an enterprise for doctors, not engineers. If such a program ever were to be established, the doctors would have to make it on their own, without assistance from the Kaiser Company. Or so they thought. "...we'd been dreaming of the possibility of a medical program like that in a permanent area, but the possibility of that seemed rather remote," said Sidney Garfield, "because of those problems of financing, getting membership, and medical opposition..."[22]

Throughout 1941, as construction of the Grand Coulee Dam neared completion and workers were dispersed to other projects, the physicians of SR Garfield MD and Associates began to seek other opportunities. Richard Moore, the first to resign, took a position at the Western Medical Clinic in Seattle, an industrial clinic with a lay board of trustees.

Cecil Cutting secured a surgical appointment at the Virginia Mason Clinic in Seattle, a private fee-for-service multispecialty clinic. Ray Gillette and Charles Olson joined the Army Medical Corps and were assigned to Spokane. Wally Neighbor remained on at Grand Coulee for a while before he too joined the Army. Gene Wiley stayed on for a year as the last remaining surgeon. He subsequently returned to Iowa, where he established a successful fee-for-service surgical practice. Sidney Garfield returned full time to Los Angeles County Hospital, where he had a specialized residency in surgery and a teaching assignment with the USC School of Medicine. Garfield joined a reserve Army medical unit then being organized at USC. When the USC unit was called up, Sidney Garfield found himself a first lieutenant in the Medical Corps of the Army of the United States. With characteristic flair, Garfield had his uniforms specially tailored. They fit him to a tee. Among his duties was the examination of civilians for military service. One of these examinees was John Smillie, a USC intern at Los Angeles County Hospital. The world was at war, and very soon, on December 7, 1941, America became involved. Garfield's unit had orders for India. Ironically, as an Army surgeon, Sidney Garfield was still in a type of salaried group medical practice outside the usual fee-for-service structure.

3

World War II and the Shipyards— 1942–1945

At each previous period of development, in the Mojave Desert and at Grand Coulee, a massive mobilization of people, material, and equipment energized the theory and concept of prepaid group medical practice. With the entrance of the United States into World War II, the industrial mobilization that sustained Garfield's program during two major construction projects would soon involve the Kaiser industries at an even more unprecedented level. Midway through the war, the physicians and support staff led by Garfield would be meeting the medical needs of more than 90,000 shipyard workers and other Kaiser employees. Two Depression-era public works projects had already proved that prepayment and group medical practice worked well in special environments. By the end of World War II, this experiment had proved itself even further and was ready to serve an even larger constituency: the general public.

In September 1940 Great Britain stood alone against the Axis Powers. Its sole source of supply was shipping convoys from the United States. In that critical month, as the Battle of Britain raged in the skies overhead, the British Admiralty sent a Technical Merchant Shipbuilding Commission to the United States to organize the construction of merchant ships in American shipyards. One contract—60 freighters for a total cost of $120 million—was won by the Todd-California Shipbuilding Corporation, which had been hastily organized in late 1940 by Henry J. Kaiser and the Todd Shipbuilding Company of Seattle. The company planned to build 30 freighters in shipyard facilities only then being organized in Richmond, California, a community a few miles north of Oakland on the San Francisco Bay. On April 14, 1941, the first keel of the first freighter, the *Ocean Vanguard,* was laid. Less then 200 days later, the ship was ready for service. That freighter was the first of 1490 vessels to be constructed in Kaiser shipyards over the next 5 years. That 197 days of construction time would soon be reduced to an average of 27 days. In the case of the *Robert E. Peary,* launched in November 1942, less than 1 year after Pearl Harbor, the time between keel laying and launching was reduced to 7 days, 14 hours and 29 minutes.

When the United States entered the war in December 1941, the Richmond shipyards added the U.S. Maritime Commission as a client. For the Commission and for other federal clients, over the course of the war, the Kaiser shipyards delivered 821 Liberty ships, as its small freighters were called, 50 small aircraft carriers, 219 Victory-class cargo ships, 24 freighters of other descriptions, 45 troop transports, 87 combat transports, 45 landing ship tank vessels, 12 frigates, and 147 tankers, for a total of more than 15 million deadweight tons of shipping: an impressive record for a group of industrialists, led by Henry J. Kaiser, who had to study a handbook of shipping terms before they made their first presentation to the British Admiralty.

Henry J. Kaiser and his young managers brought to shipbuilding the same fast-track techniques they had evolved in the construction of roads and dams in the previous two decades. In the Richmond shipyards, where the majority of the Liberty ships were constructed, techniques of prefabrication and assembly-line construction were brought to a level of high industrial art. By late 1943 some 90,000 men and women, working in three shifts, 7 days a week, were orchestrating their efforts with almost balletlike precision. Steel poured into the Richmond shipyards in carload lots. Flanged into preassembly parts, the steel was welded and riveted into ship sections, which were then trucked or lifted by crane to assembly sites. Ships took shape, section by section, assembled by teams of workers trained to perform one—and only one—task. This level of social organization and cooperation was matched by a program of medical care equally organized and disciplined. The intense social cooperation of the shipyards inspired and sustained a practice of medicine comparably characterized by innovation and social cooperation. When it was over, a new way of practicing medicine had emerged.

A mere month after Pearl Harbor, some 30,000 workers were busy in the Richmond shipyards alone. Kaiser personnel representatives had traveled the country to recruit this first battalion of what would eventually be an army of workers affiliated in one way or another with the Kaiser shipyards. This first wave of recruits arrived at Richmond from around the country by the trainload. This hastily mobilized industrial army was quartered in quickly erected barracks or later, when families arrived, in government-financed housing. This was wartime, and recruitment standards were liberal. There were no restrictions as to age, sex, or—in a still segregated America—race. Fully one-quarter of the work force, eventually, was female. A significant percentage of the male work force was either overage or in poor health. The majority of the younger men had been classified 4F by their local draft boards.

They were in indifferent or frequently poor health, and they were doing dangerous work. By October 1943, in fact, workers in American industry, operating at peak wartime levels, had sustained more than 7 million injuries serious enough to be recorded. Thousands of these accidents proved fatal. Despite every precaution, the Richmond shipyards, where tons of steel were being daily cut, shaped, welded, riveted, and swung by crane into place, were a place where accidents happened; and Kaiser's Richmond manager, Clay Bedford, the former chief engineer of the Grand Coulee project, was worried. He had 30,000 workers on his hands, and in the small city of Richmond nearby, there was only one practicing physician, L. Paul Fraser, who provided care on a fee-for-service basis. Many other physicians in the area were leaving for military service. In shipyards administered by the U.S. Navy, uniformed medical officers were assigned to care for civilian workers. Richmond, however, was strictly under civilian management.

Realizing that he had a serious problem on his hands, Clay Bedford called Sidney Garfield, who was in Los Angeles—just as A. B. Ordway had called Garfield in July 1938 when a medical program was needed at Grand Coulee. At the time, Sidney Garfield was in the custom-tailored uniform of a first lieutenant in the Medical Corps of the U.S. Army. His reserve unit, comprised of physicians from the University of Southern California Medical School and the Los Angeles County General Hospital, had been called to active duty and was scheduled to leave for India for eventual assignment to the Burma Theater to help keep the Burma Road open.

"Mr. Bedford called me up one day," Garfield later recounted, "and asked me to come up to Richmond to help them. He said they were having trouble getting the injured workers into the local hospitals, couldn't get doctors, and could I come up and help them. I told him I was in the Army and was supposed to embark for India in one month. He said, 'Well, you've got a month. Can you come up and advise me what to do?'"

Traveling north to Richmond in uniform, Garfield spent January 1942 conferring with Bedford, Henry Kaiser, Jr. (Kaiser's other son, also in the family business), and A. B. Ordway and Harold Hatch of Industrial Indemnity, regarding the establishment of a prepaid comprehensive medical program for the Richmond shipyard workers. At some point during the month, it became evident to everyone that only Sidney Garfield had the experience and talent necessary to organize and administer such an unprecedented program. In the middle of the month, Henry J. Kaiser sent A. B. Ordway to Washington with a special request for the President. When Ordway returned, he presented Garfield with a letter signed by Franklin Delano Roosevelt, the commander in chief, releasing Garfield from his military obligation so as to take over the Richmond medical program.

"He hadn't even asked me if I wanted to," Garfield later said of Ordway's action. "Of course I wanted to do it because it was a lot more interesting than going to sit around in India."

Garfield had one reservation: loyalty to the physicians of his reserve unit, many of whom were his personal friends, especially Ray Kay. However, Garfield's colonel, Clarence Berne, a surgeon, encouraged Garfield to take the new assignment. "He thought I would be doing something more important."[1] Dr. Berne was correct in his assessment. By late 1944, Dr. Garfield would be directing the efforts of more than 90 physicians and support staff in three locations: the Richmond shipyards, the Vancouver-Portland shipyards on the Columbia River between Washington and Oregon, and the Kaiser steel mill in Fontana, California.

As soon as it was clear that he would take charge of the program, Garfield began to recruit physicians. The first physician he contacted was Cecil Cutting in Seattle. In late January 1942, Cutting came down to investigate the situation at the Richmond shipyard and to hear Garfield's proposal. "The opportunity to have prepayment," Cutting remembered, "the combination of industrial and non-industrial, the opportunity to form a new group, and the fun of working with Sid...was too much to resist."[2] By March 1, 1942, Cecil and Millie Cutting were ensconced in the elegant Claremont Hotel in Oakland, and Cecil Cutting was working furiously as Garfield's chief of staff. For a month or two, Garfield and Cutting were the only active physicians in the program. Then Jerry Gill, an orthopedist fresh from his residency, joined, followed by Richard Moore, the Grand Coulee veteran practicing in Seattle, and internist Morris Collen, a friend of Garfield's from Los Angeles, who came up to assume the duties of chief of medicine. Garfield, Cutting, and Moore recruited extensively at Stanford, the University of California at San Francisco, and the San Francisco General Hospital. Three young physicians—La Mont Baritell, Norman Haugen, and Donald Grant—joined as surgical residents, completing their residency training in the wartime program. By mid-1942 a core group had been organized, including Bob King, obstetrics and gynecology, Mel Friedman, pathology, and Bruce Henley, who served as chief of surgery. Reaching back to his desert days, Garfield recruited Harry Kirby, an internist. As the program grew, Paul Fitzgibbon, a former quarterback for the Green Bay Packers who had gone into medicine, assumed major administrative responsibilities under Garfield. Like so many in the program, beginning with Garfield himself, Fitzgibbon, a neurologist, came from a residency at USC/LA County, as did Morris Collen, who would play such a major role in the organization over the next 40 years.

On March 3, 1942, Cecil Cutting opened offices at 411 30th Street in Oakland, in an area known as Pill Hill because of the proximity of Oakland's three major hospitals, Peralta, Providence, and Merritt. Cutting obtained operating privileges at Merritt Hospital where Garfield had contracted for 20 beds. With Clay Bedford's authorization and the concurrence of the Navy, Garfield went to work designing and building a small field hospital at the Richmond shipyard to back up the five existing first-aid stations. The 10-bed field hospital was ready by June 1942.

Garfield had secured the 20 temporary beds at Merritt as part of a purchase agreement. Merritt Hospital owned an unused four-story steel-and-concrete hospital structure at the corner of Broadway and MacArthur in Oakland. The structure was built in the 1920s as the maternity wing of the Fabiola Hospital, a rambling wooden building that had since burned down. The trustees of Fabiola had subsequently donated the surviving structure to Merritt Hospital when their institution went out of existence. In the early months of the war, the War Manpower Board began to renovate the structure as a dormitory but just as suddenly abandoned these plans. Harold Hatch told Garfield about the structure, and Garfield approached the administrator at Merritt about purchasing it. Garfield offered $50,000, provided that the 20 beds at Merritt Hospital could be guaranteed during the renovation program. The sale was accomplished in early March 1942.

Garfield estimated that it would take $250,000 to transform the abandoned four-story shell into a modern hospital facility. Because of the financial success of his Desert Center and Grand Coulee programs, he knew that he would have no trouble borrowing the money from Industrial Indemnity Exchange. He was already in the process of negotiating a loan, in fact, when Henry J. Kaiser himself intervened. Garfield had already taken Kaiser on a personal tour of the quasi-derelict structure. Since the elevator was out of operation, the two of them climbed to the top floor, then wended their way through a series of empty rooms, littered with the debris of a decade (the hospital had remained closed throughout the Depression) and the abandoned dormitory project. "The building was a shambles," Garfield remembered, "and I was just worried to death that he would turn it down because it looked so terrible, and we walked through it and he didn't say a word." Somewhat discouraged by Kaiser's silence, Garfield asked the older man's opinion. Kaiser smiled as he put his arm around Garfield's shoulder and asked, "What's the matter, Sid? Don't you think I have any vision?"[3]

Kaiser cautioned Garfield about becoming indebted to the very same insurance companies providing coverage for his programs. It would be better, he argued, to seek financing from a third party such as the Bank of America. Kaiser personally took Garfield across the Bay to San Francisco to see A. P. Giannini, the president of the Bank of America, who would over the course of the war extend to Kaiser Industries the longest single line of credit ever extended in American banking history. Since he already had the promise of a loan from Industrial Indemnity Exchange, Garfield felt confident as he approached the interview with Giannini. At the meeting, Garfield outlined the success of his Desert Center and Grand Coulee programs, which included the building, equipping, and financing of three hospitals. He underscored that the Mason City Hospital in Grand Coulee had operated in the black, something that hospitals rarely do. He then asked Giannini for the $250,000 loan. To his surprise, Giannini replied: "Doctor, I would not lend you one red cent on a hospital. If something happens, there is no way our bank could foreclose. What would we do with a hospital? However, if Henry here will guarantee the loan, you can have the money." Kaiser laughed at Giannini's remark, then quickly expressed his confidence in Garfield. With Kaiser's guarantee, Giannini made the loan.[4]

From the perspective of the conflicts that would later result, this entire incident is instructive. Garfield, after all, had already purchased the hospital with his own funds and arranged on a preliminary basis a line of credit from Industrial Indemnity Exchange. He did not need Henry J. Kaiser to help him finance his program. Kaiser, in fact, needed Garfield to set up the medical program. And yet Garfield permitted

Kaiser to intercede as guarantor of the loan from Giannini. Thirty years later, reminiscing on his acquiescence, Garfield was still uneasy. "I had to do what he said," Garfield said of Kaiser's decision to go to Giannini. "I really wanted to, anyway, because Mr. Kaiser controlled all the industrial work…so I said I'll just go to the Bank of America and try to borrow the money and he said, 'I better go with you.'"[5] In the midst of his massive wartime responsibilities, Henry J. Kaiser had taken the time out to inspect Fabiola Hospital and go with Garfield to see Giannini.

2

Who was this man, this Henry John Kaiser, with whom Sidney Garfield's own destiny was now being so closely linked? Born in upstate New York in 1882 to German immigrants, Kaiser left school as a teenager to become a portrait photographer. Moving to the Pacific Northwest in his twenties, he formed his own road-paving company. In this line of work, Kaiser first showed his extraordinary talent for coordinating men and machines for fast-paced construction or civil engineering projects. In 1921 he moved his company headquarters and residence south to Oakland across the Bay from San Francisco, where he coordinated a major road-paving project in Cuba. During the construction of the Hoover Dam in the late 1920s and early 1930s, Kaiser headed the Six Companies, Inc., a consortium that built this massive project. He then went on to build Parker Dam for the Metropolitan Water District of southern California. During the Coulee Dam project Kaiser first personally encountered Sidney Garfield. Kaiser spent the better part of a day inspecting Garfield's facilities. At the end of his visit he suggested that Garfield was operating a program that had implications for more than this one construction site.

The association that resulted between the lean surgeon, clear-eyed, reserved, and enigmatic, and the balding, rotund, corporate entrepreneur lasted until Kaiser's death in 1967. It was a complex relationship, to say the least. Garfield was highly educated; Kaiser was a high school dropout. Kaiser talked constantly. He lived on the telephone. During World War II, his long-distance bills frequently approached a quarter of a million dollars per year. Sidney Garfield spoke only when it was necessary and had a genius for keeping his own counsel. Kaiser regarded Garfield, in part, as a son: one of the many young men—Clay Bedford, Eugene Trefethen, Jr., and his own two sons, Edgar and

Henry, Jr., among others—whom he delighted in challenging to increased levels of performance and responsibility. Kaiser and Garfield eventually became in-laws when they married sisters.

In later years, Kaiser created for himself a mythological past—poverty, a lack of opportunity, a saintly mother dying in her son's arms without proper medical attention—another instance of Kaiser's lifelong habit of seizing upon opportunities and making them work. Kaiser left school after the eighth grade, not because upstate New York or his own family could not provide future educational opportunities, but because he was anxious to get on with it, to seek the main chance, and school had little to offer in this regard. He became a photographer because that seemed handy, and later, when roads needed paving, he got into the paving business with equal aplomb. He later entered the worlds of dam building, shipbuilding, steel making, cement manufacturing, automobiles, hotels, and real estate development, broadcasting, and prepaid comprehensive medical care with equal virtuosity. In each case, Henry J. Kaiser imagined himself in the midst of these activities, and somehow this imagining came true. The man who had to look up ship terms in the public library in 1940 was a few short years later the greatest mass producer of ships in the nation's history.

If Kaiser had one *métier*, it was the corporation. He had a genius for getting the most out of other people's talents, cooperatively organized, and giving them credit as well. Strong in ego, he was not egotistical. He shared the credit. Kaiser encountered the American corporation in the 1920s, when it was still teetering from the assaults and corrective action of the Progressive era, and he refashioned and reenergized it with a vision and a creative action that proceeded from his own uniquely American personality and point of view. Kaiser found the corporation a family factory and a company store, and he left it, in theory at least, and frequently in the practice of his own companies, a diversified and integrated social and economic environment. In this he brought to the United States a sensibility once thought to be exclusively Japanese, a concern, that is, for the totality of the work environment. Kaiser pioneered the vertical and horizontal integration of allied industries. Building dams, he manufactured cement. Building ships, he made his own steel.

Surrounding himself with talented young executives, Kaiser placed upon them responsibilities infinitely beyond their years. When his son Edgar was still in his early twenties, Kaiser thrust major responsibilities on him and on Edgar's fraternity brother Eugene Trefethen, Jr. The two of them became an effective team. Clay Bedford was barely into his thirties when Kaiser had him building Grand Coulee Dam and, later, Liberty ships. Liking young people, he had a habit of making sons of his top (and very young) executives. This largesse extended to other members of his executive team as well. The Kaiser executive dining room was part conference room, part club, part family gathering. Kaiser understood labor as well, and his successful dealings with unions were part of the total pattern of his creativity as a corporate impresario.

It must be said that Henry J. Kaiser was a dominating presence, a workaholic who tended to devour even the private schedules of his top executives. He was a lover of the good life. But he was a businessperson with unbounded energy, enthusiasm, and optimism.

3

In 1942 Sidney Garfield showed himself worthy of Henry J. Kaiser's challenge to build quickly and well. With the $250,000 secured from Giannini, Garfield went to work transforming the Fabiola Hospital into a modern facility. Amazingly, the entire renovation took only 5 months, even in an atmosphere of wartime control of materials. Forty years later, the intricacies of land purchase, architectural planning, governmental approvals, construction and equipping have pushed these 5 months to a minimum of 5 years. According to Morris Collen, who was in the audience at the dedication, Kaiser told the assembled group, "My mother died in my arms because she didn't receive adequate medical care, and I vowed that I would do whatever I could so this wouldn't happen to anybody else."[6] The 54-bed facility was dedicated by Henry and Bess Kaiser on August 21, 1942.

The renovated structure was called the Permanente Foundation Hospital because by that time the foundation concept had been adopted as the organizational strategy for the new enterprise. In the months before shipping out for India, Raymond Kay, Garfield's friend and colleague in Los Angeles, had made a study of foundations as they related to the practice of medicine. At the suggestion of Burrell Raulston, dean of the USC School of Medicine, Kay had gone to New York to investigate foundation structures and procedures and had assembled a portfolio of available literature on the subject. Kay had been severely disappointed when Garfield had withdrawn from their USC/Los Angeles County General Hospital Army Medical Unit. Before shipping out for India, Kay and his wife Martha had dinner with Sidney Garfield in San Francisco. Kay told his good friend that he would be reconciled to Garfield's leaving the unit on two conditions. First of all, Garfield should pay his physicians no more than doctors were receiving in military service. Second, Garfield should establish a foundation to set aside funds for capital to start a prepaid group-practice plan in Los Angeles after the war. With their many friends and medical associates in the Los Angeles area, Kay speculated, and with enough money put aside through the foundation, he and Garfield could ensure the future of prepaid group practice in the southland in the postwar era.

In the long run, Garfield found it impossible to meet Kay's first request. In certain cases, Garfield had to pay more than military pay schedules so as to recruit scarce categories of physicians in wartime. Kay's second request, however, the foundation, struck Garfield as a simple but elegant strategy. Garfield took the foundation idea to Clay Bedford, the chief executive officer of the Richmond shipyards. Bedford liked the idea and suggested that Garfield take it directly to Kaiser. In order to find time in Kaiser's busy schedule, Bedford had Garfield driven up 90 miles to the Sacramento train station to board the *City of San Francisco* on which Kaiser and his wife, who hated flying, were returning from Washington with attorney Paul Marrin of Thelen, Marrin, Johnson, and Bridges, Kaiser's legal counsel. During the 2-hour journey down to Oakland, Garfield outlined the foundation strategy to Kaiser.

"He was immediately sold on the idea," Garfield later recalled. "Paul Marrin, however, said 'It can't be done.' Mr. Kaiser said, 'Why can't it be done?' Marrin said, 'Well, you're not contributing any funds to the foundation. You're trying to build up a foundation out of the earnings of an operation and that's never been done. You can't build up a foundation by its bootstraps.' Well, Mr. Kaiser and I both argued with him that there had to be some way of doing it, then finally Mr. Kaiser said, 'Paul, I'm sick and tired of having lawyers tell me things we can't do. Now you tell me how we can do it. That's your job.'"[7]

Marrin took the problem to his partner Robert Bridges, a tax specialist, and within a week what Marrin said could not be done had been accomplished. The Permanente Foundation, a charitable trust, was established in Alameda County, California, with Mr. and Mrs. Henry J. Kaiser, Edgar Kaiser, Eugene Trefethen, Jr., and a number of their attorneys acting as trustees. *Permanente,* the Spanish word for *permanent* or *everlasting,* was the name given by Spanish settlers to a stream in the Los Altos Hills of Santa Clara County, south of San Francisco. Unlike most other coastal California streams, which are dry in the summer and fall, the Permanente continues to run during the dry season. In the late 1930s, Kaiser had established a cement factory on property watered by the Ria Permanente. A small canyon on the stream became a favorite spot for Kaiser to retreat to and muse upon his many enterprises. There he would dream of what could be done—from ways of building things more efficiently to making the world more peaceful through commerce. Liking the place and its romantic Spanish name, he gave it to his cement company, the medical foundation, and several other enterprises as well. *Permanente* had become Kaiser's private code word for excellence that could prove itself—and endure.

The stated purpose of the Permanente Foundation was the accumulation of funds to be used for such charitable purposes as medical research and the extension of medical services into neglected areas and sectors of the population. To initiate the Foundation, another organization, Capital Construction, was established with money provided by Kaiser. This new entity purchased the refurbished Fabiola Hospital from Sidney Garfield, who had initially bought the structure with $50,000 of his own money. It was renamed Permanente Foundation Hospital. Capital Construction also assumed liability for the Bank of America loan. Capital Construction then donated its assets and liabilities to the Permanente Foundation, a nonprofit charitable trust. Sidney Garfield, acting as Sidney Garfield and Associates, a sole proprietorship, then leased the Permanente Foundation Hospital back from the trust and operated the hospital, the health plan, and the medical group as a single entity. All physicians and staff were, in effect, employees of Sidney Garfield. There was no separation of management among the physician group, hospital administration, and health plan. Every aspect of the program came under the direct supervision of Garfield or one of his designated physicians. In the phrase of Cecil Cutting, the Permanente program was "a single ball of wax."

Garfield paid the Permanente Foundation $22,000 a month rent for the hospital. All other revenues above salaries and expenses were also turned over to the Foundation. With these monies, the Foundation was able to pay off the Bank of America loan within 9 months. (Subsequent folklore has it that Garfield and Cecil Cutting privately burnt the mortgage in the fireplace of the Cutting household on Chabot Road in Oakland.) This rapidity of repayment was possible because Garfield was a genius at keeping salaries and expenses down. He did this by convincing his core group of physicians that, by sacrificing now, by putting the program on a solid foundation, they were insuring their own future. The doctors worked for salaries in the range of $300 to $500 per month. Garfield carefully evaluated any proposed purchases of furniture or equipment before the money was spent. Garfield himself took no salary but drew on an expense account authorized him by the Foundation. In the early years of the program, Garfield lived part of the time with the Cuttings and part of the time in the Sir Francis Drake Hotel in San Francisco.

Even as he kept expenses down and paid off his long-term debt, Garfield was also building for the future. As a contingency for obligations that might continue after the war, Garfield had the insurance companies retain 15 percent of the money they had agreed to pay for industrial coverage. By the end of the war, this fund had grown to $1.5 million. After the first mortgage was so quickly paid off, the Bank of America extended to Garfield a second line of credit in the amount of $250,000 to expand the Permanente Foundation Hospital by 75 beds. This time, Giannini did not require a co-signer. Later, $1.5 million was borrowed from the government for additional expansion. By 1945 the Permanente Hospital had expanded to 300 beds, and the Richmond Field Hospital had grown from 10 beds to 75.

"We never stopped expanding," Garfield remembered. "Pretty soon we'd run short of beds even with our addition, and then we got the Navy to expand the first aid stations, and then we built about 80 beds out there, and then we applied to the government for funds to add on to the main hospital another 200 beds."[8]

This expansion involved an ongoing lobby on the part of the Permanente Foundation. First of all, it was wartime, and building materials were kept under rigid controls. It was especially difficult to secure such complex equipment as X-ray machines and sterilizers. The committee reviewing all such requests in Washington, Garfield recalled, was in the main composed of administrators of hospitals opposed to the prepaid group-practice program of the Permanente Foundation. On the home front, the other hospitals in the Oakland area began to oppose the expansion of the Permanente Foundation Hospital into a major facility.

Henry J. Kaiser took a personal interest in lobbying the necessary approvals through the wartime bureaucracy. He put his trusted assistant Eugene Trefethen in charge of procurement and permissions for the Permanente program. Trefethen also helped Garfield and Associates secure from the War Manpower Commission the services of physicians who might otherwise have been drafted. "Most of the physicians we secured were 4Fs," Garfield later explained. "People the Army and the Navy rejected on account of their physical condition or something, but there were some top men that we had to have to keep up the quality of work that we wanted to have and with his [Kaiser's] help we were able to get more manpower declared essential to our work."[9]

Garfield personally recruited most of the physicians he slated for administrative positions. He took Morris Collen, for example, to lunch at the Garden Room of the St. Francis Hotel in San Francisco. A graduate in electrical engineering from the University of Minnesota, Collen had gone on to medical school at his alma mater with a career in research in mind. When Garfield interviewed him, Collen was in the second year of a residency in internal medicine at USC/LA County Hospital in Los Angeles. Shortly after Collen's arrival in Oakland, Garfield named him chief of medicine for the growing program.

In the midst of his time-consuming obligations as one of the top half dozen industrialists involved in the war effort, Henry J. Kaiser also took more than a passing interest in the health-care program Garfield was administering. In late 1942 Kaiser revealed the range and breadth of his thought in a speech before the National Association of Manufacturers. Kaiser's stated theme was what management could do to improve the postwar world. Many of Kaiser's proposals were far ahead of their time and revealed him to be not just an industrialist of formidable energy and will, but also a social thinker—at once pragmatic and visionary—of a distinctly American style. In his address Kaiser tackled such issues as postwar employment, government debt, the need for new housing construction, and the boom in consumer demand. He emphasized health care, however, as perhaps the greatest need in postwar America. Kaiser pleaded with the corporate executives present to take a look at the program that Sidney Garfield had established at the Grand Coulee and the Richmond shipyards. Under this revolutionary model, Kaiser stated, high-quality outpatient medical and hospital care were being made available to working men and women at no capital expense to the employers. Kaiser challenged corporate America to organize, finance, and manage similar medical centers where comprehensive medical coverage could be made available to working people for a prepayment amounting to pennies a day. In his first annual report, published in the *Permanente Foundation Medical Bulletin,* Sidney Garfield proudly underscored the fact that Henry J. Kaiser had been selected in a *Newsweek* survey published in December 6, 1943, as one of the major leaders of America, with special emphasis, as Garfield put it, on Kaiser's "trail-blazing in labor/management relations and social welfare for wage earners."[10]

In his first annual report as well, issued in January 1944, Garfield took solid satisfaction in the flourishing economics of the Permanente

Foundation program. As in the case of Desert Center and Grand Coulee, industrial care was financed by a prepayment of 17 percent of the workers' compensation insurance premium. More than 90 percent of the shipyard workers also paid 50 cents a week on a voluntary basis for nonindustrial medical coverage. During the peak productive period of 1942–1943, approximately 90,000 shipyard workers were receiving comprehensive medical coverage. Comprehensive medical care was being made available at an overall cost of seven cents a day.

Initially, in 1942–1943, dependents were not covered in the program. It took the full resources of Garfield and his physicians to meet the needs of 90,000 workers. By 1944 mobilization began to decline as the inevitability of a military victory asserted itself and the efficiency of the first phase of mobilization ensured an adequate supply of ships. With fewer workers to care for, Garfield began to open the Permanente program to dependents. As shipyard employment fell off, fewer workers were covered by the industrial plan. Enrollment in the voluntary nonindustrial health plan, however, remained at a high level, suggesting possibilities for the postwar era. Some 150 infants were born at the Permanente Foundation Hospital in 1944, and 662 pediatric patients were treated. As early as 1944, families were responding positively to the Permanente Foundation program. In fact, there were so many applications for dependent care that Garfield established admission criteria—a good work attendance record, a willingness to buy war bonds, and other factors—so as to bring highly motivated clients into the program. Garfield also saw in this small but growing dependent sector a cushion for the Permanente program against the layoff of shipyard workers that was already under way.

In the innovative medical economics he was pioneering, Garfield was especially proud of the level of compensation the Foundation offered its physicians and staff. Physician salaries ranged from $3600 to $6000 a year, rising to a ceiling of $8400 by 1945, at a time when the average doctor's annual income in the United States was $5000, with 50 percent of the nation's physicians netting less than $3912 per year. Even in a restricted wartime environment, the Permanente Foundation was capable of offering qualified physicians a substantial financial incentive to enter prepaid group medical practice. Nursing and staff salaries were also highly competitive, with nursing salaries ranging from $150 to $200 per month. It was Garfield's policy each year to implement to the limit all salary increases authorized by the War Labor Board. Prudent, even obsessive, in keeping down overhead costs, Garfield departed from his more stringent salary policies of Desert Center and Grand

Coulee and was generous when it came to physician salaries during the war years—despite the fact that Ray Kay had asked him, perhaps quixotically, to keep physicians' salaries on a military scale. Garfield's salary schedules reflected, in part, the necessity to remain competitive in a physician-scarce environment; but he was also anticipating the evolution of the Permanente Foundation program into the postwar years, when the challenge to recruit and retain highly qualified physicians would become even more intense.

Throughout the program, physicians and staff more than earned their salaries. During World War II, stateside military physicians frequently experienced relaxed working conditions, especially after the draft brought stateside military facilities up to an adequate level of staffing. Duty hours frequently ended in midafternoon, and most major military bases operated, or were adjacent to, excellent recreational facilities. Wally Neighbor, for instance, assigned as an Army doctor at Fort McArthur in San Pedro Harbor, left post every afternoon at 3:00 to play tennis. At the Richmond shipyards, however, staffing was more severe, hours were longer, case loads higher, and the patients, the vast majority of them 4Fs, were in the words of Cecil Cutting, "a walking pathological museum." "We had no interns or residents," Morris Collen remembers of the first two war years at the Permanente Hospital. "We would make rounds each morning, and each one would be on all night, working all day—twenty-four hours."[11]

In order to staff their shipyards, Kaiser personnel recruited workers from around the country without regard to age or physical condition. Hernias were a common complaint. Respiratory illnesses, especially lobar pneumonia, were exceedingly common. Pneumonia cases, Cecil Cutting remembered, seemed to arrive by the train carload. On one occasion, 90 shipyard workers with pneumococcal pneumonia had to be hospitalized. It was necessary to set up beds in the corridors to handle them. In 1942–1943 the only effective antibacterial treatment for pneumococcal pneumonia was sulfadiazine, which could cause serious reactions in the blood, skin, and kidney. Only later in the war did small amounts of penicillin become available.

Morris F. Collen, who had joined the medical group in July 1942, had the distinction of treating the largest group of lobar pneumonia patients thus far to receive antibiotic therapy. In late 1943, Collen published a description of the management of 517 pneumonia cases in the *Permanente Foundation Medical Bulletin.* He later described the epidemiology and management of 864 pneumonia cases over a 1-year period. "These low fatality rates," observed the *New England Journal of Med-*

icine of Collen's experience, "suggest that conditions to which the shipyard workers were exposed did not aggravate the prognosis in those
who acquired the pneumonia. More likely, it reflects the fine type of
medical care that these patients received."[12] Hearing of the treatment
of pneumonia at Permanente, Dr. William Kerr, chairperson of the department of medicine at the University of California in San Francisco
(USCF), contacted Morris Collen to arrange a rotation of UCSF interns
through Permanente to acquire experience with pneumonia. In 1948
Dr. Collen summarized in a monograph the wartime experiences of the
Permanente physicians in the management of pneumococcal pneumonia. And then there was polio, so dreaded in this prevaccine era, and
even a half dozen cases of leprosy.

Fractures were also common, as might be expected in such an intensely industrial environment. The Permanente physicians treated
some 13,000 fractures the first 2 years. During the launching of one
ship, 50 workers climbed to the top of a shed roof to watch the launching. The roof collapsed, and nearly all of the 50 spectators suffered a
variety of broken legs, ribs, and other bones. Standing on steel plate,
some workers would suffer compression fractures of their heel bones.

Most of the knowledge, methods, agents, and equipment currently
used by physicians and hospitals have been developed since 1942–1945.
During the war years diagnoses were made primarily by history and
physical examinations, blood counts, urinalyses, and simple flat-plate X-
rays of the chest, abdomen, or extremities. Antibiotic agents were primitive, and so infectious diseases were cause for grave anxiety among
patients, their families, and physicians. Tuberculosis, typhoid fever, poliomyelitis, pneumococcal, staphylococcal, and streptococcal infections
were dreaded diseases with significant mortality. Due to the lack of an-
tibiotics and other alternatives, hospitalizations tended to be a major aspect of health care. Appendectomy patients were kept in hospital beds 7
to 10 days; hernia repair patients for 14 days; and women who had had
normal obstetrical deliveries for 7 days.

The very existence of the *Permanente Foundation Medical Bulletin*,
which began to appear a mere year after the program was inaugurated,
testified to Garfield's belief that the medical group, while remaining primarily practicing physicians, should also sponsor research and education. Amid their heavy case loads, numerous Permanente physicians
found time to write up their experiences in a series of scholarly articles
which continued to appear in the *Permanente Foundation Medical Bulletin* over the course of the next decade. "It has always been our opinion," wrote Garfield in the second annual report, "that a medical care

system worthy of perpetuation, in addition to being economically sound, must provide teaching, training, and research, all so necessary for the maintenance of high quality care."[13] The first issue of the *Bulletin*, appearing in July 1943, contained a report on 100 appendectomies without a fatality. In later issues Cutting and Henley reviewed 1001 major surgery cases and 521 minor surgical procedures. There were 11 deaths, an extraordinarily small percentage of fatalities. Clifford Kuh wrote a scholarly essay on the relative values of the periodic health examination in comparison to early sickness consultation. Other papers dealt with urethral injuries, pneumococcal meningitis complicated by diabetic coma with recovery, brachial plexus injuries, intrathoracic neoplasms, acute catarrhal hepatitis, metal fume fever, gunshot wounds, ectopic pregnancies, spontaneous retroperitoneal hemorrhage, leprosy, and of course numerous articles on pneumonia in all its variations and the developing penicillin therapy. All in all, the Permanente physicians managed to produce 67 scientific papers for the *Bulletin* between 1943 and 1945. Another 30 papers were published in other medical journals.

On August 24, 1944, the *New England Journal of Medicine* made approving reference to the scholarly articles that were appearing in the *Permanente Foundation Medical Bulletin*. The articles being produced by the Permanente physicians, the *Journal* stated, "indicate a high standard of medical practice" which was of special concern to those interested in improving the standards of low-cost medical care to low-income and moderate-income groups. The editorial went on to commend Garfield's first annual report. "This report," noted the *Journal*, "makes impressive reading and warrants more than a glance by physicians who are interested in the socio-economic aspects of medical practice. Those who are actively concerned with the problems of prepaid health and medical care insurance may find it useful to adopt some of these methods and principles in order to obtain the most effective and efficient medical service to large numbers of people at low cost—and at the same time to maintain the high standards and dignity of the medical profession."[14] Much professional and personal stress in the lives of Permanente physicians might have been prevented had the position voiced by the *New England Journal of Medicine* in 1944 been more universally accepted by the American medical establishment in the postwar period.

As it was, Garfield was forced to state in his first annual report: "Our relations with the medical profession have been poor, chiefly because of lack of understanding of our motives, distrust of our financial plan, and fear of what it might do to the economy of private practice."[15] Because the Permanente physicians were engaged purely in war work, however, and because they were bearing a staggering load compared to stateside military physicians, the medical profession had begun, Garfield admitted, to soften its initial disapproval and to allow the Foundation to secure physicians and the necessary construction permissions. All the approvals granted by the Medical Coordinating Committee, however, Garfield sadly noted, were stamped with "Approval for the Duration," indicating that the medical establishment considered the plan merely a wartime expedient.

In his second annual report, issued in the *Bulletin* in January 1945, Garfield managed to strike a cautiously optimistic note. The Foundation, he noted, had in its relationships to organized medicine moved from a first stage of antagonism to a second stage of recognition as a wartime necessity approved for the duration, to a third stage "of active support and interest by some of the leaders in medicine and some of the medical universities, who see in our plan a possible solution to medical care, a solution which could be created by the physicians themselves without the necessity of lay interference or government intervention."[16] Cecil Cutting has emphasized that the majority of Permanente physicians were members in good standing of the Alameda–Contra Cost Medical Society. Had he been so inclined, Garfield might very well have collected on his bet with Dean Chandler of the Stanford Medical School that Cecil Cutting, by going with prepayment group practice, would never be admitted to a medical society. Cutting also enjoyed operating privileges at the Merritt Hospital in Oakland, and the French and Lane Hospitals in San Francisco. Henry Kaiser helped matters along at one point by giving an elaborate dinner in San Francisco for Medical Society officers in order to win their approval of the Permanente program.

Meanwhile, the inner-core physicians, the Grand Coulee veterans and some new recruits, were experiencing some of the good times and comradeship of Grand Coulee. "There was never any time during the day for us to meet," remembered Morris Collen, "so Sid used to take all the chiefs of service to dinner at Trader Vic's for our staff executive meetings. We'd eat wonderful food and drink and discuss our concerns. The evenings were so enjoyable that any complaints faded, and we ended up feeling much better."[17] These dinners at Trader Vic's on San Pablo Boulevard in Oakland—with the Cuttings, with his chiefs, or with others—were the most remembered good times from the war years. Trader Vic Bergeron and Garfield became and remained first-name friends, and Cecil Cutting, in turn, became a recognized Trader Vic's regular at both the San Pablo Boulevard location and the later location in Emery-ville on the shore of San Francisco Bay.

Garfield remained especially close to Millie and Cecil Cutting. Vir-ginia Jackson, whom Garfield married in 1946, also found refuge with the Cuttings when she came up from southern California during the war to work as a nurse at the Permanente Foundation Hospital. When this first marriage ended, Garfield was back living with the Cuttings, this time in Orinda, from 1948 until his marriage in 1952 to Helen Chester Peterson, the sister of Henry Kaiser's second wife.

"He would come out in the morning," Cecil Cutting later remem-bered of these wartime years, "and say, 'Gee, you know what a dream I had last night—a new idea.' So this would start out and we would talk about that for a week and then often times it worked out a whole new angle. He was always thinking of new crazy approaches to problems and ideas. Many of these were genius concepts. Some of them were abso-lutely screwball. But they were always stimulating. Mr. Kaiser, Sr., was much the same way, always thinking of new ideas."[18]

Among Garfield's more Rube Goldbergish innovations was a swingout portable basin that allowed patients to wash and/or shave while remaining in bed. Another was a bedpan that emerged and re-tracted from a toilet closet in the wall, thereby allowing patients to see to their own needs.

Because drugs and medications were difficult to obtain during the war, while basic drug chemicals remained available, Garfield set up his own drug manufacturing organization, the Royfield Company, in 1943. Garfield's company was able to supply many needed drugs and medi-cations for the hospital, clinics, and first-aid stations operated by the Foundation. He eventually sold Royfield to Stayner Pharmaceuticals of Berkeley. Foreseeing the day when plastics would replace glass syringes, rubber tubing, and such stainless steel items as water carafes and emesis basins, Garfield obtained the rights to a plastic formula and founded his own plastics company, which he called Dapite Inc. In this instance, how-ever, Garfield's imagination ran ahead of technology; for the plastic sy-ringes he manufactured could not be made clear enough to see how much medication had been drawn. Garfield did introduce into the Foundation program, however, a capacity for in-house drug manufac-ture that would make the future Kaiser-Permanente Health Plan the largest private prescription drug distributor in the United States.

As she did in Grand Coulee, Millie Cutting contributed enormously to the operation of the program as an unpaid assistant to Garfield, who bore the title Executive Director. Acting as director of personnel, Millie

Cutting interviewed and hired nurses, receptionists, clerks, and occasionally a physician. When the purchasing agent was drafted into military service, she took over for 4 months as purchasing agent. A trained nurse, she organized a well-baby clinic. She helped newcomers find housing in an overcrowded wartime market. For a while she drove a supply truck between the Foundation Hospital in Oakland and the Field Hospital in Richmond. As she did in Grand Coulee, she opened the Cutting home to the staff as a social center. Millie Cutting helped organize a Permanente Medical Wives auxiliary informally dubbed "Garfield's Girls," which became famous for its rummage sales. When it was decided to change the format of the medical records at Richmond from 3 by 5 cards to 8½ by 11 sheets, Cecil and Millie Cutting and Sidney Garfield sat up nightly together, transcribing the medical record notes until the task was complete.

4

It would be inaccurate to portray these war years as an uninterrupted idyll of good feeling and cooperation. Although the core of physicians in the program were there because they wanted to be and were dedicated to quality service, some of the physicians who had been supplied to the program through Federal Procurement and Assignment were unhappy in a group-practice setting. Others had emotional, alcohol, or drug problems that had kept them out of military service. On the whole, however, given the exigencies of medical practice in wartime shipyard conditions, the caliber of physicians and medical service remained high. In 1944, Permanente Hospital received approval from the Council on Medical Education and Hospitals of the American Medical Association for intern and resident training programs. A. L.. ("Monte") Baritell, who was later to play a key role in The Permanente Medical Group, joined the staff as a resident in surgery from the University of California Hospital in San Francisco, attracted to Permanente by Bruce Henley, who had come over from UC to be chief of surgery. Two other specialists in internal medicine, Don Ash and Phil Raimondi, joined Collen, the chief of medicine. Each of these physicians remained on staff after the war and helped shape the evolving residency program.

Two other prepaid group-practice programs, meanwhile, were also developing under the sponsorship of Kaiser industries and the general supervision of Sidney Garfield. These programs served the Kaiser shipyards on the Columbia River as it passed between Portland, Oregon, and Vancouver, Washington, and the Kaiser steel plant in Fontana in southern California. The experience of the Northern Permanente Medical Foundation headquartered in Vancouver paralleled that of the Permanente Medical Foundation in Richmond and Oakland. As in the case in California, train loads of workers began to pour into Portland in early 1942, showing the same walking pathological museum characteristics — pneumonia especially — as their Californian counterparts. Henry J. Kaiser established his son Edgar Kaiser as manager of the Portland-Vancouver operation, and there existed between young Edgar Kaiser and an equally young Clay Bedford, manager of the Richmond shipyards, a competitive rivalry which the elder Kaiser no doubt intended. Point by point, ship by ship, schedule by schedule, Edgar Kaiser and Clay Bedford, friends and fraternity brothers from Cal, Berkeley, remained in competition throughout the war. Not surprisingly, then, in early 1942 Edgar Kaiser invited Sidney Garfield to come up to Oregon and establish a comprehensive medical care program for his workers as well.

Garfield initially wanted to locate his hospital in Portland. Some 50,000 shipyard workers were on the Portland side of the river, as opposed to 40,000 on the Vancouver side. Portland was also a more developed city than Vancouver. The medical community of Portland, however, opposed the establishment of any form of prepaid group practice within the city which would also include nonindustrial care. The opposition was led by Dr. Thomas Joyce, a physician powerful in Portland medical and community affairs, who was also the friend and personal physician of Edgar Kaiser. Joyce assured Kaiser that he would support a prepaid group-practice program limited to industrial medicine in the Kaiser shipyards only if its hospital were located on the Washington side of the river. Not wishing to provoke dissension, Edgar Kaiser complied. Not wishing to oppose Edgar Kaiser, Sidney Garfield also complied, although he had grave doubts about establishing a two-tier program, different on either side of the River. As a result, Vancouver was chosen as the location for the Northern Permanente Foundation Hospital. On the Washington side of the shipyards, both an industrial and a voluntary nonindustrial program were offered to shipyard workers. On the Oregon side, there was an industrial program only. Nonindustrial care for Portland workers was provided through a plan in which all Portland physicians participated.

With Maritime Commission financing arranged by Edgar Kaiser, a hospital was built a few miles east of Vancouver on a bluff overlooking the Columbia River, not far from the housing that quartered most of the workers. The city of Portland had resisted the quartering of shipyard workers on the Oregon side of the Columbia. In the case of the Fabiola Hospital in Oakland, Garfield had been forced to implement his innovative ideas in hospital design within the confines of an existing shell. In Vancouver he had the opportunity to design a completely new facility, without prior constraints. And it was in Vancouver that Garfield's ideas in hospital design, especially as they related to operating rooms, first surfaced. As design consultant, Garfield experienced the satisfactions of an avocation that would one day become his primary activity.

The Vancouver Permanente Hospital opened in June 1942 with 75 beds. Expansion was continuous until it reached 300 beds near the end of 1944. At the Richmond shipyards, the Permanente Medical Foundation operated its medical program through Sidney Garfield and Associates. By contrast, the Northern Permanente Foundation incorporated in 1942 as a nonprofit charitable foundation, operated its shipyard medical care program directly. From the start, there were serious problems of management and personnel. In Richmond, the charismatic Garfield recruited a core group of physicians who were committed to, and experienced in, prepaid group medical practice. Led by Cecil Cutting, this core group established the tone and standards of the Richmond-Oakland program. The Northern Permanente Foundation, on the other hand, secured Garfield as a hospital design consultant, but not as on-site, day-to-day administrator. Even Sidney Garfield could not be in two places at the same time. As a result, the Portland-Vancouver program suffered an initial lack of leadership. It also lacked a core group of physicians committed to prepaid group practice. Because of wartime restrictions and the general opposition of the medical community in the area, the Northern Permanente Foundation had trouble recruiting competent physicians committed to prepaid group practice, if only on a temporary wartime basis. The Seattle Medical Society controlled the allocation of physicians in the northwest region.

"I had to go to them to get physicians," Garfield remembered. "I would come up to Seattle and tell them I needed doctors. They were physicians too, and I got to know them pretty well. They were friendly to me. But they'd say, 'This guy is no damn good. You take him. We don't care what you do with him.' They gave me a couple of good men whom they wanted to keep out of the Army because they liked them so much, and felt that they wanted them to remain in the Seattle vicinity. But the majority of men they gave us were men they didn't think were worth much, 4Fs. So we had a group of men at Vancouver who really weren't interested in making out plan work. They weren't producing, and they didn't care about the utilization of the hospital. We just couldn't make the plan pay."[19]

On at least one occasion, Garfield was forced to send Morris Collen to discharge patients unnecessarily retained in hospital beds. At this point, Garfield decided to turn to his good friend from USC, the Los Angeles County General Hospital, and the Grand Coulee program, Wally Neighbor. At the time, Neighbor was a captain in the Army Medical Corps assigned to Fort MacArthur in San Pedro where he had the leisure to work on his tennis game. Pulling strings in Washington, Garfield and Edgar Kaiser succeeded in getting Neighbor released from the Army in 1943 to become chief executive officer and medical director of the Northern Permanente Foundation. "We took him out of the beautiful job he had," Garfield remarked slyly. "He was in medical administration in San Pedro with no problems at all....First thing he knew he was discharged for our services. Of course, he went along with it....He landed in that horrible mess of making that plan work, and I guess it gave him a mild heart attack once in a while during the job. That was a terrible experience."[20]

Wally Neighbor brought much needed discipline to the Portland-Vancouver program. From this experience, Garfield also learned an important lesson. "No matter how the principles of our plan are meant," Garfield later said, "if you don't have the physician group who have it in their hearts to make it work and who believe in prepaid practice, it won't work. This is the thing that makes me wonder about HMOs all over the country. They aren't going to work unless they get men in those operations who really believe in giving service to the people."[21]

Under Neighbor's direction, the Northern Permanente Foundation provided care until the close of the war. The clinical experiences paralleled those of California. As in California, there was a high incidence of pneumonia. Dr. C. M. Grossman contributed a review of 440 pneumonia cases to the *Permanente Foundation Medical Bulletin*. Interestingly enough, there was another prepaid group-practice program in the area serving a secret war project conducted by the DuPont Company at Hanford in central Washington. Secret from 1942–1945, the Hanford project was a component of the Manhattan Project to develop the atomic bomb. At Hanford, a medical care program provided both industrial and nonindustrial care for the employees. Similar in many respects to the Permanente programs for shipyard workers, the Hanford program involved group practice, a company-owned and company-operated hospital, and salaried physicians. Its medical director was

Ernest Saward, an internist trained at the University of Rochester School of Medicine and the Peter Bent Brigham Hospital in Boston. Before coming to Washington, Saward had been practicing his subspecialty of pulmonary medicine on the staff of the Mary Imogene Basset Hospital in Cooperstown, New York. Like Garfield, Saward was committed to the notion of preventive care as being both medically and economically beneficial. At Hanford, for instance, he instigated public health measures that helped control an epidemic of meningitis which was causing a panic in the work force. When the Hanford project began to wind down in 1944 and its medical program phased out, Saward started to look for a permanent position that would be professionally satisfying. He visited Neighbor in Vancouver several times and was offered a position as chief of medicine. Joining the Northern Permanente staff in June 1945, Saward would play a key role in the evolution of the program in the postwar years.

Both the Richmond and the Portland-Vancouver shipyards were black holes for the consumption of steel. By late 1942, the Kaiser shipyards were building Liberty ships so quickly that it was difficult to get steel plate in a timely fashion. Receiving permission from the government to build a steel plant at Fontana, California, Kaiser sent a contingent out across the country scavaging the components and spare parts of steel manufacture. It was a next-to-impossible task in wartime. Kaiser chose the town of Fontana as the site of his new steel mill because it was near the junction of two important railroad lines: one bringing iron from Iron Mountain near Desert Center in the Mojave Desert, the other bringing coal from a Kaiser-operated mine in Carbon County, Utah. Forty miles east of Los Angeles, Fontana was also far enough from the California coastline to be considered safe from enemy attack. Six months into operation, the Fontana management found that it was experiencing problems in getting adequate medical and hospital care for its employees. Sidney Garfield was brought in as a consultant. "Already we had our hands full in Vancouver and Richmond," Garfield later said. "Taking on another area was just more headaches for us. But it also gave me an opportunity to get my foothold in the south. I remembered my commitment to Ray Kay that eventually I would have a plan in Los Angeles."[22]

Recruiting Al Sanborn as medical director, Garfield converted an administration building into a 60-bed hospital. (Sanborn, incidentally, was another USC/Los Angeles County Hospital resident who had trained there with Ray Kay, Morris Collen, and Wally Neighbor.) The program at Fontana offered industrial care primarily. Only some 25 percent of the steel plan employees enrolled in a voluntary prepaid nonindustrial health plan. Dues for the voluntary program were 60 cents per week for adults and 30 cents per week for children. Physician staff size varied between 6 and 10 doctors. These physicians did not keep extensive records, and so it is impossible to compare the health needs of the steel workers to those of the shipyard workers in northern California and Oregon-Washington. It is not known, for instance, whether pneumonia was as pervasive a problem as in the north. There was no Foundation in Fontana, either. Dr. Garfield provided medical and hospital services as the sole proprietor of what was eventually named the Kaiser Fontana Hospital Association. As small an operation as it was, however, the Fontana program in its close association with the steel workers' union foreshadowed the postwar evolution of prepaid comprehensive medical care.

5

By late 1944, approximately 100 physicians and their support staff were caring for 200,000 workers and their dependents in northern California, the Pacific Northwest, and southern California. By the spring of 1945, as World War II drew to a close, program facilities consisted of the 100-bed Richmond Field Hospital, the 300-bed Permanente Hospital in Oakland, the 330-bed Northern Permanente Hospital in Clark County near Vancouver, and the 60-bed hospital at Fontana. Taken in its entirety, it was the largest civilian prepaid medical program ever achieved in American medical history.

Not surprisingly, Garfield and others pondered the future of this program in the postwar era. As early as his first annual report published in the *Permanente Medical Bulletin* of January 1944, Garfield was envisioning the future of his program in a brief but pertinent essay. Delicately, Garfield acknowledged the resistance that he and his colleagues were experiencing, but he attributed it to the concern that all physicians have for the proper care of the patient. He did not back down, however, from the three major principles of medical care—prepayment, group medicine, and adequate facilities—which he considered the building blocks of medical care in postwar America. Garfield demanded nothing less than an acknowledgment by the medical profession that group medicine was the best possible medicine. "This has been proven in the universities and the large clinics throughout the country," Garfield argued.[23]

It was now time to take group practice to a large public. It was time as well to introduce preventive medicine as a major factor in both the practice and the economics of medical care. "How much wiser to transfer the economy of medicine to payment for keeping the patient well!" Garfield enthused. "Such becomes the case with prepaid group medicine operating in efficient and adequate facilities. Under these conditions, the fewer the sick the more the remuneration; the less serious the illness, the better off the patient and the doctor."[24] For the postwar era Garfield envisioned the rise of medicine that would emphasize, not sickness, but health.

Far from restricting physicians' incomes and talents, the medicine of the postwar era — prepaid, preventive in orientation, organized as group practice — would ensure incomes and outlets for talent for a new generation of physicians. "Well-trained young men under the private practice system," Garfield wrote, "spend the best years of their lives waiting to be discovered. During this period they are disillusioned and often are forced to step beyond their fields and ability because of financial reasons. Such a man entering a group could immediately be used to his full capacity, because under such a system the group sponsors the young man."[25] Garfield proposed a three-tier medical system that would allow for full-time private practice, full-time group practice, or a mixture of the two. To service the medical needs of the postwar era, Garfield envisioned for California a system that would be organized for social good while remaining nongovernmental and under physician control.[26]

Such a heroic envisioning of the future, however, confronted a far different reality a year and a half later as the war ended. As rapidly as they were organized, the shipyards closed down. Within a few months, the 90,000 workers at Richmond dropped to 13,000 and the medical group collapsed from 75 physicians to a dozen as doctors left the program for fee-for-service practice.

"I never thought they would shut the shipyards down overnight," Garfield later admitted ruefully. "I didn't think that was possible. I thought the government was smart enough to slowly let the people go, but, bang, they just shut the shipyards down. We lost our membership. Most of them returned from whence they came, from all parts of the country."[27]

At the Permanente Foundation, there was talk of closing the program down for good. In Vancouver, the medical staff expressed every intention of terminating the group and the health plan. At a meeting convened to vote on dissolution, Saward moved to table the motion to dissolve, appealing for more time to consider the action. The motion to table carried. At a subsequent meeting held a week later, most of those intending to vote for dissolution had already departed. Those who wished to continue the plan and the medical group voted affirmatively to open the health plan to the communities of Vancouver and Portland. A similar decision was made in northern California. But by late 1945, with only a handful of physicians committed to the prepaid group-practice ideal, Garfield's dreams seemed a long way from fulfillment. As in the case of Desert Center and Grand Coulee, prepaid group medical practice seemed, once again, to be—in the words of the wartime bureaucracy—stamped "for the duration only."

4

No Blueprint to Follow— Survival and Reorganization in the Postwar Era

At the conclusion of the Los Angeles Aqueduct and Grand Coulee projects, Garfield's program had disestablished itself. As World War II began to draw to a close, Garfield and a core group of Permanente physicians began seriously to consider continuing the program in the postwar era. Similar conversations had occurred at Grand Coulee as that program moved toward termination. In the case of the conversations that began toward the end of the war, however, aspiration would become reality.

Discussions began in late 1944 as Kaiser's shipbuilding program peaked and layoffs began. As cutbacks mounted, the Permanente physicians experienced an early premonition of postwar conditions. They were of necessity challenged to think of the future.

The war ended as abruptly as it had begun. By October 1945, the voluntary nonindustrial plan members whose monthly dues provided the financial resources necessary to operate the program were suddenly reduced from 60,000 to fewer than 10,000 enrollees. In Vancouver-Portland, only 3000 members remained by April 1946. In Fontana enrollment remained stable at 3000. If the plan were to survive, massive adjustments would be necessary.

The first such adjustment—in physician staffing—was automatic. The disaffected or uncommitted physicians departed. Some of them left because they no longer needed draft exemptions. Others, while committed to the program as an emergency wartime measure, did not see in it a viable method of medical practice in peacetime. In northern California, for example, the wartime roster of some 100 physicians rapidly consolidated itself to 13 doctors committed to the idea of prepaid group practice in the postwar era. The doctors shared the views of Garfield and Cutting, who throughout 1945 had been discussing the future as they had at Grand Coulee in the late 1930s. This time, however, they would not only envision the future, they would also make it happen. With the concurrence of the core group of physicians committed to prepaid group practice, Garfield and Cutting approached Eugene Trefethen, upon whom Henry J. Kaiser depended for many organizational decisions, to discuss taking the Permanente program public after the war.

Trefethen saw in the program a way to continue medical coverage for the remaining Kaiser workers, and so he agreed. In September 1945, as massive layoffs began in the shipyards in Richmond and Vancouver-Portland, as well as in the steel mill at Fontana, the Permanente Health Plan, a nonprofit trust, was established to take the program into the postwar era. This new nonprofit organization was chosen instead of a corporation in order to avoid the charge of corporate practice of medicine, which was at the time an unthinkable alternative. Under the nonprofit trust strategy, the Health Plan enrolled members and collected membership dues. The Permanente Foundation continued to own the hospitals and to carry all indebtedness. Sidney Garfield remained sole proprietor of the medical group and continued to operate the entire program as executive director. Garfield leased the hospitals from the Foundation. All personnel, including physicians, remained Garfield's employees. The medical group, the hospitals, and the Health Plan, while legally distinct, operated as a single organizational unit under Garfield's direction. In current terminology, the Permanente Health Plan resembled a staff model Health Maintenance Organization (HMO) with its own hospitals.

Whatever model was chosen, there had to be a strong membership for the health plan to succeed. Two important factors, the locale of California and the emerging concept of employee benefits, were even then working to create a new postwar membership. It was initially assumed that, once the war was over, the shipyard workers would return to their homes in the east and the south. This did not happen. Despite the shipyard layoffs, there was still plenty of work for skilled industrial workers in the San Francisco Bay area; and besides, having experienced life in California, the majority of the shipyard workers were reluctant to leave. Deciding to remain, they, together with returning veterans who had made the same decision, created a postwar boom in California, whose population doubled over the next 15 years.

During the war, some economists had predicted that the Depression would reassert itself with the coming of peace. The exact opposite occurred, especially in California. In this economic and demographic boom, a climate favorable to the growth of the Permanente Health Plan was created. Just as there was a core group of physicians committed to prepaid group practice, there was also a core group of former wartime workers who had experienced the benefits of prepaid comprehensive coverage and desired to continue these benefits in peacetime. This satisfied membership constituted an informal but effective network of recruitment for new Health Plan members in the postwar era.

The physicians, staff, and trustees of the Permanente Health Plan now faced the challenge of making their program work in new circumstances. Energetic, innovative, charismatic, Sidney Garfield remained both in fact and through the consent of the governed the principal leader and executive authority. For many outsiders, Sidney Garfield *was* the program. For the time being, Garfield's unquestioned leadership provided continuity between the war and the postwar periods. Within a few short years, however, as opposition by the medical establishment fixed on Garfield personally, the conspicuousness of the founder became, even in Garfield's opinion, a liability. In 1945–1946, however, Garfield's continuing presence as an administrator, as liaison to Henry Kaiser, as innovator and public spokesperson, provided for the program and its core physicians a leader around whom they could rally as they struggled to implement their innovative health plan.

By the end of the war, Cecil Cutting, by now a 10-year veteran of prepaid group practice, had emerged as Garfield's close friend and second-in-command. It was to Cutting that Garfield first turned for preliminary discussions about continuing the program after the war. Cutting joined Garfield in taking this idea to Trefethen and the Kaiser organization. For the time being, however, Cutting stayed out of administration and spent his professional time on surgery. "I was able to branch out into other areas in which the other surgeons weren't comfortable,"

Cutting later remembered of the 1940s. "For a while, I did all the intervertebral discs, mainly because I didn't like the way one of our early orthopedists operated on a patient. I did the first lung resection and did a lot of thoracic surgery. When new surgeons came aboard who had special residency training, I moved to cardiac surgery. I went to Western Reserve in Cleveland and learned a technique of anastamosing a vessel from the aorta to the coronary sinus, reversing the direction of flow in the heart in patients with restricted coronary artery flow."[1] As happy as he was in surgery, however, Cutting also was developing his executive and personnel skills and in time would be called upon by his peers for an expanded leadership role. Meanwhile, Cecil Cutting continued to operate and to find time for publication. In May 1945, *California and Western Medicine* published a survey of over 13,000 fractures of every variety, jointly authored by Cutting and two other Permanente physicians.

Also prominent in the group, its third leader in fact, was Morris Collen, whom Garfield had recruited from a USC residency at Los Angeles County Hospital early in the war. By 1945 Collen had established himself as a national authority on the management of pneumonia, a field in which he continued to do research after the war. In 1945–1946 Collen authored or jointly authored four major articles and one monograph dealing with pneumonia treatment. Amiable in personality, committed, and hard-working, Collen concealed behind his unassuming friendliness an element of iron in his make-up that would come to the fore in 1948 during the second postwar reorganization of the program. Among the core group of physicians, Collen was the practical planner and intellectual: the continuing realist in dialogue with Garfield the visionary and Cutting the trusted colleague.

Also remaining with the program were the young physicians recruited in 1944 and 1945: A. La Mont Baritell, Norman Haugen, Donald Grant, Thurman Dannenberg, Clifford Kuh, Richard Moore, Donald Ash, James Basye, Peter Baroni, Paul Fitzgibbon, and Alex King and Robert King, who were unrelated. Born in China in 1910, Beatrice Lei joined the program in 1946 as assistant chief of pediatrics at Richmond and was the first woman physician in the medical group. In the early spring of 1948 Wally Neighbor, who had been with Garfield at Grand Coulee, resigned as executive director of the Northern Permanente Foundation and rejoined the staff in Oakland.

Other early staffers included Clyde Diddle, a pharmacist at Oakland; William Price, accountant and controller; Dorthea Daniels, a nurse administrator; and Albert Brodie, who monitored enrollments for the

Health Plan. The general manager of the Permanente Health Plan was Jack Baird, who had been hired at the urging of Trefethen. On Baird's staff were two critical support personnel: Avram Yedidia, an economist specializing in consumer, employer, and union relations, and Thomas K. McCarthy, staff legal counsel, a former partner with the firm of Thelen, Marrin, Johnson, and Bridges, the firm that had handled the establishment of the Permanente Foundation in early 1942. Yedidia had gone to work for the Kaiser shipyards in 1941, in charge of receiving steel shipments. While there, he had encouraged a 100 percent voluntary enrollment of his division in the Health Plan and had over the course of the war become quite familiar with its intricacies. In May 1945 he lunched with Garfield, who offered him a position with the Health Plan after the war. In the financially precarious early postwar years, Yedidia made a major contribution toward keeping the Plan solvent and financially competitive by developing comprehensive benefit schedules and initial rates based upon experience with the shipyard population and best guesses about unknown variables.

Health Plan trustees consisted of Kaiser executives Eugene Trefethen; Todd Inch, who handled industrial relations for the Kaiser industries; G. G. Sherwood, a financial officer; Harry Morton, a labor negotiator; and the lawyer Thomas McCarthy. Henry J. Kaiser did not join the board. Eugene Trefethen also chaired the Permanente Foundation, which was supervised by trustees Trefethen, Inch, McCarthy, William Marks, another lawyer with the Kaiser organization, Henry J. Kaiser, and Edgar Kaiser. These high-powered trustees, however, met only six times between 1945 and 1948. The actual management of the Health Plan might be envisioned as a circle with Sidney Garfield in the center. Around Garfield rotated the various trustees, with some closer to him than others and with Trefethen the dominant presence. "So he wasn't just out there running loose," was how Trefethen later remembered this informal arrangement.[2]

2

In discussions regarding the future of prepaid group practice, three barriers to success were continually raised. First of all, organized medicine would inevitably oppose the program. Second, it would be difficult to market a program of medical care that was little known or understood, especially since medical ethics precluded advertising. Third, the creation of a prepaid comprehensive program for the general public would involve enormous start-up costs as new facilities were constructed. As was feared, each of these difficulties did indeed arise.

Opposition from organized medicine escalated overnight. It was one thing to conduct prepaid group practice among restricted groups and their dependents in remote rural regions or during a wartime emergency, but the war was now over, and the Permanente Health Plan was now seeking an expanded membership in a highly desirable urban environment. From the point of view of fee-for-service physicians, the special need for prepaid group medicine had now evaporated with the return of hundreds of physicians from military service. Not only did the Permanente program pose an economic threat to returning veterans anxious to resume old practices or launch new ones, but it also threatened established physicians in the community, who were competing with each other as well as with the returned veterans. In southern California the Ross-Loos Medical Group had avoided hostility from the medical establishment by promising not to seek a membership beyond already enrolled employees of the Metropolitan Water District and the city of Los Angeles. In New York, the Health Insurance Plan (HIP) established in March 1947 for city employees limited itself to medical services only. Hospital care was to be financed through Blue Cross. The Permanente Health Plan, by contrast, was offering a prepaid comprehensive program centered in its own hospitals. It was also actively seeking an expanded membership.

Then there was the question of third-party control of medicine. Since the Permanente Health Plan involved a lay board of trustees, it appeared to violate a principle of physician independence that American physicians had established over a century of struggle. According to this philosophy, the sole allegiance of the physician must be to the individual patient. Should the physician be paid by anyone other than the patient, then this necessary allegiance would be diluted by the demands of the payer, demands that might not be in the best interests of the patient. This question of third-party interference was an especially sensitive point with a generation of physicians who had served in the military during World War II and remembered how they often had to make decisions "for the good of the service." Such decisions frequently interfered with the doctor-patient relationship.

Given this climate of opinion, it is not surprising that physicians in the Alameda–Contra Costa Medical Society soon became outspoken opponents of the Permanente Health Plan. An article in the local medical society journal suggested that the Permanente hospitals be turned over to Alameda County for the care of public charges. It was mistakenly perceived that the Permanente hospitals in Oakland and Richmond had been built at taxpayers' expense. Actually, the financing of these facilities had been through a combination of private and government loans, the original debt of $700,000 having been retired in 1944 and a later and larger loan being then in the process of rapid liquidation.

The Medical Society soon had two points for contention. The first involved a slightly irregular temporary appointment. Among the returning veterans who presented themselves to Sidney Garfield for consideration was Lt. Col. Clifford Keene, a highly experienced combat surgeon with extensive operating and medical experience in the Pacific. Arriving in Oakland from Camp Stoneman on the morning of January 3, 1946, Keene was wearing his khaki uniform and was still smelling, by his own admission, of the rice paddies of Korea, where just a few days earlier he had been winding up his Army career as medical consultant to the commanding general of the XXIV Corps. When asked by Garfield if he had done much surgery, the lieutenant colonel, exhausted and underweight from nearly 4 years of operating under combat conditions in the Pacific, replied that he had performed just about every kind of surgery that he could imagine. An honors graduate from the University of Michigan School of Medicine, Keene had before the war become chief resident in a pyramid system surgical residency at the University of Michigan Hospital in which only one resident survived for the fourth year. He was also among the first American surgeons to be certified by the American Board of Surgery. This had been followed by his extensive experience as chief of surgery in several Army hospitals and field commands during the war.

In the course of their first interview, Garfield told Keene that the Kaisers were starting an automobile factory at Willow Run, Michigan, and were looking for a director of medicine for the facility. Garfield urged Keene to visit Willow Run after he had been reunited with his family in Detroit. Keene replied that he preferred to establish himself in California, at which point Garfield mentioned that there might be an opening on the surgical staff at the Permanente Hospital in Oakland. Keene then told Garfield that he did not have a California license. Garfield did not anticipate this as a difficulty. Keene, he said, could serve as a resident in surgery until he obtained California certification.

A month later, in February 1946, Garfield contacted Keene in Detroit, offering him a temporary appointment in Oakland as a try-out for the Willow Run position. Keene again reminded Garfield that he had no California license. Garfield reassured Keene by telegram that it would make no difference. He could work as a resident until he took his examinations in California. Anxious to obtain a California license and to practice there if possible, but wanting to keep the Willow Run option open, Keene accepted a temporary appointment as a surgeon at the Oakland hospital from February 11 until April 8, 1946, when he returned to Willow Run. Keene later testified that he felt uneasy as an ostensible resident, having finished his residency in Michigan before the war; but since he was obviously being looked over, either for Oakland or the Willow Run appointment, he acquiesced. Keene was right. He was being looked over. "Edgar [Kaiser] had asked me to find a physician to run the industrial health care at the Kaisers' automobile factory in Willow Run," Garfield later stated. "I wanted Cecil [Cutting] to check him out on his capabilities as a surgeon before he went east."[3] Garfield employed at least one other physician under similar circumstances.

Learning of these irregularities, the Alameda–Contra Costa Medical Society complained to the California Board of Medical Examiners. Summoned to a hearing, Garfield defended himself on the grounds that it was a common practice in teaching hospitals to employ residents whose licenses had not yet been processed by the State Board of Medical Examiners. Rejecting Garfield's defense, the board suspended Garfield's license to practice medicine. Garfield contested the suspension in superior court, which decided against the Board of Medical Examiners' action. This decision, in turn, was appealed to the court of appeal by the medical examiners. Keene, meanwhile, returned from Willow Run to take his general medical examinations for California licensure in San Francisco on June 8 and 9, 1946. Sitting for 2 days before his two examiners, Keene was given what he later considered the most difficult examination of his life. "They didn't think well of Sidney Garfield and they didn't think well of what he was trying to do," Keene recalled of his examiners, Herbert Chapman of Stockton and Joseph Zeiler of Los Angeles. "I believe they were determined that I would fail. But I didn't fail, and I was given a license, because I did pass the examination. They'd ask me a question and I'd write it down and then I'd give them an answer, because I realized that I was being examined by a hostile board of examiners."[4]

With the granting of a California license to Keene and Keene's removal to Michigan where he remained for the next half dozen years, *Garfield v. the Board of Medical Examiners* became moot and was eventually dropped. Garfield was ill-advised in seeking to bypass state requirements, especially in the case of a surgeon as qualified as Clifford Keene. On the other hand, the matter would ordinarily have been quietly corrected had not Garfield and his program posed such a threat.

The fact that Garfield, the executive director of the Permanente program, lost his license, even temporarily, was at once an embarrassment to the Permanente program and testimony to the level of opposition that existed to prepaid group medical practice.

The Board of Medical Examiners also questioned the status of another Permanente physician, Thomas Flint, Jr. Prior to coming to Permanente, Flint had been put on probation for administering narcotics to himself to counteract a painful orthopedic condition. By the time he presented himself to Permanente, Flint had conquered his addiction; but since he was on probation, Cecil Cutting, who had great faith in Flint as a physician, sought and received verbal permission from the chairperson of the Board of Medical Examiners to hire him. This permission, however, was never formally ratified by the entire Board of Medical Examiners and it thus became a second cause of action against Garfield. The action was eventually dropped when it became established that permission had been sought and received in an appropriate manner. Subsequently, Thomas Flint enjoyed a distinguished career as a Permanente physician. As a specialist in emergency medicine, Flint wrote the protocols for the management of emergency care in Permanente hospitals. In 1954 he published *Emergency Treatment and Management* with W.B. Saunders Company, the well-known medical publisher. *Emergency Treatment and Management* gained a widespread reputation and was translated into several languages.

Aside from these dramatic actions taken against Garfield personally because he was still the sole proprietor of the medical group, there also occurred in these postwar years a pattern of rejection of Permanente physicians by local county medical societies that was gratuitously hurtful. Permanente physicians who applied for membership in local county medical societies were routinely denied acceptance. Although Permanente physicians did not need such memberships to practice medicine in Permanente hospitals, such exclusions affronted their professional pride. Since membership in the California Medical Association and the American Medical Association depended on membership in local county medical societies, Permanente physicians were also precluded from participating in medical affairs on the state and national levels. Not only did such exclusion discourage Permanente physicians, it also precluded any dialogue on the state and national level between fee-for-service physicians and prepaid group practitioners.

Local medical societies also discouraged physicians who were considering association with Permanente. Such physicians were warned that should they ever choose to leave Permanente and return to fee-for-service private practice, they would be stigmatized and would encounter difficulties in getting hospital privileges or attracting referrals. On an even more intense level of persecution, potential Permanente physicians were told that they would not get their board certifications if they joined Permanente. Even non-Permanente specialists, such as neurosurgeons or plastic surgeons, who were considering working for Permanente on a fee-for-service or retention arrangement, were quickly warned that they should not work for Permanente or they would not receive referrals from other fee-for-service physicians. Fortunately, Cecil Cutting very quickly developed an in-house surgical capacity at Permanente, including the services of a neurosurgeon who remained with the program for 5 years before going into fee-for-service practice in Walnut Creek.

By June 1948, aside from the Keene and Flint cases already mentioned, Sidney Garfield was also the object of further charges by the Council of the Alameda–Contra Costa Medical Society. Garfield was accused of advertising and soliciting patients for the Health Plan. He was accused of placing mass production techniques ahead of the health needs of individual patients. He was accused of preventing patients from having their free choice of physicians, of rendering inadequate service at an understaffed hospital, of channeling unethical and illegal profits into the Foundation and Health Plan. As if these charges were not enough, there was also a blanket charge that Garfield and his physicians were rendering medical services under conditions which made adequate medical care impossible. As far as can be determined, the Council listed these charges without investigating whether or not they were accurate. No one from the Council had visited the Permanente Hospital in Oakland to review administrative, financial, or professional records or to interview Health Plan members, patients, or members of the staff.

Deciding that truth was the best defense, Garfield invited delegations from the local medical society to visit the Permanente hospitals. A number of delegations accepted the invitation and examined the facilities and the program. They found no significant cause for complaint. A number of the delegates, in fact, became supporters of the program. In general, however, despite the friendly attitude of these few fee-for-service physicians, the Medical Society leadership continued to nurture a free-floating opposition to the Permanente Health Plan that was ever on the lookout for damaging evidence.

Henry J. Kaiser, himself no stranger to unfounded charges during the war (among other things, Kaiser had been accused of dealing in black market steel), suggested to Garfield that he openly invite representatives of the Council of the Alameda–Contra Costa Medical Society to visit the Permanente Hospital, investigate its program, and either substantiate or withdraw the charges. Throughout the last months of 1948 and the first months of 1949, investigating committees from the Medical Society made a number of visits to the hospital and the Health Plan. As a result of these inspections, the charges of the Council of the Alameda–Contra Costa Medical Society were found to be without merit—with one exception. The financial records of the Health Plan did disclose that in 1945, $61,000 had been allocated for "promotion and selling," which was contrary to medical ethics. This activity, however, had not been budgeted after 1945 and was thus moot as a point of contention.

"They sent committees, several times," remembered Cecil Cutting, "to look us over. But one thing they never could find was poor quality. They couldn't get us on quality. They would come and look over our emergency log and see if we kept nonmember patients who had come in emergency, or if we would refer them to their own doctor on the outside. They found that we did call him up, and if the doctor wanted to see him, fine. If the doctor didn't want to come out that night, why, we'd take care of it and keep him."[5]

Cutting also recalled that it was repeatedly pointed out to him that all problems with Permanente would cease if non-Permanente physicians were allowed to treat Health Plan members on a fee-for-service basis, to be reimbursed by the Health Plan. Such a suggestion, aside from being a less-than-subtle form of shake-down, was inconsistent with the basic principles of prepayment and group practice and was thus rejected.

In the public relations war, Sidney Garfield was not without resources. One of his staunchest supporters was the medical journalist Paul De Kruif, whose son David was a Permanente physician. During the war, De Kruif had written a series of laudatory articles on the Permanente program for the *Reader's Digest,* which were published in book form in 1943 under the title *Kaiser Wakes the Doctors.* In 1948 Garfield invited De Kruif to come back to Oakland and do a similar series on the warfare being waged against Permanente by the Council of the Alameda–Contra Costa Medical Society. De Kruif produced a series of spirited defenses which appeared in the *Reader's Digest* and were later included as two chapters in his 1949 book *Life Among the Doctors.*

In a flamboyant, emotional style, De Kruif defended Garfield as a medical man of destiny, a Good Samaritan, smeared and harassed by petty-minded opponents. "How could they lick Sid Garfield?" De Kruif intoned. "He did not deal in the fine art of the smear. He did not argue.

His books were open to any responsible medical man who asked to see them. His medical care at his hospitals was there to be seen. They kept trying to wreck him and he kept beating them simply by what he did."[6] Given the enormous circulation of the *Reader's Digest,* De Kruif was able to defend the Permanente program to an audience of millions, which infuriated Garfield's opponents but also may have tempered their attacks.

Garfield also received encouragement from another quite unexpected quarter: from the very heart of the American medical establishment itself. Dr. Ray Lyman Wilbur had served successively as professor of medicine at Stanford, dean of the Stanford Medical School, president of Stanford University, secretary of the interior in the administration of his Stanford classmate Herbert Hoover, and president of the American Medical Association. It would be hard to imagine a more strategically placed physician. In 1947, as the attacks of the Council of the Alameda–Contra Costa Medical Society were gaining in intensity, Garfield found himself at a cocktail party in San Francisco honoring Wilbur. "I went to the party and I had a few cocktails," Garfield later recalled, "and all of a sudden I found myself in the corner with Ray Lyman Wilbur and I remember I started complaining to him about why the Medical Society was giving us such a bad time. I said: 'We're carefully following the ethics of the Medical Society. We're doing a good job for the doctors as well as for the people. I just don't understand what their thinking is that they should do this sort of thing. They really ought to be supporting us.'"

As he was making his lament, however, Garfield noticed that Wilbur was growing impatient—although Garfield also admits that he could not stop talking. Wilbur at last brusquely interrupted Garfield and said, "Young man, you are not wearing a crown of thorns. Nothing new or good has ever been achieved without strong opposition. If you were not opposed, it would be because you were not contributing anything worthwhile. You are very fortunate. Not only are you doing something new and good for the people, you are doing something new and good for the doctors of this country, and you should be very happy."[7]

Coming as it did from a physician at the core of the American medical establishment, Wilbur's encouragement galvanized Garfield, staving off any temptation to self-pity. In the years to come, as the Permanente program began to win acceptance in the medical community and as active opposition began to die off, Wilbur's encouragement seemed to Garfield a prophetic statement. Told and retold, the story of this encounter became part of the Permanente folklore: a memory that bridged, if only in retrospect, the painful gap between Garfield's aspiring medical group and fee-for-service medicine.

3

In these early years, operating capital was as hard to come by as approval from the medical establishment. During the war, capital had been needed to renovate Fabiola Hospital, to build the Richmond Field Hospital, and then to expand both to a combined capacity of 425 beds. Dues from an expanding membership had generated the capital necessary to pay off the loans from the Bank of America and to meet obligations on the loan from the federal government. But with membership stabilized at 10,000 in 1946, it was not clear just exactly how many doctors, nurses, technicians, and administrative staff 10,000 enrollees could support. This question was even further complicated by the fact that in order to compete with Blue Cross at the prepayment level, the Health Plan was forced to reduce its rates. A subscriber with three dependents, for instance, was paying $8.45 a month in the fall of 1945 but was paying only $5.25 in March of 1946. To offset the effects of this rate reduction, the Health Plan was forced to introduce a $1 office visit charge, a $2 house call charge, and a $60 maternity fee.

Fortunately, Permanente still possessed the contingency fund that the insurance companies had created by retaining 15 percent of the monies payable to Dr. Sidney Garfield and associates during the war. The purpose of this retention was to set aside money to meet continuing obligations for workers' compensation cases after the war and to service the debt on outstanding loans. The fund—which had grown to $1.5 million by 1945—was also intended as a survival kit during the transition from an industrial to a community-based plan. Without it, there was no way that the program could have made the transition into the postwar era; but even with its help, it was necessary to operate the program in a stringently cost effective manner. Operating expenses and debt service quickly depleted this survival kit. It was also necessary to upgrade hospital facilities to accommodate changes in medical technology. It was no longer possible to say, "There's a war on," as an excuse for deferred maintenance or a new purchase.

The most significant way to control expenses remained salaries. Permanente physicians were compensated in the range of $400 to $800 per month, which was not competitive with the growing prosperity of fee-for-service physicians in the San Francisco Bay Area. A key Health Plan representative worked for $350 per month. Nurses received about $1400 per year. Combined with medical society opposition, these stringent salaries constituted a further barrier to recruitment.

In the immediate postwar years, as Garfield struggled to retire the government debt and to keep the program alive on its 10,000 membership base, what Garfield called "the economy of shortages" came into effect at Permanente. "The shortage of anything produces economy," was the way that Wally Neighbor described this philosophy of austerity. "If you don't have enough beds in a hospital, you are going to use them more perfectly. If there are more beds than you need, you're going to let patients languish in hospitals. If there aren't enough outpatient visits, a doctor is going to fiddle away his time. If he's pressed for time, if his appointments schedules are full and overflowing, it's a more efficient operation."[8]

The economies of these years have become legendary. Furniture was repaired, and renovation and remodeling were performed by a staff carpenter who had stayed with the program after Grand Coulee. (His son later went to medical school and became a Permanente physician.) Niceties such as carpets and draperies were deferred. Spartan furnishings remained spartan. A deposit was taken for crutches as a means of having them returned. As executive director of the program, Garfield examined every bill and signed every check. He abhorred cellophane or Scotch tape, allowing it to be used only on patients allergic to regular adhesives. In order to draw a new pencil from supply, Permanente employees had to turn in a pencil stub ground down to at least 3 inches. Whether this device saved much money was in Garfield's mind immaterial; it did, however, function as a teaching device to make the organization cost conscious. In later years, a Pencil Stub Club was established to honor Permanente employees of 35 years of service. Their reward, a lapel pin in the shape of a pencil stub. This period of stringent economy established a pattern of frugal allocation of resources that persisted even into more prosperous years. Formed by these early economies, the physicians and staff at Permanente, as a matter of institutional culture, continued to abhor waste.

Control of spending, however, could only do so much toward generation of operating capital. It would have been logical in these early years to increase available capital by increasing total membership; but the third major difficulty confronting the struggling Permanente program was the question of marketing. Medical custom forbade direct promotion and sales of medical services. Group health insurance was almost unknown. Most employers provided no health insurance for their employees. If an individual employee wished to purchase health insurance, he or she had "consumer choice" of plans that were willing to provide individual coverage. Those employers who did provide some health insurance often limited coverage to employees. Dependents might in some cases receive elective coverage for which the employee bore the full cost. A favorable group premium rate depended on at least 75 percent of the employee group being covered by a single plan. The employee in such a situation rarely had a choice. In the mid-1940s, Blue Cross and California Physicians Service (Blue Shield) were the two major plans.

Aggressive unions and groups with politically liberal leadership were wary of the Permanente plan because of its relationship with Kaiser, an industrialist who was perceived to have reaped profits from the war. Other unions and employer groups with politically conservative leadership were equally wary, because medical care in which the fees were prepaid to a closed panel of physicians appeared to them to be socialized medicine. Many Bay Area residents continued to regard the Permanente plan as limited to Kaiser employees, not understanding that subscription was open to the public. Of those who knew, few wanted to be associated with the enrolled members, whom they perceived as the "riff-raff" Kaiser had imported to work in the shipyards. It was not a favorable market for growth, nor was it immediately apparent how recruitment could be carried on in a manner acceptable to the medical profession.

Take the matter of the so-called collectors in the early phases of postwar recruitment. Discharged shipyard workers working in other industries after the war included many who had become accustomed to getting medical and hospital care in the prepaid plan and wished to continue. Some of these enthusiasts organized collector groups among their fellow employees. They volunteered to enroll workers they could persuade to join the plan. The collectors also maintained the list of enrollees and dependents, collected dues from them, and transmitted the dues to the health plan. Some of these collectors became overzealous at times and used solicitation methods that would not have been approved by the physicians providing medical care. Permanente physicians became sensitive to criticism from their fee-for-service colleagues about the ethics of solicitation. Care was taken that a Permanente Health Plan representative did not approach a prospective group until a written letter of inquiry had been received from that group.

One particularly successful marketer of the Health Plan was Aloysius Brodie, who had been manager of the Health Plan during the war.

Harold Hatch of Industrial Indemnity had originally suggested Brodie to Garfield as a recruiter for the nonindustrial program in the Richmond shipyards. Brodie had proved an energetic salesperson, although on one occasion Garfield had to warn him that he could not sell vitamins on the side to shipyard workers or recommend Health Plan members to a dentist in Richmond. Brodie performed yeoman service in enrolling a large number of civilian workers at the naval shipyards in San Francisco and Vallejo into the Permanente program as well as marketing the nonindustrial program to Kaiser shipyard workers and, later, their dependents. After the war, Brodie branched out to enroll other federal government employees in the San Francisco Bay Area. He received 60 cents per family subscriber unit until 7500 subscribers had enrolled and 40 cents per subscriber over the 7500 mark. These fees were paid Brodie from surcharges above the standard dues rate. From this income, Brodie hired his own staff and paid all his own office and administrative expenses. He was running, in effect, an auxiliary health plan. "He did very well," said Garfield of Brodie's efforts. "He probably earned more than our doctors at the time. It was a very good incentive."[9]

4

The establishment of The Permanente Medical Group in 1948, the most significant development of this period, was the direct result of the pressures, tensions, and possibilities of these uncertain postwar years. In February 1948 the medical care program, which had been operating as a single entity, was restructured into three components: the Permanente Health Plan, Permanente Hospitals, and The Permanente Medical Group. The Permanente Foundation and the Northern Permanente Foundation in the Oregon-Washington region continued to own the hospitals that Permanente Hospitals ran. Established in 1945, the Permanente Health Plan continued as a nonprofit trust, presided over by lay trustees. The Permanente Hospitals and The Permanente Medical Group constituted new entities.

The Permanente Hospitals were incorporated on February 20, 1948. The Henry J. Kaiser Company made a $150,000 non-interest-bearing loan to help the new corporation get started. For his interests and assets in the hospital operations, Garfield was compensated for an aggregate of $257,500, of which $142,500 was paid in 10 monthly installments with interest at 3 percent. This transaction removed Garfield in a curious way from the dominant position he had occupied in the program since its inception.

As Paul De Kruif wrote in *Life Among the Doctors*, "Sid Garfield was Permanente. That was maybe the weakness of this experiment in prepaid group specialist medical care."[10] As sole proprietor of Sidney Garfield and Associates, Garfield was psychologically and legally the embodiment and guarantor of the medical group. This condition befitted the small-scale programs of the Mojave and Grand Coulee. During the war, however, Garfield had of necessity become increasingly aligned with the Kaiser organization. The administrative structure adopted in 1945 formalized the control of the Henry J. Kaiser Company over the program. Kaiser executives held the final responsibility for the Plan, the hospitals, and the Foundation that owned the hospitals. Sidney Garfield held final responsibility for the medical group, which he owned. Between 1945 and 1948, the lay trustees of the Plan and the Foundation were content to allow Sidney Garfield to run the operation as a single entity. They were willing to do this because Garfield, Henry J. Kaiser, and the Kaiser management team had devised a workable means of sharing authority and responsibility in the developing program.

There was no way, however, that this informal, intensely personal arrangement could withstand the stress and strains of an expanding and vulnerable program. When the Council of the Alameda–Contra Costa Medical Society went on the attack, it was Sidney Garfield, sole proprietor, whom they named in their allegations and complaints. At the same time, as a matter of internal organization, it was implausible that a growing, increasingly complex medical enterprise involving physicians, support staff, hospitals, an actuarily intricate health plan, and an increasingly sophisticated network of relationships with insurance companies, unions, employee organizations, and other group subscribers, could continue to come under the supervision of one physician, Sidney Garfield, however talented and charismatic he might be.

Other factors urged a reorganization as well. For tax reasons, it was necessary to establish clear-cut distinctions between the Foundation, a nonprofit trust, the hospitals, a charitable corporation, and the medical group, a profit-making partnership. Since Garfield had a proprietary interest in both the hospitals and the medical group under the previous organizational structure, it was necessary to buy him out of the hospitals, which Henry J. Kaiser did, and to restructure his proprietor-employer relationship to the other physicians.

Sidney Garfield thus found himself on the receiving end of pressure from a number of quarters. The Henry J. Kaiser Company, first of all, needed further legal and administrative clarity; otherwise, the tax-exempt aspects of the program were sure to come under question by the Internal Revenue Service (IRS). Garfield enjoyed an extremely close relationship with Henry J. Kaiser. A number of times, Garfield described this relationship as that of a son to a father. "Sidney was a dreamer, and Henry Kaiser was a dreamer," Eugene Trefethen, Kaiser's chief administrative deputy later remembered, "so they dreamed together."[11] On the other hand, Kaiser executives such as Eugene Trefethen wanted the program to be less dependent upon one dominant personality. The Permanente physicians, for their part, could not be expected to continue in their dependent status as employees of Sidney Garfield. It was time for the next stage of evolution.

The announcement of the partnership came casually, unexpectedly to Morris Collen. Eating lunch at the doctors' dining room at the Permanente Hospital in Oakland, he ran into Garfield. "Morrie," Garfield announced, "we have decided to set up a partnership for our physicians, and we would like to know if you would be willing to be a partner."

"Well," replied Collen, "I don't know all the implications, Sid, but if you think that's best, I'd be very happy to." It was that simple.[12]

The Permanente Medical Group was established as a partnership February 21, 1948. The seven original partners were Sidney R. Garfield, Cecil C. Cutting, A. LaMont Baritell, Morris F. Collen, J. Paul Fitzgibbon, Robert W. King, and Melvin Friedman. The partnership agreement called for a capital investment of $10,000 from each partner with the exception of Garfield, who invested $20,000. Garfield asked nothing and received nothing from the new partners for their shares in what had been up until then a solely owned medical practice. This point, however, should not be exaggerated, for Garfield had been fairly compensated by the buyout of his hospital assets arranged by Henry J. Kaiser. Two months later, at a meeting held on Saturday afternoon April 10, 1948, the seven original partners determined that, eventually, there would be three categories in The Permanente Medical Group: senior partners, junior partners, and physician employees. Senior partners would be expected to put up capital according to a certain formula, would participate in income according to a certain formula, and would participate in the decisions concerning the rendering of medical service. All heads of large departments would be expected, eventually, to become senior partners. Junior partnerships would require a smaller initial investment in the partnership and would yield less income. Junior partners would participate in the decision-making process in an advisory role. Heads of small departments and senior physicians who had been with Permanente for at least 5 years were classified as junior partners. Unlike the heads of large departments, however, they did not have to apply for this status.

"The idea of the partnership was that there would not be employees," Garfield later said of this first agreement. "Because in general physicians have been trained and taught to be their own bosses as much as possible, we wanted to preserve the feeling that they were their own bosses and controlled their own destinies."[13]

Even this arrangement, however, kept Garfield in a condition of possible conflict of interest. As a partner in The Permanente Medical Group, Garfield was participating in a profit-making enterprise. As the executive officer of the Health Plan and the hospitals, he was administering a charitable corporation and a nonprofit trust. Upon the advice of George Link, Kaiser's tax attorney, Garfield withdrew completely from The Permanente Medical Group. A second partnership agreement, superseding that of February 21, 1948, became effective on July 1, 1949. Six of the original partners signed the second agreement, joined by Alexander King. Sidney Garfield did not sign the agreement. He was out of the partnership. "With that change," Garfield remembered, "I divested myself of ownership and became an employee of the medical group, the health plan, and the hospitals, as the medical director of all three. I did this with complete faith—I guess you would call it blind faith—that these changes would not alter the situation that existed when I owned it. We doctors had conceived the plan, developed it, sacrificed for it, made it work, and believed that it was going to remain our operation. We felt that the non-profit health plan and non-profit hospitals made up a suitable framework in which we would continue to carry on our ideals."[14]

In removing himself from the partnership he had founded, Garfield firmly believed that he was deescalating the attacks of the medical profession upon the Permanente program. As Garfield later stated, "As soon as I got out of that position, being the boss of the medical group, which I continued to be on an unofficial basis, I had no official status. Then there was no longer any real reason for their attacking me. When you attack fifty different doctors, you are getting into a different sort of deal than when you are attacking only one person."[15]

The format and much of the wording of the Articles of Partnership of June 29, 1949, governed The Permanente Medical Group until it became a professional corporation on January 1, 1982. These articles established an executive committee to carry out the business affairs, management, and administration of the partnership. The executive committee consisted of six permanent members — Baritell, Collen, Cutting, Fitzgibbon, Robert King, Neighbor — and two other members elected from the physician membership. The six permanent members were to serve continuously until death, retirement, or voluntary resignation. In the event of a vacancy, the committee itself possessed the power to appoint a successor who would thereupon become a permanent member. The two elected members of the executive committee served for a 2-year term, as did their replacements. Garfield as sole proprietor was replaced by a small centralized executive committee directorate. Continuity was further established by the fact that Sidney Garfield was remaining on not only as executive director of the Health Plan and hospitals but also as the de facto executive director of The Permanente Medical Group as well. Garfield attended all partnership meetings, reported on financial affairs, appointed persons to positions, and made most of the major decisions. From this perspective, Garfield's renunciation of his partnership had little effect as far as his relations with the other Permanente physicians was concerned. At the meeting of April 10, 1948, for instance, in which the executive committee established the senior partner, junior partner, and employed physician categories, the doctors also noted that Garfield should obtain the approval of the partners for expenditures "on anything of significant amount." It was left to Garfield, however, to decide what amount of expense would be significant. Yet Garfield's hegemony could not continue indefinitely to remain in effect. In the partnership agreement and the executive committee structure, the Permanente physicians now had in hand the legal instrument with which, in Garfield's own words, they might seize control of their destiny. Time would bear this out.

In the meanwhile, the executive committee of the partnership, meeting with Garfield in his de facto director status, carried on the day-to-day, week-to-week, month-to-month business of the medical group. A committee was appointed on November 8, 1949, for instance, to improve the Health Plan coverage sheet. At this and following meetings other additional committees were established covering better service, the better use of supplies and equipment, house call policies, and the supervision of interns and residents. Other committees formed over the next few years included bed allocation, economy, the library, research, grievances and complaints, housekeeping, staff education, and entertainment. As these committees functioned, they diffused authority and responsibility throughout the physician membership. By the early 1950s, self-governance, under the guidance of the executive committee, had become a habit.

In 1949, Garfield hired an internist, Dr. Richard Weinerman of Yale University, to be the medical director of the Permanente Health Plan. A personable and articulate advocate of prepaid group practice, Weinerman did not become a partner of The Permanente Medical Group. He did, however, attend the meetings of its executive committee so as to keep the physicians and the Health Plan in continual contact. Weinerman initiated seminars on medical economics and practice for the medical staff. He started consumer health councils and health education programs for Health Plan members. He sought foundation grants to support the gathering and analysis of statistical data on the performance of the program. Weinerman functioned, in effect, as the key medical intellectual, a concept developer and a problem solver, coordinating the efforts of the physicians and the Health Plan. In May 1951 Weinerman reported that some Plan members had complained about the waiting time to schedule appointments in the clinics. He also advocated a systematic study of the use of facilities and reported that membership representatives had requested meetings with staff physicians to discuss topics of mutual concern. Lastly, Weinerman discussed the need for the in-service training of both medical and nonmedical staff and the need for a health education outreach program aimed at the Health Plan membership. Weinerman also reported to the executive committee that the physicians in Vallejo were concerned about administrative decisions affecting patient care.

Based only in the Health Plan, Weinerman found it difficult to work on medical matters from outside the partnership. In September 1951 he resigned, and authority in the Health Plan reverted exclusively back to Garfield who, while not a member of The Permanente Medical Group, was paradoxically its founder, and thus the person who had recruited and selected the original partners. The impasse that resulted in Weinerman's departure suggested that the doctors considered themselves equal in authority to the Health Plan and the hospitals. Much unfinished business remained in the matter of authority and governance among the entities of the Permanente medical program.

Nor was the executive committee of the medical group always correct in its decisions. In July 1951, for instance, a young black physician was appointed as an intern. Although segregation by race was not allowed in assigning patients to hospital rooms (the Permanente hospitals were among the first in the community to have such a policy), the executive committee decided that it did not wish to assign a black intern for in-patient care without the patient's consent. It was then believed that such a unilateral assignment could in some cases cause resentment. The executive committee decided to assign the black intern only to services where patients would have an opportunity to choose another intern instead. This decision and this policy caused serious adverse reactions in both the Oakland community and the Health Plan membership, with its significant number of black enrollees. The policy was dropped—and never repeated.

5
Regaining Momentum

1

With only 10,000 members in mid-1945, Permanente physicians had every reason to become discouraged. Many did, and they left the program. Within 2 years, however, enrollment had increased to some 60,000 members, representing some 200 groups under contract. By April 1948 membership had risen to 72,000, approaching the peak wartime enrollment of 90,000. Despite the problems and challenges facing the Permanente physicians and their program in these postwar years—attacks by the medical establishment, the shortage of capital, the difficulties of properly marketing the program, the absence of appropriate organizational structures—the sine qua non of success, a committed membership for the Health Plan, was solidly present. The program was succeeding because the membership, the majority of them working men and women, gave to the physicians of Permanente and to prepaid group practice an overwhelming vote of confidence.

First of all, Permanente made medical care affordable. Of importance to members in an era when employees rather than employers paid for their own health insurance, Permanente eliminated the wide swings of high and low expenses characteristic of medical care in fee-for-service arrangements. One steady rate covered all contingencies. One place, moreover, provided the full spectrum of medical services, including X-rays and laboratory tests. Many members had moved to California from elsewhere during or after the war, dissolving their ties to physicians in their previous places of residence. Perceiving themselves to be receiving quality care at Permanente, they bonded with the doctors of The

Permanente Medical Group. The fact that 72,000 other people had made the same decision reinforced them in their newfound allegiance.

Even before the war was over, decisions were made and forces were set in motion that would foster growth. During the war, in an effort to accommodate organized labor, the wage and price control authorities of the Roosevelt administration determined that fringe benefits such as retirement plans and health insurance provided by an employer were exempt from wage controls. This meant that despite wartime restrictions, organized labor was able to negotiate higher benefit packages, including health care. The Internal Revenue Service ruled that such fringe benefits were deductible by the employer and were not taxable to the employees. These de facto administrative decisions were formalized after the war. In the Revenue Act of 1945, Congress approved the fringe benefit exemptions. Wage and price controls ended late in 1946. In 1948 the Supreme Court ruled that bargaining for fringe benefits was legal under the National Labor Relations Act. Thus the stage was set for unions, flourishing in the postwar boom economy, to begin to campaign for health benefits as part of their contracts.

Other positive factors were also coalescing. The postwar period witnessed the rise of other organizations, such as faculty and civil service associations, anxious to establish health-care programs for their memberships. Teachers' associations and academic faculties were among the first groups to be attracted to Permanente after the war. The University of California faculty was an early "collector" group, which meant that the enrollment of members and the collection of dues was handled by the faculty itself. Many Berkeley professors elected the Permanente program. On one occasion, Avram Yedidia, the Health Plan representative, observed a distinguished looking man working quietly on some papers while waiting for an appointment with his physician at the Permanente Hospital in Oakland. Sensing that the gentleman had been waiting for some time, Yedidia asked him if he were satisfied with the medical attention he was receiving from the Plan. The gentleman said that he was. Yedidia then asked if he minded the waiting. No, he did not, the gentleman replied. He understood how busy the doctor was. Yedidia then introduced himself, and asked the man's name. He was Enrico Fermi, a professor of physics at UC Berkeley and a winner of the Nobel Prize.

Three major decisions strengthened the ability of unions and other employee associations to choose the Permanente Plan on favorable terms. The first decision diminished Blue Cross's monopoly on employee enrollment. In 1946 Blue Cross threatened to cancel any group whose enrollment fell below 75 percent as a result of the introduction of the Permanente Health Plan as an alternative choice. Permanente appealed this decision to the state of California. The California insurance commissioner ruled that Blue Cross could not cancel its contract if 75 percent of the eligible employees were distributed among the several plans offered. This did not mean, however, that at least 75 percent must belong to one dominant plan, such as Blue Cross. Those who elected Permanente were to be counted toward the total 75 percent.

In 1947 the United Steelworkers of America selected Permanente as an alternate plan and requested that the companies employing union members provide payroll deductions. The companies refused. In arbitration, it was decided that employers must offer health insurance payment by payroll deduction even when the group health plan was unilaterally selected by the union. This second important decision further strengthened the right of working men and women, operating through their unions, to select their own health-care programs.

The third decision introduced the concept of dual choice, which involved the issue of the free choice of physicians. In 1948 the Health Service System of the city and county of San Francisco chose to offer Permanente as an alternate choice for city employees. The Retirement Board refused, noting that the patient's choice of physician in the Permanente program was restricted to Permanente physicians. The Health Service System sued the Retirement Board over this matter. The dispute was finally resolved by the California Supreme Court which upheld an administrative ruling that free choice had been offered to the employees because they could enroll either in Permanente or at least one other indemnity plan that allowed them to choose their own physicians. Thus their choice of physicians was not being limited to the closed panel. This concept of dual choice—which is to say, a choice between Permanente and a program allowing the individual choice of physicians—would grow by the end of the 1940s into an important component of the Permanente Health Plan. The physicians insisted that no one should ever be forced to join Permanente. There should always be an alternative. There should always be dual choice.

Energized by its growing membership, the Permanente Health Plan began to expand beyond its East Bay locale. In 1946 Permanente came to San Francisco when civilian workers at the Hunters Point Naval Shipyard enrolled in the program. It was not feasible to ask these workers to commute 12 miles to the Permanente Hospital in Oakland, 8 of these miles being on the busy San Francisco–Oakland Bay Bridge. The Industrial Indemnity Exchange asked Permanente to assume direction of a small outpatient rehabilitation clinic it had sponsored during the war on the third floor at 515 Market Street. Garfield asked Cecil Cutting to serve as director on this first San Francisco facility. Cutting and a few colleagues began seeing Permanente Plan patients there in 1946. The name Permanente was not displayed on the clinic door since it was feared that the San Francisco medical authorities would use such a designation as evidence of the corporate practice of medicine. Instead, "C. C. Cutting, MD and Associates" was painted on the door. Thus, almost surreptitiously, Permanente slipped into San Francisco at a time when, across the Bay, the Alameda–Contra Costa Medical Society was arming itself for a prolonged attack.

The building at 515 Market Street was ancient and somewhat shabby. Each elevator ride to the clinic on the third floor was an adventure, made even more so by the erudite elevator operator, Eric, a refugee from Nazi Germany. The staff and many Health Plan patients, including a sizable contingent of faculty from San Francisco State College, learned to savor Eric's informed conversation between floors. They also learned to deal with the difficulties of a building that was not designed for the practice of medicine. The allergy department, for instance, established by Dr. Benjamin Feingold in 1951, had to be located in the loft of the building, accessible only by stairs or the freight elevator. "We often served as elevator operators for our allergy patients who were unable to climb the stairs," remembers Florence Owyang, an early staffer. "On rainy days we had 'canned music' as buckets of all sizes were placed strategically in the waiting area to catch the rain drops. Often we were tempted to rotate the buckets to get a new tune."[1]

In 1948 at Garfield's recommendation, the Permanente Foundation purchased for $125,000 a 35-bed hospital in the Bayshore District of San Francisco near the Hunters Point Naval Shipyard. Located at 331 Pennsylvania Street, this facility was also an aging structure, having previously been owned by an ambulance service. Garfield refurbished the facility and named it Permanente Harbor Hospital. Intended as a temporary expedient, the Permanente Harbor Hospital had as its most important advantage its proximity to the Naval Shipyard and to the ambulance company next door. A small clinic was also opened in the city of South San Francisco to take care of workers and their families at nearby Bethlehem Steel.

In 1948 Garfield also assigned Wallace Neighbor, who had returned to Oakland from Vancouver the previous year, to take over the San Francisco clinic from Cutting. Garfield wanted Cutting back in Oakland to devote more of his energies to surgery. Cutting was disappointed by Garfield's request that he step aside in favor of Neighbor. He had thrown himself into the establishment of the San Francisco program and had built a high level of morale among the five other Permanente physicians. Nevertheless he complied with Garfield's request. "A very loyal friend he's always been," Garfield later said of Cecil Cutting. On the other hand, Garfield also believed that bringing Cutting back to Oakland had been the right decision, since it turned out that Cutting eventually became the executive director of The Permanente Medical Group.[2]

After the turmoils of directing the embattled Vancouver program, Wally Neighbor was glad to be back in a flourishing group practice. The stress of Vancouver had given him pseudo-angina. In San Francisco, by contrast, Cecil Cutting and his fellow physicians had achieved a remarkably high level of team spirit. "It isn't the bricks and the stones and the mortar that make a hospital," Neighbor later commented of the San Francisco facilities. "It's the people in them and the kind of care that they give.... It was a happy time again. We were small enough that we all knew each other. We got together, we worked closely and hard, and we finally got Saturday afternoons off."[3]

By this time the first generation of Permanente doctors to complete their residency training program at Permanente Hospital—A. L. Baritell, Wallace Cook, A. J. Sender—were coming into the system as trained physicians. Interns, residents, and specialists were also being recruited from medical schools and university hospitals. Every effort was made, Cecil Cutting remembers, to try to ascertain the suitability of a candidate for group practice. One of the young physicians interviewed by Paul Fitzgibbon, director of the entire Oakland–San Francisco medical group, was the author of this history, John Smillie, a USC-trained pediatrician who had completed his residency at the Los Angeles County General Hospital after wide experience as an Army medical officer in the Pacific. At Los Angeles County General Hospital, which had exercised such positive influence on Garfield, Collen, Neighbor, Kay, and Fitzgibbon, Smillie also experienced a high quality of medical practice in a grouplike setting. Offered an association with a prosperous fee-for-service practice in Hollywood, Smillie chose Permanente instead. In the vocabulary that was only then emerging, he was "group suitable," which is to say, he wished to enter immediately into as challenging a practice as possible in a group setting without spending long years building up a practice. Prior to being retained for the San Francisco Clinic in 1949, Smillie was briefed by Fitzgibbon on both the advantages and disadvantages of prepaid group medical practice. This orientation was continued by Wally Neighbor, then director of the San Francisco Clinic, as the two doctors commuted by car from the Market Street clinic and the Permanente Hospital on Pennsylvania Street. In personal sessions such as these, the Permanente philosophy was communicated to Smillie and to other young physicians by the generation who had helped found the program.

The physicians chosen for San Francisco — Wally Neighbor, Bill Hunter, Joe Thal, Phil Perloff, Cecil Aker, Robert Cogswell, and John Smillie, together with Cecil Cutting who still came over from Oakland to do surgery — knew that Permanente had a solid future in that city. In the meanwhile they worked 5½-day weeks getting the program established. When Dr. Alice De Kruif was reassigned to Oakland, Smillie found himself the only pediatrician in San Francisco, responsible for covering the clinic, the Harbor Hospital, and making house calls. The next year, another Los Angeles County General Hospital resident, Irving Klitsner, joined Smillie as the second pediatrician in San Francisco. Klitsner later returned to southern California for a distinguished career with the Southern California Permanente Medical Group. In 1951 a third pediatrician, Catherine Haney, joined the San Francisco staff, further adding to its capabilities.

A Permanente program in Vallejo was likewise showing strong growth. In the summer of 1945 the tenant council of the Vallejo Housing Authority requested that Permanente establish a medical center to provide medical care for tenants and employees living in eight large government housing projects on Vallejo 20 miles northeast of Oakland across the Carquinez Bridge in northern San Francisco Bay. In this case the request to provide medical care for shipyard and arsenal workers came not from the government or from the unions, but from a tenants' group. The following January, the Permanente Medical Center opened in a former U.S. Public Health Service Infirmary at the corner of Sonoma Boulevard and Maryland Street in Vallejo. Two doctors and five support personnel served a Health Plan membership of approximately 1500 persons. When membership was opened to employees of Mare Island and Benicia Arsenal, the Health Plan increased so rapidly that it became necessary to obtain larger facilities. A large cantonment-style government hospital, considered war surplus, was leased from the Federal Works Agency and began operating on April 1, 1947. By this time the Health Plan membership in Vallejo had increased to 8000 members. The Vallejo Hospital facility was subsequently purchased by the Permanente Foundation, with all lease payments applied to the purchase.

Between 1947 and 1954 membership in the Vallejo program more than tripled. Members came from employer groups such as the Vallejo and Napa school districts, the City of Vallejo and the Solano County Employees Association, the Vallejo Housing Authority, and the American Smelting and Refining Company. Members of the Painters Union, the Retail Clerks Union, the Teamsters and Chauffeurs Union, and the Machinists Union also joined the plan, as did federal employees from Mare Island, Travis Air Force Base, the Benicia Arsenal, and the local Postal Employees Association. By 1954 there were 30,000 members in the Permanente Vallejo area. A three-doctor clinic in Napa served approximately 5000 members.

As in the case of Oakland and San Francisco, many younger physicians were recruited from their residencies to join the medical staff. One very senior physician, however, Donovan J. McCune, an often published professor of pediatrics in the College of Physicians and Surgeons of Columbia University, also joined the Permanente Medical Group in 1951 for service in Vallejo. After a 20-year career in academic medicine, this energetic graduate of Johns Hopkins Medical School, with an impressive record behind him of teaching, publication, and consultantships in the United States and Latin America, was anxious for a midlife career change involving a more active practice of pediatrics. Over the next 25 years, until his death in 1976, McCune played an important role in the development of the Vallejo Permanente Hospital, where he eventually became chief of staff. An avid collector of rare books, a classicist, and a fine printer, McCune donated his 1000-volume library, including a leaf of a Gutenberg Bible, to the Vallejo Public Library, which established the Donovan J. McCune Room in his honor.

Also joining Vallejo, in July 1950, was Jun T. Ajari, a Japanese-American pharmacist who had recently graduated from the University of California School of Pharmacy in San Francisco. "There was much discrimination going on during those years before and after Pearl Harbor," Ajari remembers, "so I was indeed surprised when Julian Weiss, later vice president of all pharmaceutical operations in the Northern California regions said to me, 'Jerry, could you come tomorrow?' Looking back to those formative years, little did I dream that one day our Pharmacy Department would grow from a staff of two, one pharmacist and one clerk, to a total complement of 40 persons, and little did I dream that our form of prepaid health care would turn out to be the world's biggest and best health maintenance organization!"[4]

2

An important if temporary catalyst behind the rise of Permanente in Vallejo was the Kabat-Kaiser Institute. During the last year of the war,

Henry J. Kaiser, Jr., the younger of Kaiser's two sons, became ill with multiple sclerosis. Cecil Cutting made the diagnosis. Cutting also had to explain to Henry Senior and his wife Bess the prognosis for their son's disease. Initially depressed by his son's plight, Kaiser Senior soon became characteristically forceful. He became determined to find someone who could arrest or even reverse the inevitable downhill course of his son's illness that Cutting had outlined to him. Soon after Cutting made his diagnosis, Kaiser Senior read an article in the *Reader's Digest* by Paul De Kruif concerning Dr. Herman Kabat, a neurophysiologist and clinical neurologist. Working alone in his home in Washington, D.C., Kabat had treated a woman with multiple sclerosis with the drug prostigmine. Prostigmine was known to help victims of a muscle-weakening disease called myasthenia gravis. It also seemed to help the residual muscle spasm of paralytic poliomyelitis. Kabat was also using an innovative program of passive and active exercise. According to De Kruif, the multiple sclerosis victim treated by Kabat with prostigmine improved dramatically. Kaiser Senior asked Garfield to go to Washington and check out the story.

"I talked with his patients," Garfield remembered, "who were enthusiastic. The prostigmine apparently relieved their spasms, which could then be treated with physiotherapy."[5] Under Kabat's guidance, Garfield treated Kaiser Junior with prostigmine, and the younger Kaiser showed marked improvement. He even resumed the dancing he had so much enjoyed before being stricken.

What Henry J. Kaiser Senior liked, he organized. Not surprisingly, given his son's progress, he became a devoted advocate of Kabat's rehabilitation program. At Kaiser's request, Garfield sent Richard Moore, a Grand Coulee veteran, and Rene Cailliet, a young internist, to Washington to learn the rehabilitation program from Kabat and his physical therapist, Maggie Knott. In 1946 the Kabat-Kaiser Institute was established in Washington, D.C.

Kaiser, however, wanted the Institute brought to the West Coast. It was first moved to a former beach club in Santa Monica, with Richard Moore as director, then brought to Vallejo in 1948 when the purchase of the hospital there made available more space than the Vallejo health plan needed. The Institute treated patients with multiple sclerosis, post-poliomyelitis and residual weakening from strokes. It also formed an affiliation with the United Mine Workers of America to care for their members with spinal cord injuries. The United Mine Workers had previously invited Permanente to survey several hospitals in West Virginia and Kentucky, with the possibility of establishing a prepayment system in that region. Garfield went back to West Virginia and Kentucky with Todd Inch, a trustee of the Foundation. "We looked it over," Garfield later said, "and came back with the recommendation that we take the offer. But Mr. Kaiser was not pleased with the association with John L. Lewis, so he turned it down. Later, he became friendly with Lewis. By that time Lewis wanted to do the hospital and medical care himself."[6] Lewis did, in fact, establish a health plan under the auspices of the United Mine Workers' Welfare and Retirement Fund, which employed a combination of medical groups and solo practitioners under the supervision of regional medical officers. Despite this program, however, the United Mine Workers had several hundred members with spinal cord injuries who were getting little or no rehabilitative care. Signing an agreement with the Kabat-Kaiser Institute in Vallejo, the United Mine Workers sent these injured miners to California for rehabilitative care.

Had not Henry J. Kaiser, Jr., contracted multiple sclerosis, it is highly unlikely that Permanente would have become so actively involved in the maintenance of a long-range rehabilitation program such as the Kabat-Kaiser Institute. As worthy as this program was, it represented a distraction to the developing prepayment program.

Another experiment, a school of nursing, lasted 29 years with highly beneficial results. During the war, Permanente had trouble competing for qualified nurses because so many were in the armed forces. As a resident in surgery at the Los Angeles County General Hospital, Garfield had been impressed by that institution's nurses-training program. In exchange for their training and frequently subsidized room and board, student nurses provided hours of nursing services in the course of their 3-year program. When a scarcity of nurses continued in the postwar market, Garfield became determined to establish a Permanente training program under the auspices of the Permanente Foundation, which as a tax-exempt entity could offer such an educational program. Upon Garfield's recommendation, the Foundation purchased a small hotel near the Permanente Hospital in Oakland. In 1947 the first class of 40 student nurses began their training. No tuition was required. Room and board were furnished free in addition to a monthly stipend ranging from $10 to $20. The Permanente Foundation Hospital School of Nursing was the first in California consistently to recruit minority students.

Within the first year, the assistant director of the school, Dorothea Daniels, became the director. A medical professional of great force and character, Dorothea Daniels—whom Garfield later described as the "Henry J. Kaiser of nursing"—soon put the program on a solid basis. At the Permanente Foundation Hospital School of Nursing, students followed a 3-year curriculum leading to a diploma as Registered Nurse (RN). The first class graduated in 1950. Because of the standards established by Dorothea Daniels, graduates of the School of Nursing regularly received high scores on the state licensing examinations. In 1967, for instances, graduates of the school placed first among 65 nursing schools, including 4-year universities giving baccalaureate degrees, in three subjects: medical nursing, surgical nursing, and pediatric nursing. Graduates were eagerly sought by other community hospitals. Daniels encouraged her RNs to continue with their educations at colleges and universities. In many cases the Foundation or Daniels herself provided financial assistance.

Within a few short years, graduates of the School of Nursing permeated the nursing staffs of the various Permanente Hospitals. One graduate, Susan Tucker, wrote a respected medical text, *Patient Care Standards*. Another, Gretchen Karnish, became the medical center administrator at Walnut Creek in the mid-1950s and, later, vice president of the Health Plan for quality assurance. When the Permanente program expanded to Los Angeles, Dorothea Daniels herself transferred there in 1954 as the hospital administrator.

The very fact that Dorothea Daniels encouraged her students to continue on to the baccalaureate underscored the changing nature of nursing education. During the 1950s and 1960s, more and more nursing programs became affiliated with 4-year colleges or universities. In 1965 the Permanente Foundation Hospital School of Nursing became the first nursing school in California to offer the junior college Associate of Arts degree; but even this measure could not compete with a growing tendency to professionalize nursing education as a 4-year discipline. Garfield considered student nurses a valuable source of inexpensive labor and compassionate bedside care. In time, however, nursing educators, most of them university-based, began to shift the educational emphasis from practical experience to classroom instruction and supervised clinical internships. This was part of a transition in the nursing profession itself as it struggled to shed its traditional role as handmaiden to doctors and become instead an integral component of the medical care delivery team. Given these changes, it became increasingly difficult to recruit student nurses to 3-year hospital training programs. It also became more difficult to retain graduates within the Kaiser Permanente program once they received their RNs. Faced with these factors, together with the rising costs of nursing education, the Foundation closed the school in 1976 with the graduation of that year's class. The school was an experiment that had run its course, but it had also enriched the Permanente philosophy with a sympathy and respect for the nursing profession as an essential component of group-practice medicine.

3

Another major development of this period, the move to Los Angeles in 1950, was destined to yield permanent results. Two unions, the International Longshoremen and Warehousemen Union under the leadership of Harry Bridges and the Retail Clerks, Local 790 in Los Angeles, under the leadership of Joe De Silva, brought Permanente to the Southland. Despite Henry J. Kaiser's initial suspicion of John L. Lewis, Kaiser was not an antiunion industrialist. On the contrary, Kaiser believed that strong unions were an essential element of a flourishing industrial economy. Unions had demanded comprehensive prepaid coverage at Grand Coulee, and now unions were bringing the Permanente program to a new plateau of growth. In late 1949 Avram Yedidia approached Garfield with the dramatic news that the entire International Longshoremen and Warehousemen Union (ILWU) was ready to join the Permanente Health Plan. Union leader Harry Bridges had been attracted to the plan because of its comprehensive coverage but had initially held off because of his reluctance to deal with a major industrialist, Henry J. Kaiser, on this issue. Becoming convinced upon closer scrutiny that the medical program offered benefits comprehensive and economical enough to offset the Kaiser association, Bridges asked Yedidia to talk to Garfield.

Before enrolling his 5894 workers as members, however, Harry Bridges laid down two conditions. First of all, all ILWU members had to be accepted into the Plan, including those at greatest risk for health problems. Within the union membership itself, there would be no alternative choice for health care. Bridges believed that some of his union members would not enroll unless the union gave them no alternative. Bridges was quoted at the time saying that he did not want his longshoremen dying in the county hospital. Although Bridges's first requirement violated the philosophy of dual choice that was then emerging, Garfield was willing to live with it on a temporary basis.

As long as the longshoremen and warehousemen had no choice regarding their prepaid care, they nurtured a grudge against what they considered Kaiser's program. Sometimes they expressed their resentment in the language and gestures of the waterfront. To counter this behavior, the administrator of the clinic at 515 Market Street hired two airline stewardesses as receptionists and facilitators. Presenting themselves for care to the beautiful young women, even the roughest longshoreman settled down and became polite. Relations were also strained from the Permanente physicians' point of view because Harry Bridges retained his own personal fee-for-service physician, Asher Gordon, thereby suggesting to his men and their dependents that he did not have full confidence in the Permanente panel of physicians. Not until 1954 was Avram Yedidia able to convince the ILWU to offer alternative programs. When dual choice was implemented, relations between Permanente and its ILWU patients improved considerably. All in all, the ILWU brought 14,700 workers and dependents into the program.

Bridges's second requirement was more complex. He demanded that the contract with the Health Plan must cover the entire Pacific coast from Seattle to San Diego. Since Permanente operated programs only in the Portland-Vancouver area and the San Francisco Bay Area at the time, Bridges's second condition required the establishment of new Permanente Plans in Seattle, Los Angeles, and San Diego. Seattle, however, already had a prepaid group-practice plan, the Group Health Cooperative of Puget Sound, founded in 1946 by 400 families in association with a 15-physician medical group. In 1947 the cooperative purchased its own clinic and hospital. Deciding not to open in the Seattle area, Garfield arranged for the Group Health Cooperative of Puget Sound to take the ILWU contract. The ILWU represented the first expansion of the cooperative beyond its original cooperative membership. Garfield also arranged for the Northern Permanente Medical Group to cover the Portland-Vancouver region, although the director there, Ernest Saward, considered the longshoremen a high-risk group. Garfield promised to subsidize Northern Permanente if there was overutilization and did so for a number of years.

Saward was having his own problems. Health Plan growth was much slower in Oregon-Washington than in the Bay Area. The hospital that served shipyard workers during the war was not conveniently accessible to the postwar population. It was 3 miles east of Vancouver, a city that did not have a population large enough to support the Permanente Plan. Residents of Portland, Oregon, were reluctant to join a program that required crossing the Columbia River to get hospital care. Oregon families did not like the idea of their babies being born in another state. In 1945 membership was about 15,000 and plunged to 3000 in April 1946. It grew slowly—agonizingly so—to 14,000 in 1950. By 1955 it had only reached 23,000.

As in the case of Oakland, the local medical society went on the attack. In 1945 the Washington State Medical Society declared that the Northern Permanente Foundation Plan was unethical. Saward (the only Permanente physician member of the society) appealed to the AMA Judicial Council. The charge was withdrawn in June 1946. Employment of physicians, however, by the Foundation, a lay organization, continued as a point of dispute. To obviate this charge, the physicians organized The Permanente Clinic, a medical group partnership, in late 1946.

If all this were not enough, Vanport Hospital, a public housing authority hospital on the northern edge of Portland, which the Northern Permanente Foundation acquired in 1947, was swept away by a flood in May 1948. Fortunately, it was empty at the time. Given all these difficulties, Saward entertained Garfield's ILWU proposal with some reluctance.

The health needs of ILWU members in the San Francisco Bay Area could be covered by the existing Oakland, San Francisco, Richmond, and Vallejo facilities. Only the small port at Stockton presented a problem. It was 60 miles east of Oakland, and there never had been any serious intent to establish the plan that far from the major hospitals. Goldie Krantz, an officer of the ILWU, informed the San Joaquin County Medical Society that unless they came up with an acceptable plan, the ILWU would bring Permanente to Stockton. Thus challenged by Krantz's less-than-veiled threat, a group of Stockton physicians, led by Donald Harrington, an obstetrics-gynecology specialist with a natural gift for leadership, established the San Joaquin Foundation for Medical Care, a prepaid plan in which the physicians maintained their separate offices but handled the health care of ILWU members and their dependents on a cooperative basis. Hospitalization for the ILWU in Stockton was subcontracted to the Pacific National Life Insurance Company. Stockton offered a dramatic contrast to the behavior of the Alameda–Contra Costa Medical Society. Rather than oppose Permanente, the physician group headed by Harrington formed it own regional Independent Practice Association prototype, among the first of its kind. Eventually, the Health Maintenance Organization Act of 1973 provided for Independent Practice Associations (IPAs), HMOs—foreshadowed by the San Joaquin Foundation for Medical Care, which originated from Krantz's threat to bring the Permanente version of prepaid group practice to Stockton. Similarly, in San Diego, a small existing health plan agreed to assume responsibility for the longshoremen. That left Los Angeles.

Although flourishing with 8500 members, 8 physicians, and a 60-bed hospital, the program at Fontana, 45 miles east of Los Angeles, was too far away to offer any effective coverage of the Los Angeles waterfront. Nor could ILWU dependents be expected to travel out to Fontana for their medical needs. From Sidney Garfield's perspective, the ILWU contract offered a welcome opportunity to bring the Permanente program into Los Angeles itself. In a very important way Sidney Garfield had remained a citizen of that city. He had gone to school there. He had served his surgical residency there at the County Hospital, where he first developed a taste for group practice. He had returned to Los Angeles after the Mojave and Grand Coulee programs had ended. He had business interests there. His family still lived there, and it was in Los Angeles that he had formed some of his most enduring friendships. One such friendship was with Raymond Kay, then at Fontana, whom Garfield had promised in early 1942 that they would, together, bring prepaid group medical practice to southern California after the war. And now, the prospect of covering the ILWU at the Los Angeles harbor in San Pedro offered an opportunity to expand the program to the city where the ideas behind the program had been so strongly nurtured.

Kaiser and Trefethen, however, had no desire to expand into the southland; and because both the Hospital and the Plan itself were under the control of a lay board of trustees whom these two controlled, Garfield was unable to act without their consent. Without a Permanente Hospital, a successful Permanente Plan in southern California would be impossible. Before the ILWU offer surfaced, Kaiser and Trefethen had expressed reluctance about moving the program into the Los Angeles area. "You know," Garfield said of the situation, "San Franciscans don't like Los Angeles. I would talk to them and work on them every time I saw them and I was getting no place fast. They just weren't interested in the Los Angeles area."[7]

Trefethen later denied that he had ever opposed the southern California expansion. He said that he was only concerned that the ILWU wanted special treatment. In any event, once the contract was signed with ILWU in 1950, the point became moot. Permanente was now committed to Los Angeles.

The building of a hospital remained an open question. The Foundation rented space in a medical office building in San Pedro and established a clinic there with Ira ("Buck") Wallin as physician in charge. The building was owned by several fee-for-service physicians who had offices there and agreed to provide some specialist referral services. An arrangement was made with a local hospital to admit southern California Permanente Health Plan patients. Unfortunately, opposition from the medical establishment soon surfaced in the Wilmington–San Pedro medical community. Pressured by their colleagues, the fee-for-service physicians who owned the medical office building declined to provide the speciality services they had initially promised. They also served an eviction notice on their prepaid group-practice tenants. New quarters were not found until a week before the eviction. This experience helped to reinforce one of the emerging principles of the Permanente program: the ownership and integration of hospital facilities. For the Permanente program to function properly, hospital, clinic, office space, and laboratory had to be in a single or adjacent buildings under Permanente ownership where all medical services could take place. Not only was such an arrangement more efficient, it also protected Permanente from outside interference or, in some cases, outright harassment by a hostile medical community.

Within 7 months of establishing the San Pedro clinic, Sidney Garfield received a telephone call from Joe De Silva, head of the Retail Clerks' Union Local 770 in Los Angeles. De Silva told Garfield that he wanted a comprehensive health-care program for the 30,000 members of his union. De Silva was convinced that the Permanente program would best meet his union's needs. He even offered several months of dues in advance as an inducement. In 1951 this large, well-managed union joined the Permanente program. Renting space in the Rexall Building on La Cienega Boulevard, Garfield established a second Los Angeles clinic under the direction of Ray Kay, who moved to Los Angeles from Fontana. Health Plan trustee Todd Inch arranged for 30 beds at the Los Angeles Methodist Hospital. The enrollment of the Retail Clerks' Union convinced the Foundation that it was time to build a Permanente Hospital in Los Angeles. Property was purchased on Sunset Boulevard near Vermont, $5 million in financing was arranged, and planning and construction began on the first phase of the 200-bed Sunset Hospital in Los Angeles, which opened in February 1953. Permanente was in the southland to stay.

By contrast, Permanente was in Utah on a temporary basis. During the war, Kaiser Steel operated a coal mine in Utah. Medical facilities at Dragerton in Carbon County included a 35-bed hospital built under the auspices of the War Production Board. After the war, a local physician purchased the facility as war surplus property and began providing medical coverage to the miners. Complaints surfaced, however; and Dr. William Dorsey, regional medical director for the United Mineworkers' Welfare and Retirement Fund, and his assistant, Ada Kruger, a registered nurse, began an extensive investigation. They discovered, among other things, an unusually high number of surgical operations. Despite the fact that he was not a trained surgeon, the Dragerton doctor was refusing to refer major surgery cases to Salt Lake City. Owning the hospital, the doctor preferred to operate himself whenever possible and to prescribe long hospital stays for which his billing practices were frequently suspect. Himself the son of a coal miner, the Dragerton doctor had earned a statewide reputation by being willing to do down into the mines in emergencies to treat injured men. Thanks to his hospital, he had become a wealthy man with excellent social connections in the mining and medical establishments. Confronted with the report of Dorsey and Kruger, the Utah State Medical Society returned a de facto whitewash, recommending that the Dragerton doctor take a refresher course in surgery and update his bookkeeping, which he did not do. When the abuses continued, Dorsey and Kruger convinced the local union leadership that only a strike against the coal operators could force reforms at the Dragerton hospital. The strike occurred.

To reopen the mines, the major operator, U.S. Steel, asked Henry J. Kaiser if the Permanente Foundation would take over the hospital. Kaiser agreed. The articles of incorporation of the Utah Permanente Hospital were signed on February 26, 1952. Dr. Wally Cook, then finishing his fourth year of surgical residency at Oakland, left immediately for Dragerton to provide emergency medical and surgical care for the community. Less than 2 weeks later, Cook was joined by five other Permanente physicians: Steven Thomas, Lloyd and Jane Owens (a married couple), Willard Carmel, and Jack Smillie. Although they did not possess Utah medical licenses, the Medical Society in Salt Lake extended them verbal permission to practice at Dragerton while their applications were pending. Felix Day, a veteran Permanente administrator who had been with Sidney Garfield since Grand Coulee, became hospital administrator. The strike was called off.

Initially, the physicians wanted 24 hours to get organized, the hospital being in complete disarray. However, the word quickly spread that there were doctors at the hospital and patients began to knock on the door. At approximately 10:00 A.M., a union leader who called himself "Alabam" emphatically demanded that the doctors open the facility. It opened at 10:10 A.M. Many people in Dragerton were sick. There seemed to be two epidemics, one of measles and one of severe streptococcal pharyngitis. In addition, rheumatic heart disease and acute rheumatic fever were common. Many patients had surgical scars as the result of the unqualified operations of the previous medical director.

After several days, a telegram came from the Department of Business Regulation commanding the Permanente physicians to cease and desist from the practice of medicine since they were not licensed in Utah. The physicians called Dr. Garfield and returned to Salt Lake City to the Registration Division. There they learned that it might take several weeks to get licenses. But suddenly and without explanation the Department of Business Regulation announced that the "Kaiser" physicians had been cleared to practice in Utah and would receive their licenses in the mail. An unverified report had it that Henry J. Kaiser had telephoned the Governor of Utah.

The Permanente medical team stayed in Dragerton for 4 months, during which time their replacements were recruited. Wally Cook stayed only 1 month, replaced by Miles Fellows, a surgeon from Southern California Permanente Medical Group at Fontana. James McClintock, the chairperson of the department of surgery at the Veterans Administration Hospital in Grand Junction, Colorado, relieved Fellows. (McClintock took the position himself instead of sending along one of his graduating senior residents.) Several other physicians arrived to replace the departing Permanente doctors in July 1952. A prepaid Permanente health plan was never established in Utah. The hospital, however, owned by the Permanente Foundation, continued as Utah Permanente Hospital until 1966.

4

By 1952, the year of this emergency sortie to Utah by the Permanente physicians, the program was 10 years past its organization in Oakland in 1942 and nearly 20 years since the time that Sidney Garfield first went out to Desert Center. In the Mojave, at Grand Coulee, at Richmond, Oakland, San Francisco, Vallejo, Fontana, Los Angeles, and even the embattled program in the Vancouver-Portland region, certain concepts and principles had asserted themselves. Ernest Saward was later to call these principles the genetic code of the Permanente program. As early as April 4, 1945, Sidney Garfield outlined them in a speech to the Multnomah County Medical Association in Portland, Oregon. At that time Garfield cited four principles, which were later expanded to six. These were prepayment, group practice, adequate facilities, and what Garfield called a new economy of medicine.

"The thing to remember about prepayment," Garfield told the Multnomah County Medical Association, "is that it brings the patient to the doctor earlier in his illness and more often, which is one of the most important effects of a health plan because it permits the practice of true preventive medicine. Any plan which sets a barrier between the patient and the doctor by eliminating the first two or three visits, by covering the patient only for hospital or surgical care, or by limiting this coverage in other ways, in our opinion defeats its purpose and is not good."[8]

The preventive care made possible by prepayment to providers of professional services had asserted itself in the desert, at Grand Coulee, and at the shipyards. It also emerged most dramatically when Permanente assumed the care of the longshoremen of the ILWU. Union officials had so much trouble getting the rank and file to visit the doctors at a hospital or clinic that they asked the doctors to go down to the docks. A crew of Permanente physicians and nurses traveled from dock to dock conducting multiphasic health examinations at the working site: blood pressure, chest examinations, and other routine testing. In this way, numerous problems among the hard-working, hard-living longshoremen were detected. Encouraged by these results, Sidney Garfield asked Morris Collen to start a program of regular multiphasic health checkups at the various Permanente facilities. Multiphasic health testing was incorporated into all regular medical appointments beginning in November 1951 in Oakland and extended to San Francisco 2 months later.

The second of Garfield's four principles, group practice, had proved itself again and again over the past 20 years. Medicine, Garfield believed, was by its very nature a cooperative enterprise. "It has always seemed a paradox," he told the Multnomah Medical Society in 1945, "that in the universities which teach us medicine, we learn medicine under the highest form of group practice; but when we go out into practice, we revert to the old type of individual private practice."[9]

Garfield's third principle, adequate facilities, also referred to as integrated facilities, was the material equivalent of group practice among physicians. By bringing all facilities together under one ownership and under one roof, physicians were enabled to practice medicine more efficiently and hence more to their own satisfaction. Group-practice physicians who enjoyed integrated and adequate facilities not only practiced better medicine, they also enjoyed their lives more. Doing more and better work in less time, they escaped the burden of overwork which constricted the lives of so many fee-for-service physicians.

By the new economy of medicine, Garfield meant the reversal of traditional medical economics inherent in the fee-for-service system. When only the sick paid for themselves, a constricted payment base forced medical costs to soar. By having the healthy pay to maintain their own health, capital coalesced with which to care for the sick.

The experience of Permanente with the ILWU affirmed the fifth principle in the Permanente genetic code, voluntary enrollment with dual choice. The ILWU demand that 100 percent of its membership enroll in the Permanente program did not prove advantageous to either party. Many longshoremen had experienced bitter labor disputes with employers, and resentment still smoldered in them toward the employer class. Physicians and other health professionals disliked providing service to patients who felt forced to see them instead of choosing to do so. In addition, the lack of dual choice gave effective ammunition to charges of "captive" patients. In 1954 the union accepted the concept of dual choice for each subscriber: the option of Permanente or an alternate choice, an indemnity plan. Given dual choice, only 10 percent of the longshoremen chose the indemnity plan.

Dual choice was thus added to the operating principle of voluntary enrollment that had been an important feature prior to the ILWU experience. Dual choice meant that each individual employee subscriber would be given the opportunity to choose a plan such as Blue Cross, Blue Shield, or an indemnity plan that offered the choice of an open panel of all physicians in the community, as an alternative to Permanente. If the alternate plan favored by an employer or union was a plan that also limited the panel of physicians from which the subscriber could choose, such a plan was not acceptable to Permanente for purposes of dual choice. Furthermore, once an employee had made a choice, periodic open enrollment gave the subscriber the opportunity to change plans. Open enrollment periods tended to occur annually at the time of contract renewal. Both dual choice and annual election proved to be features favoring Permanente as membership satisfaction stimulated new enrollments.

The sixth principle of the Permanente genetic code, physician responsibility in management as well as medical matters, was inherent in the other five. The exact parameters of the responsibilities and authority of the Permanente physicians vis-à-vis the Hospitals and the Health Plan as of 1952 were still emerging toward a more explicit definition. The direction of that movement pointed to the shores of Lake Tahoe, where Henry J. Kaiser maintained his summer residence, but relations between the Kaiser organization and the physicians of Permanente had yet to be tested.

6
Who Is in Charge?
1952–1955

_____ 1 _____

In the August 1952 tenth anniversary issue of the *Permanente Foundation Medical Bulletin,* Sidney Garfield assessed the Permanente program in California, Oregon, and Washington and found much in which to take satisfaction. Having dropped to 30,000 just after the war, Permanente was now serving 250,000 members. By 1952 the membership in northern California had passed the 160,000 mark. One hundred and twenty-five physicians were practicing with The Permanente Medical Group. The Permanente Hospitals, a nonprofit corporation, was operating four successful facilities with a total bed capacity of 500. Clinics were operating in Walnut Creek, Redwood City, and Napa. Three major new hospitals – in Los Angeles, San Francisco, and Walnut Creek – were in the planning or construction stages. The Permanente Hospitals maintained a thriving nursing school and an approved intern and residency training program. There was even talk of establishing a medical school in San Francisco after the Stanford Medical School moved south to Palo Alto. A quarter of a million dollars of the 1952 budget had been appropriated for research, including the acquisition of a basic research laboratory building in the suburban town of Belmont, south of San Francisco. Relations between Permanente and the medical societies of Alameda–Contra Costa, Los Angeles, and San Bernadino County were showing some signs of improvement. "Opposition to change is natural and healthy," Garfield graciously stated in his report; "the effect of this opposition was to stimulate us to do a better job."[1]

Nowhere was this effort to do a better job more evident than in the hospitals being planned for San Francisco, Los Angeles, and Walnut Creek. The 35-bed Permanente Harbor Hospital in San Francisco soon proved too small to accommodate the growing Health Plan membership in the city. Most San Francisco patients had to be referred to the Permanente Hospital in Oakland for admission, an inconvenience to San Francisco members and an irritation to personnel on both sides of the bay. With funds provided by a $4.5 million loan from Bank of America arranged in September 1951, a major property on Geary Boulevard near Divisadero was purchased as the site for a new San Francisco hospital. Likewise in Los Angeles, the hospitalization of Health Plan members at Methodist Hospital or other hospitals throughout the Los Angeles basin was proving increasingly unworkable. With funds made available by the same Bank of America loan, a tree-covered property previously part of Barnsdall Park was acquired for a new hospital to serve the rapidly growing Health Plan membership in southern California and to create a presence in the Los Angeles community that would aid marketing and enrollment.

In planning the Los Angeles and San Francisco hospitals, Sidney Garfield worked closely with the architects to implement the design features he had been evolving for much of his medical career. Instead of the usual central corridor, for instance, used in common by patients, staff, and visitors alike, Garfield called for three corridors, each of them serving distinct traffic. The central service corridor served patients and staff. It featured decentralized nursing stations, supply cupboards, medical records units, and microwave ovens to assure hot meals. Walkways outside patients' rooms on both sides of the building provided visitor access through sliding glass doors. Thus Garfield separated the medical activity of the hospital from the flow of patient visitor traffic. On the obstetrics floor, Garfield arranged each mother's room adjacent to a small soundproofed one-bassinet nursery. Each newborn infant was housed adjacent to its mother while also remaining under the supervision of the medical staff. A mobile bassinet, set in a standard metal file drawer, was placed in the wall between the mother's room and the nursery. The infant's mother merely had to pull the mobile bassinet into her room to enjoy the company of her child. A light signal system in the nursery indicated whether a baby was in the nursery or in its mother's room. There was also a viewing window in each mother's room that allowed her to see her child at will without disturbance. Garfield believed that the earliest contact between mother and infant was crucial and should be fostered in the hospital environment. Permanente Hospitals eventually showed high statistics of mothers choosing to breast-feed.

Each room in the new hospitals had a maximum of two beds. The top floor of the hospital was reserved for ambulatory patients. Here an effort was made to create a hotelstyle atmosphere. Patients took their meals from a dining room buffet, were allowed to sleep late in the morning, and were encouraged to participate in planned recreation and social activities.

2

Behind the optimistic surface of Garfield's Tenth Annual Report, however—his belief, as he wrote, "that the accolade of 'mission accomplished' cannot be too far off"—there were serious problems developing within the Permanente community. Most of them revolved around problems of governance. Who exactly was in charge? The Medical Group held jurisdiction over medical programs. At the same time, the medical program operated within financial strictures and facilities under the jurisdiction of Health Plan and Hospitals. Decisions made by lay administrators frequently impinged upon or directly affected medical practice. As long as Sidney Garfield, a physician, was serving in a tripartite capacity as de facto executive director of the Medical Group, Hospitals, and Health Plan, the issue of physician control could be held in abeyance; but in the early 1950s Sidney Garfield's single ball of wax had begun to melt in three directions as the Medical Group, the Hospitals, and the Plan each began to assert separate needs, jurisdictions, and prerogatives. The Plan was a nonprofit corporation, and Hospitals was a charitable trust. The Medical Group, by contrast, was a profit-making partnership. Many Permanente physicians were beginning to perceive that their incomes were being constrained by the cost of hospital expansion. This expansion, in turn, was empowered by Bank of America loans that were guaranteed, not by the Medical Group or Health Plan, but by Kaiser Industries. The Bank of America considered hospitals in and of themselves a poor credit risk and would only establish a line of credit for their construction because of the Kaiser Industries guarantee. Kaiser Industries became of necessity concerned with the financial solvency, even the day-to-day operations, of the program. From the point of view of physicians, it was their program. The Health Plan enrolled the members, received monthly dues from consumers, and paid for their medical care by prepayment instead of fee-for-service. Hospitals provided the necessary workshop in which physicians practiced. From the point of view of Kaiser Industries executives who owned and controlled the Health Plan and Hospitals, the program was theirs, with doctors serving only as professionals with the responsibility to provide the medical care. It took more than a decade to work out this problem of governance. But it was worked out. Both the Medical Group and Health Plan struggled for control, sharing the clear goal that the medical care enterprise was an important social contribution and should continue.

It was not this way in the beginning. At Grand Coulee and during the busy war years, Henry J. Kaiser had too much else on his mind — the construction of a great dam — the production of warships — to involve himself in the minutiae of the health program serving his employees. Kaiser wanted the program to work, and when it did, he was satisfied to leave its supervision to Sidney Garfield. During those years, Kaiser and his executives and attorneys functioned primarily as advisors, not managers, to the program. With the exception of a non-interest-bearing loan of $150,000 to cover the initial operations of the Permanente Health Plan in 1945, neither the Kaiser family nor Kaiser Industries provided financial subsidies to the Plan.

Between Sidney Garfield and Henry J. Kaiser, however, there continued throughout the postwar period a close physician-patient relationship and a strong idiosyncratic friendship. Garfield frequently compared his relationship with Kaiser to that of a son to his father. In one way or another, the dynamic young executives who surrounded Kaiser from the 1930s onward were all his sons.

Sidney Garfield had a habit of referring all his major decisions to Kaiser, even though he was simultaneously capable of arguing with Kaiser on medical matters. For Garfield, the industrialist was, quite simply, the Boss. As long as Garfield was primarily serving Kaiser employees, this designation was accurate and appropriate. When the Permanente program assumed the dimension of a major development in American medicine, however, having a nonmedical industrialist as the Boss created difficulties.

Such difficulty first surfaced when Ray Kay urged Garfield to make good on his wartime promise to expand the program into southern California. With his Fontana steelworkers adequately covered by Permanente physicians, Kaiser was in no mood to help the program extend itself to non-Kaiser employees in greater Los Angeles. Garfield needed Kaiser, however, to guarantee the line of credit the Los Angeles expansion required. "They were the original board of directors," Garfield later said of Kaiser, Trefethen, and the other executives and attorneys. "Once we set it up that way, they controlled the decisions. They let me operate pretty much the way I wanted to....I ran it and Trefethen was the man I worked with most of the time."[2]

Garfield thus acknowledged the ultimate control of the Kaiser organization while at the same time insisting that he, a physician, ran the show. In the immediate postwar years, this working solution, despite its intrinsic contradictions, succeeded in great part because of the implicit trust between Kaiser and Garfield, because of Kaiser's noninterference, and because of Garfield's personal style. Dapper, assured, by turns spontaneous and restrained, Garfield functioned not so much as the chief bureaucrat of the organization but as its chief source of instruction, encouragement, and, when necessary, chastisement. Off the job, Garfield could be as genial and outgoing as he was demanding during work hours. He delighted in entertaining at Trader Vic's in Oakland, a habit begun during the war, and on many occasions would present each female guest with an expensive Trader Vic's recipe book. Every Christmas Garfield would send by special messenger to the homes of his administrative staff an expensive silk Hawaiian shirt. After the holidays, staff members would compare notes as to whether they had made Dr. Garfield's Shirt List. Whatever economies Garfield imposed on the Permanente physicians in order to make the program self-sufficient, he was willing to use his own personal resources to maintain the morale of key people. He was a generous and supportive leader.

Garfield personally chose the key physicians and lay staff of the organization. They in turn granted him, initially, a level of personal loyalty that glossed over the question of whether such a personalized style of leadership could direct a multimillion dollar medical enterprise caring for the needs of a half million patients. In the meanwhile, Garfield's personalized leadership seemed to work. One loyal staffer was Dorothea Daniels, dean of the School of Nursing. When the scheduled Permanente Hospital in Los Angeles required an administrator, Garfield dispatched Dorothea Daniels to the southland. With the exception of Roman Catholic nursing sisters, few women were given the opportunity to administer major hospitals in the early 1950s. Garfield's choice proved to be the perfect solution. Her little dog Snuffy tucked into the opened bottom drawer of her desk, Dorothea Daniels revealed herself as a crackerjack administrator: a trained nurse with a highly informed sense of medical responsibility, and a no-nonsense, sometimes stern matriarch ruling physicians, nurses, and staff with total authority.

Daniels's style, charismatic but highly individual (Snuffy was the only pet allowed in the hospital), reflected the leadership style Garfield himself pursued.

Similarly, no one pursued a more personalized leadership style than Henry J. Kaiser himself. Trait for trait, action for action, Henry J. Kaiser defied the stereotype of the corporate smoothie, bland and efficient. He was a self-made megaindustrialist, the founder and energizer of vast enterprises; and he incorporated within his character and personality (indeed in his very physical self) capacities and contradictions that raised him above the level of ordinary people. Roads, dams, ships, steel, cement, aluminum, aircraft, automobiles, and hotels: Henry J. Kaiser loved nothing so much as to organize massive manufacturing enterprises, which he then turned over to trusted young individuals to run on a day-by-day basis. Peripatetic, driven by inconceivable energy, requiring little sleep, Kaiser moved from place to place, enterprise to enterprise, organizing, cajoling, creating. Day and night he kept in contact with his subordinates by long-distance telephone, running up astronomical bills. "Rome wasn't built in a day," Kaiser was fond of saying, "because the Romans didn't give us the contract."

Born in the late nineteenth century, Kaiser sustained throughout his twentieth-century career a Victorian optimism, enlivened by an evangelical faith in people and events and the possibilities of the human spirit, that hovered on the borderline between the trite and the sublime. He loved the poetry of Alfred Lord Tennyson and Rudyard Kipling, whose moralistic poem "If" served Kaiser throughout his life as a constant call to action. He was at once a member of the elite (by the early 1950s, he was one of the wealthiest individuals in the United States) and a thoroughgoing democrat given to reciting a poem about a young man wanting to speak to God:

> I climbed the highest steeple.
> And God said, "Go down, young man,
> I live among the people."

Kaiser was quick to take up new projects, especially construction projects, and equally quick to walk away from them when they were complete. His ever active intellect was constantly devising new solutions to old problems. No solution gave him more pleasure than those which made labor easier and more efficient, such as the rubber balloon tires he had placed on the wheelbarrows at his construction site so as to make pushing a load easier. Henry J. Kaiser had little capacity for chitchat or small talk and was on the job, or so it seemed, for the 20 hours a day he was usually awake. He could be impatient. A former photographer, he bought every new camera that came on the market but did not read the attendant instructions. The camera usually jammed, so he gave it to a subordinate to figure out. He was happy when constantly surrounded by an entourage, and he was greatly dependent upon his wife Bess. He also had a hunger that he could not satisfy. "My only affliction," Kaiser said of himself, "is that I suffer from stomach trouble. I never can get enough in it."[3]

Lithe and athletic as a young man, Kaiser grew heavy in middle age. By his sixties he was noticeably overweight, although his physical energy never diminished. At restaurants he would order double portions of food, unless prevented from so doing by his wife or Sidney Garfield. Cecil Cutting, who lived with the Kaisers for 6 months during Bess Kaiser's last illness, remembers him constantly barbequing hamburgers. When Permanente physician Fred Pellegrin visited Kaiser at his home in Lafayette, the two men sat down to a luncheon of superbly grilled New York steaks. The telephone rang just as the two men sat down to eat. Pellegrin was wanted at the hospital. As Pellegrin left the dining room, he saw Kaiser spearing the physician's steak over to his own dinner plate.

Sidney Garfield was constantly working with Kaiser to keep down his weight. Kaiser lived to 85, but Garfield believed that he would have lived to 100 had he cut back the double portions. Later, in Hawaii, Garfield put Kaiser on another diet, allowing him to snack between meals only on shark-fin soup. Kaiser had a huge kettle of shark-fin soup sent over to his home from the Golden Dragon Room at the Hawaiian Village Hotel and would sip it constantly during the day. A chain smoker of cigars, Kaiser gave them up on doctor's orders.

Henry J. Kaiser was devoted to Bess Kaiser and dependent on her as well. Whenever possible, he wanted her to travel with him. Unlike many men of his generation, Kaiser was in the habit of keeping his wife fully informed regarding his business life and decisions. Bess Kaiser would personally assess candidates for promotion within the organization or for joint ventures with the Kaiser Companies. She was the only human being who could exercise authority over her husband's impulses. She took personal pride in keeping house and cooking, and like her husband she grew heavy in her later years. Her two interests outside the home were horse races and the Women's Athletic Club in Oakland, of which she was an active member. In her household and among the top executives she was known as Mother Kaiser.

3

Kaiser's enormous drive and energy and his need to control everything with which he was actively involved are of critical importance in the history of The Permanente Medical Group because, starting in 1952, he began to try to control the program, including its physicians. Kaiser's energy, vision, will, and obsession with growth and construction, and his new and compelling interest in medicine as he understood it, brought him into a decade-long conflict with the same physicians whose medical care program he had supported in the previous decade with a minimum of interference. The stage was set for a titanic battle of wills. The major casualty of this battle would be Sidney Garfield.

Sometime in the summer of 1950 Bess Kaiser, who throughout her life had suffered from high blood pressure, became weaker and weaker with chronic nephritis. By the fall it was obvious to Garfield, the Kaiser family physician, that Bess Kaiser was in a serious, possibly terminal condition. Garfield sent Albert Bolomey, a cardiology and renal disease specialist in The Permanente Medical Group, to a number of major medical centers to study the latest treatments. Since artificial kidneys were primitive and untested at this time, renal dialysis was not a realistic option. Garfield also asked Cecil Cutting to take a leave of absence and move into the Kaiser penthouse on Lake Merritt as Mrs. Kaiser's personal physician during her final ordeal. During the next 6 months, Cutting practically lived with the Kaisers. Bess Kaiser trusted no other doctor to carry out the procedures her declining condition made necessary. Garfield also sent over a Permanente nurse, Alyce Chester, who moved into the Kaiser apartment to provide continuing nursing care for Mrs. Kaiser.

Tall, athletic, and attractive, Alyce Chester was a divorcee in her early thirties and the parent of a son. Her younger sister Helen, equally attractive, was also in the process of a divorce, which had become delayed when her husband contracted polio. In the late 1940s Alyce Chester had joined the Permanente staff in Oakland as a nurse. She attracted the attention of Sidney Garfield, who became her mentor, promoting her to positions of increasing responsibility. Intelligent and committed, Alyce Chester soon became part of the executive team that revolved around Sidney Garfield. "She was very close to Sid," Dr. Wallace Cook later remembered.[7] Outgoing and gregarious, Alyce admired physicians but was not intimidated by them. They, in turn, found her sympathetic. She was often invited to join the younger doctors at bridge during their off hours.

Bess Kaiser died on March 15, 1951. Three months later on June 10, 1951, Henry J. Kaiser, aged 69, married Alyce Chester, some 35 years his junior. The wedding was held in Santa Barbara with a reception in the Biltmore Hotel. Kaiser's two sons, their new stepmother's contemporaries in age, opposed the marriage, which they considered precipitous, as did some Kaiser executives. Henry J. Kaiser, however, dreading the prospect of living alone, insisted on his right to marry the dynamic and sympathetic young nurse. Sidney Garfield agreed with Mr. Kaiser's decision.

Less than a year later, Sidney Garfield, by then divorced from his first wife Virginia, married Alyce's sister Helen Peterson, whose divorce from her first husband had become final. Toward midnight, after a long day spent salmon fishing with the Wally Neighbors outside the Golden Gate, the Cuttings received a telephone call.

"Mr. Kaiser wants you down at the airport right away," came the unidentified voice. "Sid's getting married."

Garfield, who was living with the Cuttings at the time, then got on the phone and asked the Cuttings to meet him at the Oakland Airport in an hour and bring along his best suit and a clean shirt. "We're going to Reno to get married," Garfield told Cutting.

Within the hour the Cuttings and Neighbors joined Henry J. Kaiser and Alyce Kaiser, Helen Peterson, and Sidney Garfield for the flight to Reno on Kaiser's private plane. On arrival at Reno City Hall, it was discovered that Garfield had no ring for the ceremony. Wally Neighbor loaned Sidney Garfield his wedding ring. After the ceremony, the party flew back to Oakland.[8]

Sidney and Helen Garfield moved next door to Henry J. and Alyce Kaiser in Lafayette. Garfield and Kaiser were now brothers-in-law, married to sisters who were extremely close to each other, visiting back and forth every day. In the evenings, the two couples would gather for cocktails and conversation. Sidney Garfield was now the brother-in-law, physician, and close personal confidant of Henry J. Kaiser.

Alyce Kaiser was an energetic and intelligent woman who was not satisfied to be limited to the social activities of the wives of other Kaiser Companies executives. She needed an activity that kept her involved in medical care. And besides, Kaiser's sons, representing the sentiments of the upper echelon of Kaiser Industries management, wanted their father, now 70, to begin to ease himself in the direction of semiretirement. Wasn't it time for Edgar Kaiser to take over? The newlyweds determined upon another activity into which they could channel their energies and find identity as a married couple. Since Alyce Kaiser was a nurse by training, and since Henry J. Kaiser had helped sponsor a pioneering medical plan, it was only natural that the couple—some 35 years apart in age, each seeking a common ground of interest and activity with the other—should turn to medicine. Having married a beautiful young nurse, Henry J. Kaiser decided to build her a hospital. Garfield went along with the idea.

During Bess Kaiser's last illness and the early months of Henry J. and Alyce's marriage, Garfield and his staff were carefully planning the multimillion dollar San Francisco and Los Angeles hospitals. Throughout the lean postwar years, Garfield set aside money from the organizations for these facilities. The Permanente physicians considered that they had donated considerable sweat equity so that the program might have major hospitals in San Francisco and Los Angeles. Even as the bulldozers were clearing the two sites, Henry J. Kaiser unilaterally announced that he was building a new Permanente hospital in Walnut Creek, a suburban community in a warm valley 20 miles east of Oakland not far from the Kaiser-Garfield homes in Lafayette. Never in any discussions regarding growth had there been the slightest mention of a hospital in Walnut Creek. Not only was money needed for Los Angeles and San Francisco, but the facilities at Oakland and Vallejo were also in need of refurbishment. There were fewer than 5000 Health Plan members in the Walnut Creek area, in contrast to the 160,000 members being served in other Bay Area hospitals. In retrospect, Henry J. Kaiser correctly anticipated the growth of the Concord–Walnut Creek area, where by the late 1980s there would be 300,000 members in the Health Plan. But from the viewpoint of the Permanente physicians of 1952, Kaiser's decision to siphon off sorely needed funds for expansion into what was then a rural area, constituted an unconscionable interference in the ability of the physicians to determine their own destinies. It was also perceived as a serious appropriation of funds they had helped earn by providing good-quality, cost-effective care. They sensed that they had been moved from principals in the medical care enterprise they had started to employees ignored in the decision-making process.

Whatever Henry Kaiser did, he did in a visionary manner and on a large scale. Typically, he determined that the Walnut Creek hospital would be a showcase, the hospital of the future. Not only would it serve Health Plan members in Walnut Creek, it would also be available to fee-for-service physicians since no other community hospital was then available. Kaiser was using revenues—some of which were generated by Permanente physicians—to subsidize a luxury hospital for fee-for-service physicians in the Walnut Creek area. It was a bitter pill for Permanente physicians to swallow.

As the site for his hospital, Kaiser chose the Art and Garden Center owned by the former mayor of Walnut Creek. In the preliminary negotiations, the owner was told merely that a group of doctors were interested in the property. The asking price was then $80,000. But Kaiser, as usual, became impatient and while negotiations were under way, personally went out to inspect the property. Garfield cautioned him to keep his name out of it, but Kaiser replied, "The hell with it. Let them know it's me. I don't like doing anything sub rosa anyway."[9] When it was reported that the great Henry J. Kaiser himself had inspected the property — two adjacent sections each with a home, one with an elegant swimming pool — the price escalated to $100,000.

Working together, architect Clarence Mayhew and Sidney Garfield created a luxurious 100-bed ranch-style facility that incorporated all of Garfield's innovative design and planning ideas: the central work corridors, the decentralized nursing stations, the innovative maternity ward arrangements. Patient rooms each had a ground-level outside access, although at certain times this allowed undischarged patients to wander into town for an unauthorized visit. The hospital was initially planned for 70 beds, but during construction Henry J. Kaiser, frequently on the scene, ordered an increase of 30 beds. In the construction of the San Francisco and Los Angeles hospitals, construction costs were clearly monitored. In Walnut Creek, the sky was the limit. In the early phases of clearing the site, Kaiser personally operated a bulldozer. Supervising construction, which like everything else he did he put on a fast-track basis, Kaiser donated $700,00 to the project. The Bank of America, on Kaiser's say-so, loaned the project another $885,000. As if in further affront, the Walnut Creek hospital, resentfully dubbed the Country Club by many in the Permanente community, opened in September 1953, 6 months before the San Francisco and Los Angeles hospitals were ready.

Unconsulted in the matter of building the Walnut Creek hospital, The Permanente Medical Group executive committee was now ignored in the matter of its staffing, which the executive committee considered its prerogative. Operating as de facto administrator of the Walnut Creek facility, Alyce Kaiser personally selected the medical staff on her own authority and without consultation. The emergency room nurse had herself become the de facto administrator. To be Physician-in-Chief Alyce Kaiser chose Wallace Cook, a 31-year-old fourth-year resident in surgery whom she promoted over the heads of all the other physicians, some of whom had been associated with the program since Grand Coulee and others who were veterans of the war and postwar years. She also chose Fred Pellegrin in internal medicine, Steven Thomas in obstetrics-gynecology, and James Flett in pediatrics. At the time, Flett was teaching at the University of Colorado. "Aly chose us," Wallace Cook later recalled. "In some people's perception, she was butting into the Medical Group's business; in other people's perceptions she had taken the best and the brightest, so to speak—some people said that, and I'm not going to say it, because you can't say that about yourself."[10]

It was also rumored among the Permanente physicians that the Walnut Creek physicians were to receive higher salaries than their Permanente Medical Group colleagues. Wallace Cook was personally invited to meet with the executive committee to discuss the pay scales of the Walnut Creek doctors. While compensation was comparable, Cook was himself being paid a supplement by the Walnut Creek hospital for hospital duties, in addition to his Permanente salary. This supplement was later built into his basic salary.

The Walnut Creek hospital did indeed become a showcase. "I was as much an entertainer as an administrator," Wallace Cook later remembered. "I was touring people very, very frequently, because we were the new hospital, before San Francisco opened. Also I guess, ours was thought to be a little bit more unique insofar as its gardenlike setting. I know we were called the Country Club for years, and may still be called the Country Club. That was a pejorative term, everyone else feeling that we were the playboys, playgirls, or whatever. Actually our statistics were as good as anybody else's, but we were treated as the Kaiser family showplace, to some extent."[11]

Henry and Alyce Kaiser involved themselves intimately with the day-to-day administration of their showplace. One Sunday morning in early 1953 Kaiser called an 8:00 A.M. meeting at the hospital for the physicians and administrative staff. He wanted to know what type of filing system was being used in the clinic records department. When told that it was a terminal digit system, in which the last two numbers of the medical record number functioned as the key to the numerical filing system, Kaiser exploded that he did not want his patients to be treated as numbers. He demanded that the filing system be put on an alphabetical basis.

In an alphabetical system, it would be quite difficult to locate a misfiled chart, it was pointed out.

How are you going to solve that problem? Kaiser retorted.

Someone suggested that a different color be assigned for every letter of the alphabet.

Are there 26 distinct colors, someone else asked?

My daughter has a giant box of Crayolas, someone else interjected, and it probably has 26 colors.

With that, Kaiser seized a piece of chalk and began writing the letters of the alphabet on the floor. He then had everyone gather the medical files, form a large circle, and walking around the circle of letters, drop the files alphabetically on top of the corresponding letters. These letters were then color-coded. Implemented at the time to placate Kaiser, this peculiar color-coded system was later abandoned as unworkable.

In 1952, the Health Plan and the Hospitals formally adopted the name *Kaiser*, further testimony to Henry J. Kaiser's growing identification with and involvement in the program. From that time onward, the program encompassed the Kaiser Foundation, the Kaiser Foundation Health Plan, a nonprofit corporation, and the Kaiser Foundation Hospitals, a charitable trust. Garfield had himself proposed the use of the name *Kaiser* just after the war. The name *Permanente*, the Spanish language designation of a creek running near the Permanente Cement factory in Los Altos, was strange, difficult to pronounce, and without significance to anyone outside the Kaiser organization. The name Kaiser, by contrast, was easy to pronounce and had high name recognition throughout the United States. The designation Kaiser connoted stability, energy, productivity, creativity, and strength. This postwar suggestion was dropped, however, in part because of the controversial nature of the program. A number of top Kaiser executives and their wives had close social contacts with fee-for-service physicians and their spouses. To attach the name Kaiser to a controversial program being bitterly opposed by the Alameda–Contra Costa Medical Society would have strained, even sundered, important social relationships. And besides, Kaiser executives pointed out, if the program failed (as many of them expected it would) and was named Kaiser, this would injure the reputation of the companies. Ironically, of all the industries these executives were running, only the Health Plan would survive and thrive in anything resembling its original form.

In 1951, with Kaiser's growing involvement in the program, the proposal to name it Kaiser once again surfaced, advanced this time by Stubb Stollery, a public relations executive in Kaiser Industries. The proposal also had Garfield's approval. Garfield later contested Stollery's claim regarding the revival of the suggestion. "The Kaiser-Fraser automobile business," Garfield later recalled, "was going down hill. I was anxious to be helpful. I had all our doctors driving Kaiser cars. I suggested to Mr. Kaiser that we change the name to Kaiser. We had several hundred thousand members. I thought that people, knowing they were members of Kaiser Health Plan, would be interested in buying Kaiser cars. I even wanted to have them put their models on display in the clinics. The Kaisers accepted the name change."[13]

The Permanente Medical Group, however, refused to change its name. To call themselves the Kaiser Medical Group, the physicians argued, would create the impressions that they were employees of Henry J. Kaiser rather than an autonomous medical partnership. Already, too many fee-for-service physicians regarded the Permanente doctors as salaried employees of Kaiser Industries. By refusing to take on the name Kaiser, the Medical Group also underscored its resentment over the Walnut Creek hospital and other aspects of what it considered Henry J. and Alyce Kaiser's unwarranted intrusion into physicians' prerogatives. Garfield, meanwhile, was lobbying his fellow physicians for the name change. When it became clear that they would not cooperate, he asked Ray Kay to explain their refusal to Henry J. Kaiser himself. Entering the board room in Oakland, Kay sat across a long table opposite Eugene Trefethen. At one end of the table was Henry J. Kaiser and at the other was Sidney Garfield. Trefethen invited Kay to explain to Kaiser the reason why the physicians did not want to use his name.

When Kay was finished, Trefethen said, "Well, Mr. Kaiser, I think there's some merit in what Ray is saying."

Henry J. Kaiser, then said, "Of course, of course, I wouldn't let him [Kay] use my name. I don't want them to use my name. I wouldn't let them use my name."

It was, as Kay later recalled, "just as if we'd taken candy away from him."[14]

In response to the hostility of the Medical Group to Walnut Creek and its refusal to change its name, Kaiser began openly to advocate that the Medical Group break up into separate partnerships. At the time, May 1952, The Permanente Medical Group consisted of 101 full-time physicians, 29 of them partners, 11 of them participants or prepartners, and 61 of them salaried employees. Kaiser thought that each facility should have its own separate medical partnership. The Medical Group easily perceived this as a divide-and-conquer tactic and mounted strong opposition to the proposal. Only a large and strong medical group, they correctly believed, had any chance of standing up to Henry J. Kaiser. Discreetly, Kaiser had articles of incorporation prepared for a separate Walnut Creek medical group, one that he and Alyce could control. For the next year and more, this threat of a breakaway partnership hung over the Permanente Medical Group. Critically, Wallace Cook and the other Permanente physicians at Walnut Creek remained within the partnership. Their withdrawal, taking with them a major hospital facility, would have changed the course of the Medical Group.

Morris Collen was dispatched to the Kaiser home in Lafayette to communicate the unequivocal resistance of the Group to this idea. At a tense meeting in the Kaiser living room, Collen handed him the Executive Committee's negative report.

"What's all this gobbledygook?" Kaiser snorted, throwing the report down on the coffee table. "Can we start a separate partnership or can't we?"

Informed by Collen that he could not, Kaiser stormed out of the room. He was unaccustomed to opposition, especially from "his" physicians.[15]

4

Sidney Garfield found himself increasingly caught in the middle of this conflict between Henry J. Kaiser and the Permanente doctors. As Kaiser's brother-in-law, personal physician, next-door neighbor, and confidant, Garfield had backed the Walnut Creek venture. He had sought to convince the Medical Group to change its name to Kaiser. During the height of McCarthyism and on the explicit order of the Kaiser organization, Garfield became involved in the firing of three physicians suspected of being Communists.

Engaged in a controversial experiment in cooperative medicine under private auspices, Permanente physicians were especially sensitive to charges that they were Communist; indeed, such charges were frequently made in the late 1940s and intensified during the McCarthy era. At the same time, as Ernest Saward later made clear, the Permanente organization did include a few left-leaning physicians for whom group practice was charged with ideological overtones. Saward himself later admitted to forcing a few left-leaning activists out of The Permanente Clinic in Oregon because in his judgment they were casting discredit upon the organization. In The Permanente Medical Group, Dr. Leslie Collins, medical director at Vallejo during the war, was a member of the Communist party. In the postwar era a few other Permanente physicians were openly sympathetic. Under a vague pretext of community relations, Collins went so far as to induce Garfield, Cutting, and Collen to attend a meeting from which the trio fled when people began chanting, "I'm a red! I'm a red!"

"It just scared the hell out of me," Collen later remembered.[16]

Kaiser and his top executives were especially sensitive to charges that the Health Plan and Group Medical practice had Communistic overtones. For a while in the early 1950s Kaiser had the FBI run security checks on potential Permanente physicians. "It was policy," Collen later recalled, "and Dr. Garfield supported it. Dr. Garfield always supported whatever Mr. Kaiser wanted in those years."[17]

The concern of the Kaiser organization about employing Communists or sympathizers in the McCarthy era cost Herman Kabat, Wendell Lipscomb, and Richard Weinerman their positions. Ironically, at the time Kabat was treating Henry J. Kaiser, Jr., for his multiple sclerosis.

A second physician to be let go was Wendell Lipscomb, a black intern who was not granted a residency because of his alleged Communist affiliations. In applying for an internship after his graduation from the University of California at San Francisco, Lipscomb had not included his photograph in his application, evidently fearing that he would be turned down because of his race. Lipscomb was accepted as an intern. Hearing that Lipscomb had belonged to a Los Angeles group calling itself the Little Red Church, the Kaiser organization used the fact that Lipscomb had apparently deceived Permanente on his application to order him fired from his internship. "That caused even more consternation in the house staff," Wallace Cook later remembered, "and a threatened strike and so forth. So Henry J. Kaiser got into it, and he was much more conciliatory, and the ultimate decision was that Lipscomb retained his internship, stayed with the group, and was not accepted for residency...." Cook also insisted that the firing was not based on race ("We had black doctors in the Group; I hired black doctors when I came to Walnut Creek") but on Lipscomb's alleged Communist affiliations.[19] The ILWU, however, considered the refusal to grant Lipscomb a residency an act motivated by racial prejudice. An angry rally on Lipscomb's behalf was held in the ILWU hall in Oakland on February 20, 1952, dealing with this and other alleged discriminations.

Another physician fired by Garfield in 1951 during the McCarthy era was Richard Weinerman, medical director of the Health Plan, a liberal activist whom Garfield had hired from Yale University in the late 1940s because of his enthusiasm for group medical practice. The alleged reason given for Weinerman's forced resignation was administrative incompatibility with Garfield. On the surface, this charge had some credibility. Weinerman's dramatic, flamboyant style contrasted radically with Garfield's quiet, personal, behind-the-scenes way of operating. The Permanente physicians, however, suspected that Weinerman's resignation had been forced by the Kaiser organization. At a meeting of the partnership called to discuss the ouster, Morris Collen presented a four-point program. The partnership, first of all, should seek to become of one mind regarding the crisis. Second, it needed to be reemphasized that direction of the medical group should be entirely in the hands of the doctors and free from outside interference. Third, the executive committee needed better communication with the partners, participants, and employed physicians. Fourth, The Permanente Medical Group should have no loyalty policy nor require any loyalty oaths. The business of the medical group was medical care, not politics.

This confrontation over Weinerman's departure (he returned to Yale where he had a distinguished career in academic medicine) was an important early skirmish in the war to come. Realizing that Weinerman had been sacked for political reasons, the Medical Group was beginning to speak up on its own behalf. This growing resistance to Kaiser interference would gain force and momentum after 1952. A number of major issues were emerging as points of contention between the Medical Group and the Kaiser Foundation/Hospitals/Health Plan.

First of all, there was the question of the ownership of the program. Physicians of the Medical Group felt that the program was their medical practice. Its difference from traditional practice resided only in the fact that fees were prepaid on a regular basis. The Medical Group considered the Kaiser Health Plan as an adjunct agency intended to provide a mechanism to enroll members, set rates, and collect prepaid fees. The physicians considered the Kaiser Hospitals as workshops intended to provide them an adequate setting for the practice of medicine. In the Kaiser conception, on the other hand, the Foundation and the Health Plan were regarded as the driving force of the program. Members belonged, not to the physicians, but to the Plan, and the members in the Plan were the ultimate source of money. From this perspective the Plan enrolled the members and paid the physicians' group and hence the Plan was the matrix agency in the organization. The Foundation and the Plan, furthermore, had a major amount of capital tied up in the Hospitals. Therefore, the Foundation and the Plan, and not the Medical Group, bore all the responsibilities of ownership and indebtedness. While physicians were necessary to provide medical practice, it would be better if that were all that they did. Businesspeople, not physicians, should run the business of the program.

The Medical Group disputed this theory of management. Between 1945 and 1952, the doctors argued, Sidney Garfield and other physicians had managed the program, and it had survived and grown to a multimillion dollar per year business under physician leadership. On the other hand, the Kaiser people replied, growth demanded further facilities, and this in turn necessitated further debt. Financial institutions would be more likely to react favorably to requests from responsible businesspeople like those employed by Kaiser, accustomed to the management of large enterprises.

The Permanente Medical Group especially resented Kaiser's attempt to fragment it into separate groups competing with each other for the same Health Plan memberships. Kaiser replied that competition between smaller groups would improve medical services. The Medical Group believed that it should be consulted on any new expansion and/or construction project. The Kaiser organization replied that since it had the financial responsibility, the Health Plan had to have the decision-making authority. The Medical Group resented the allocation of scarce monies for what it considered luxury aspects of the Walnut Creek Hospital, which ran counter to the prudent allocation of resources, a basic principle in prepaid group practice. The Kaiser organization replied that Walnut Creek served as a symbol of excellence for the entire program. *Architectural Forum* had awarded architect Clarence Mayhew a prize for the building, which had also been publicized as Hospital of the Month in *Modern Hospital* magazine and had been featured in *Look* magazine and showcased by Universal Newsreel in thousands of movie theaters.

Much of the dissension came down to money. In the early 1950s the Medical Group was compensated with a percentage of Health Plan dues. In reality, this so-called percentage was deliberately modified to adjust for the expenses of the growing program. As chair of the Medical Group executive committee, Morris Collen would meet with Eugene Trefethen, representing the Kaiser Foundation Health Plan, to negotiate compensation rates for the Medical Group. Neither the Medical Group nor the Health Plan found this informal, noncontractual method entirely satisfactory. The matter of surcharges for certain services was also proving troublesome. Flat fees, for instance, were assessed for maternity care and tonsillectomies. These fees, however, were collected by the Kaiser Hospitals instead of by The Permanente Medical Group. The Permanente physicians felt that the one dollar surcharge that most patients paid on registration to see a physician, together with charges for laboratory and X-ray services, should be returned to the Medical Group as income.

These policy and procedural difficulties, exacerbated by Henry J. Kaiser's growing personal involvement, were rapidly bringing the Permanente experiment to a point of crisis. No one realized this more than the founder himself, Sidney Garfield, caught as he was between the Scylla of Permanente and the Charybdis of the Kaiser organization. The crisis would be successfully coped with; but in the process of negotiation and compromise, founder Sidney Garfield would prove expendable as the program evolved into a more satisfactory organizational form.

7

Toward the
Tahoe Agreement

Despite the issues that divided the Permanente Medical Group from the Kaiser organization, the years of 1952 to 1955 were years of impressive growth. Membership in the Health Plan increased from 200,000 in northern California in 1950 to more than 300,000 by 1955. Clinics opened in Napa, Redwood City, Pittsburgh, and San Leandro. The Walnut Creek Hospital opened in September 1953, and in March 1954 a seven-story ultramodern $3.25 million Kaiser Foundation Hospital incorporating many of Garfield's ideas opened at 2425 Geary Street in the Anza Vista District of San Francisco. Each patient room was served by both a central access corridor and a glass-walled outside visitors' corridor. The sliding glass doors opening onto this second window corridor were covered by power-operated drapes which the patient could open or close from his or her bed. Operating and delivery rooms extended radially from central staff work and preparation rooms. The maternity floor featured the personalized bassinet drawer system. On the seventh floor, ambulatory convalescent patients returned to health in a hotellike atmosphere. All medical equipment and technology were state of the art. By this time, 1 out of every 10 San Franciscans was a member of the Health Plan.

During this period, property adjacent to the Walnut Creek Hospital was purchased for subsequent hospital expansion and for a clinic building. The property had a large swimming pool, which soon became very popular among physicians and staff. A Permanente physician's teen-aged son, who later became a physician himself, was hired as lifeguard. The administrator of the Walnut Creek Hospital was made responsible for the maintenance and safety of the pool. The Executive Committee of the Medical Group appointed several physicians to serve on a Walnut Creek pool committee. The alleged country club aspects of the Walnut Creek Hospital thus achieved a measure of reality. Within 2 years, the pool had become an administrative headache. Fortunately, it became necessary to fill in the pool to prepare the site for the construction of additional medical care facilities. As much as they loved the pool, the physicians and staff of Walnut Creek were even more upset over the loss of a fine large old oak tree that had to come down during site preparation.

During this period, Permanente Services, Inc., was established to provide certain administrative services for the Hospitals and the Medical Group. Initially, the responsibilities of Permanente Services, Inc., were limited. For example, the Medical Group chose to retain its own purchasing function. The executive committee of the Medical Group designated Morris Collen as the physician member of the Permanente Services board. Eventually, Permanente Services provided a wide range of accounting, purchasing, warehousing, data-processing, employee and community relations support, together with the operation of the pharmacies and the management and repair of facilities.

To keep up with the growth of the early and mid-1950s, the Permanente Medical Group added physicians. By March 1953 there were 125 career physicians in full-time service in northern California. Forty of these were partners, 5 were participants or prepartners, and 85 were physicians employed by the partnership. Forty of the 125 Permanente physicians held certifications from specialty boards; 9 had passed one part of the board examination; and 51 were eligible by residency training to take the examination. At the time, these were impressive figures and offered a measure of defense against attacks by the fee-for-service medical establishment. Between November 1953 and May 1954 alone, The Permanente Medical Group added 31 physicians. This improved the doctor-member ratio to 1:1190. This improved ratio represented only part of the goal of 1:1080 adopted by the Medical Group. Because of the difficulties of recruiting well-qualified physicians committed to prepaid group practice, efforts at recruitment continued vigorously throughout this period.

It did not help such recruiting efforts, however, that organized medicine still continued its opposition, despite the program's impressive growth and quality of medical care. Wallace Cook later remembered

.

that even at Walnut Creek, where the Kaiser Hospital extended privileges to local physicians, opposition continued. Before the Walnut Creek facility was constructed, local physicians had been forced to go to Oakland to find a proper hospital. The convenience of Kaiser Hospital in Walnut Creek, however, in no way implied detente on the part of the fee-for-service physicians who used it. "Your reception at times could be terrible," remembered Cook of meetings at the California Medical Association. "You'd be introduced, and they'd say, 'Well, where are you?' And you'd say you're at Permanente, and some people would turn around and walk away. And others would say, 'Oh!' in such a way that they couldn't think of anything else to say. Our reception at Walnut Creek was very traumatic. They'd call us communists."[1] People would even come up to Cook and ask him if his doctors were interns or if they had finished medical school. It hurt.

2

An important new personality, meanwhile, was entering the Kaiser-Permanente picture. In September 1953 Clifford Keene, realizing that the Kaiser Motors Corporation would soon be discontinuing automobile production at Willow Run in Michigan, began looking for new employment. Keene had been serving as medical director at Willow Run for the past 6 years. In the *Journal of Occupational Medicine* he learned that the U.S. Steel Company was seeking a physician to set up an industrial health-care program in the United States and in its foreign subsidiaries. Writing U.S. Steel, Keene was invited to Pittsburgh for interviews, including lunch at the exclusive Duquesne Club, the *sanctum sanctorum* of steel company executives. For someone who had worked as a steelworker during his summer vacations while in college and medical school and kept his Steelworkers Union card framed near his diplomas in his study, lunching at the Duquesne with the upper management of U.S. Steel was a gratifying experience. Here in no uncertain terms was evidence of the good life that could be his as an executive of U.S. Steel. As Keene move closer to being offered and to accepting the U.S. Steel position, one question continued to surface: would the Kaiser organization be making him a counteroffer? Keene told U.S. Steel that no discussions had been forthcoming. He determined, however, to bring the matter up personally to Edgar Kaiser at Willow run. Presenting himself to Edgar Kaiser in Kaiser's oak-paneled office on the second floor of the Willow

Run administration building at 11:00 on a Monday morning in early November 1953, Keene put the matter on the table.

"Edgar got very, very quiet," Keene later remembered. "Edgar was an incessant smoker. He smoked and inhaled and looked at me and got up and walked around the desk and grunted and shook the change in his pockets a couple of times, and said, 'Well, you're a good doctor; you're a pretty good doctor; you've done an excellent job here; yes, you have. I can write him a letter and tell him you're real good. I could call him up too. But I'm not going to do a goddamn thing. You just get out of here and go downstairs and go back to work.'"

The following Wednesday morning Keene received a call from Edgar Kaiser's secretary, inviting him and his wife Jean to a dinner party that night in honor of Henry J. Kaiser at the Barton Hills home of Edgar and Sue Kaiser in Ann Arbor.

"Sue and Edgar come to the door," Keene describes the event, "[and] greet us effusively. The last time I talked to this fellow he threw me out of his office! That was forgotten. The old man is there, Mr. Henry Kaiser, big as God."

Throughout the dinner party, Henry J. Kaiser carried on a ceaseless monologue on how the Health Plan in northern California was in a mess. Kaiser was especially troubled by the bad relationships with local medical societies. He also wanted to bring a more systematic, businesslike administration to the Health Plan, the Hospitals, and even the Medical Group.

"You organize to do just that," Kaiser told the listening table. "You establish a financial organization to provide facilities and equipment and convince doctors to work together as a real organization, just as if you're going to build steel or cement or aluminum or whatever and put it together and make it work."

Kaiser was especially critical of what he considered Sidney Garfield's haphazard style of management. Kaiser complained that his top executives had trouble dealing with Garfield. The physicians of the Medical Group were also rebelling against Garfield, Kaiser continued. A good part of the conversation, in fact, revolved around criticisms of Sidney Garfield's management style.

At 11:00 o'clock, aware that he had surgery the next morning at 7:00, Keene tried to excuse himself from the dinner party. The conversation seemed irrelevant to his interests. He had all but accepted the offer from U.S. Steel. As a parting remark, however, Keene asked, "What's all this got to do with me?"

Henry J. Kaiser looked at Keene in astonishment. "What I'm trying to tell you," the Boss expostulated, "is that, in the first place, you wouldn't like U.S. Steel. They aren't our kind of people. The other thing is, I want you to come out there to the West Coast and run this thing."

"Mr. Kaiser, run what?" Keene asked.

"Do what I just told you about. Put together a medical program and make it go. We need some business principles."

After some further discussion, Keene agreed to fly out to the San Francisco Bay Area and to Los Angeles to look over the situation. He was coolly received by the Permanente physicians in northern California. His reception in southern California was overtly hostile. The Permanente physicians did not want an outsider, especially a board-certified surgeon who was not a member of the partnership, put into a position of authority over the entire program.

Discouraged by this negative reception, Keene decided to accept the U.S. Steel offer. Understandably, Keene did not wish to be caught between the Kaiser organization, its Health Plan and Hospitals, and the opposing forces of the Permanente Medical Groups, where resistance to Kaiser domination was mounting. But then none other than Sidney Garfield invited Keene to breakfast at the Mark Hopkins Hotel in San Francisco on the morning of Saturday, December 5, 1953. The breakfast meeting was at first quiet, even stilted. Keene decided to press the situation.

"Sid," Keene told Garfield, "in my opinion, the whole medical program is in a hell of a mess, and I don't know how one would solve all its problems. The medical program is your baby, and if anybody should attempt to correct it, it should be yourself."

Garfield continued for a moment to eat his grapefruit in silence. He then replied, "Mr. Kaiser doesn't have any confidence in my ability to manage the program, and everyone agrees the program needs some kind of leadership, strong leadership, and strong leadership hasn't emerged yet."

Garfield then surprised Keene by speculating that perhaps he, Garfield, did not have the ability to run things and perhaps Keene should come out and take a job in the administration of the medical program and see if he could help turn it around. An awkward silence of 2 or 3 minutes ensued, then Keene said, "Sidney, that changes the whole aspect of the situation. If you want me to come and Mr. Kaiser wants me to come, I would guess that there is enough chance for success for me to try it."

Following the breakfast, Keene called Henry Kaiser. "Sidney says he can't provide leadership for the program," Keene informed Kaiser, "and he has asked me to come and I accept your offer."[2]

By January 1954 Clifford Keene was working out of a desk in Garfield's suite of offices at the former Piedmont Hotel near the Permanente Hospital in Oakland. The Nursing School was located there as well. Garfield and Keene shared the same assistant, Jack Chapman. "I was given an office in the rear overlooking a neighbor's washline," remembered Keene, "and started to become acquainted with the Kaiser Permanente Medical Care program."[3] Keene had no precise title, nor were his responsibilities and authority clearly described. It was an awkward situation, and it would continue to get worse.

3

At the annual meeting of the American Medical Association held in San Francisco in June 1954, the New York delegation introduced Resolution 16, aimed directly against the Health Insurance Plan (HIP) of New York City. Resolution 16 affirmed "the unrestricted freedom of a patient to choose his own physician." In certain cases, the resolution continued, "a third party has a valid interest when, by law or volition, the third party assumes legal responsibility and provides for the cost of medical care and indemnity for occupational disability." Thus far, Resolution 16 in no way opposed programs such as the Kaiser Health Plan. At this point, however, Resolution 16 continued in such a way as to cut to the core of prepaid group medical practice as it was being carried on by Kaiser-Permanente. "If, however," Resolution 16 continued, "the third party be an organization or corporation which agrees to provide medical and/or surgical services through the medium of individual or group practice, payment to the physicians under contract being either on an indemnity or a per capita basis, a requirement restricting choice of physician to either individual or group practitioners under contract vitiates the subscriber's right to free choice of physician. This is contrary to the best interests of the public and of the medical profession."[4]

In short, Resolution 16 stated that plans such as the Kaiser Health Plan, which limited the choice of physician to a panel of physicians in group practice, were unethical. Had Resolution 16 been adopted by the House of Delegates, it would have made recruitment of physicians for the Permanente Medical Groups and other prepaid medical groups impossible. Fortunately, Resolution 16 was not voted on immediately but was referred to the Judicial Council of the American Medical Association. After a decade of harassment by local medical societies, Permanente Medical

Groups and the Kaiser Health Plan now faced condemnation by the most powerful organization in American medicine.

To complicate matters further, The Permanente Medical Group and the Kaiser Health Plan were divided as to just exactly who should speak up on behalf of the entire program. When Resolution 16 went before the Judicial Council of the American Medical Association, Morris Collen and Ray Kay objected to Clifford Keene's speaking on behalf of the program because he was not a member of The Permanente Medical Group but was an employee of the Kaiser organization. Keene could speak for the Health Plan and the Hospitals, Collen and Ray stated, but not for the Permanente Medical Groups. Keene, however, did speak spontaneously from the floor on behalf of the program at the San Francisco meeting of the American Medical Association and was quoted in *Time* magazine. Keene had the right to speak because he was still a member in good standing of the Wayne County, Michigan, Medical Society. From the floor, Keene asked for an amendment recognizing that freedom of choice would be satisfied in situations where the subscriber elects of his own volition to be treated by a group or a single doctor within a group. It was Keene's proposal that got Resolution 16 referred to the Judicial Council without a vote. "If I didn't do anything else all year in 1954," Keene later remembered, "that was worth my salary."[5] Resisted, even rudely treated by the Permanente physicians who saw him as Kaiser's tool, Clifford Keene had forestalled a potential disaster. Even the Permanente physicians who were opposing him must have begrudgingly acknowledged Keene's contribution.

In September 1954 a brief responding to Resolution 16 was prepared on behalf of the Kaiser Foundation Health Plan. A meeting was planned with other prepaid group-practice health plans, to be held in Buffalo, New York, on October 11, 1954, to prepare a joint brief that would be forwarded to the Judicial Council of the American Medical Association. Collen and Kay objected to Keene representing the views of the Permanente Medical Groups at the Buffalo meeting. After a meeting among Collen, Keene, and Garfield, it was agreed that Garfield, and not Keene, would serve as spokesperson along with Dr. George Baehr of HIP and Dr. Russell Lee of the Palo Alto Clinic in discussions with the AMA. If the AMA could not be dissuaded from Resolution 16, the strategy was then to appeal to the Anti-Trust Division of the Department of Justice. The Board of Trustees of the AMA had meanwhile appointed a Commission on Medical Care Plans chaired by Dr. Leonard W. Larson. The Commission was asked to inquire into three points: the nature and methods of operation of the various types of plans through which persons received the services of physicians; the effect of these plans on the quality and quantity of medical care provided; and the legal and ethical arrangements used by the various plans. The AMA also agreed to defer action on Resolution 16 pending the completion of this study by the Commission on Medical Care Plans. Thus the matter was effectively tabled—for 5 years as it turned out—and The Permanente Medical Group was allowed to continue its program of expansion and recruitment without operating under the stigma of an AMA condemnation.

As if Resolution 16 were not trouble enough, harassment of the program continued on the local level as well. In the summer of 1952, as war raged in Korea, a number of Permanente physicians—including Sidney Garfield and Morris Collen, a 4F in World War II—were ordered to report for their draft physicals. Correctly assessing this as a ploy of the local medical society working with the draft board, Henry J. Kaiser wrote a vigorous letter of protest on Garfield's behalf. Not until the following summer were the 44-year-old Garfield and the 39-year-old Collen out of danger of being called up along with a number of younger physicians who actually went into uniform. Garfield was forced to argue at length with Local Board 49, Alameda County, on behalf of himself, Collen, and others, including the 53-year-old M. Coleman Harris who had served in both World War I and II.

Permanente physicians continued to be denied membership in local medical societies. Even Clifford Keene, a board-certified surgeon, a fellow of the American College of Surgery, was rejected for membership in the Alameda–Contra Costa Medical Association because of his association with the program. In August 1953, Paul Foster, president of the Los Angeles County Medical Association, issued a condemnation of the Kaiser-Permanente program as being de facto unethical. Foster sent out an inflammatory letter and slanted questionnaire asking southern California MDs to gather evidence against the program. In January 1954, the AMA sent out a similar appeal to its members to help it gather evidence against all prepaid group-practice programs. Stung by the southern California attack, the Health Plan considered a personal libel suit against Paul Foster. Infuriated by the AMA attack, Henry J. Kaiser personally drafted a "Declaration of War" against the AMA and drew up plans to take his case directly to the American people. Only with some difficulty was Kaiser dissuaded from making himself the national point man against the AMA on behalf of prepaid group medical practice. Kaiser wanted prestige from his association with the program, not notoriety. That is why he had asked Clifford Keene "to help make us respectable."

Clifford Keene, meanwhile, devoid of title or specific assignment beyond "making the program respectable," began to take on the problems no one else wished to deal with. The Kabat-Kaiser Institute, for example, had fallen into disrepute because of Herman Kabat's rumored Communism. Todd Inch, the Kaiser organization's top attorney, gave Keene the mission of cleaning up the Kabat-Kaiser Institute. After Kabat had been fired, Keene brought in Dr. Sedgewick Mead of St. Louis to head the Institute and changed the name to the California Institute of Physical Medicine and Rehabilitation.

Keene also involved himself in trying to improve relations with local medical societies and intensifying academic standards at the Kaiser Foundation Nursing School. Attending commencement exercises in February 1954, Keene was called to the platform when a delayed Sidney Garfield could not arrive on time to make the commencement address. Keene spoke at every graduation exercise for the ensuing 22 years. He also appointed a new Nursing School director, Josephine Coppedge, who intensified the academic program.

Believing that respectability is gained through academic and professional circles, Keene established the Kaiser Foundation Research Institute at the Richmond Hospital, with William Caulkins, a retired Navy captain, as administrator. Keene sought consultation with Professor Hardin Jones, associate director of the Donner Laboratory at the University of California at Berkeley (UC Berkeley). Jones joined the Institute as advisor for grants and programs. Jacob Yerushalmy, a professor of biostatistics at UC Berkeley, secured a major federal grant for the study of human growth and life cycle. "I don't want any budget," Yerushalmy stormed one day when Keene cautioned him about expenses. "I just want some money to spend when I need to spend it."[6]

The Kaiser Foundation Research Institute also began to sponsor symposia and lectures that were open to the public. Environmental writer Rachael Carson spoke at one of these forums. Gradually, the research at the Institute, together with its public programs, helped alter the image of Kaiser-Permanente.

All this activity was being carried on by Keene on behalf of the Foundation, the Health Plan, and the Hospitals. The Permanente Medical Group remained more or less aloof from these programs. Keene was never invited to join the Group. He became more and more, in fact, a Kaiser executive and was considered as such by the Permanente physicians. Reluctantly, Keene, a board-certified surgeon, gave up the practice of surgery for administration. Part of the problem, aside from the time involved in his new duties, was the fact that Keene, a Kaiser appointee, perceived as Kaiser's point person in an effort to assume control of the entire organization, would have to be accepted by the Medical Group for practice in the Kaiser Hospitals. The Medical Group refused to extend this courtesy. This conflict between Kaiser and Keene on the one hand and The Permanente Medical Group on the other intensified throughout 1953, 1954, and 1955, as Henry J. Kaiser continued to speak for and attempt to run all aspects of the program.

Just exactly when did Henry J. Kaiser take it on himself to speak for the doctors of The Permanente Medical Group as well as for the Health Plan, for which he had already served as an intermittent spokesperson since 1942? Ray Kay and Wally Neighbor felt it began with an incident in 1948. Faced with a condemnation of the Permanente program in Portland and Vancouver by the Washington State Medical Society, Kaiser took Neighbor, then the director of the Northern Permanente Medical Group, to the Chicago headquarters of the American Medical Association and there confronted Dr. Morris Fishbein, the executive director. In the course of the discussion, Kaiser, taking affront at something Dr. Fishbein said, mistakenly grabbed Wally Neighbor's hat, jammed it on his head, and began to stalk about the room, shouting that he would not be treated this way and would start his own medical society. The problem was, Wally Neighbor's hat size was three sizes smaller than that required by the taller, greatly more rotund Kaiser.

"This great huge man paced up and down the office with this little gray fedora on his head," Wally Neighbor later remembers, "the funniest picture you could imagine..."

Apparently, Kaiser's ploy worked, for Fishbein leapt from behind the desk and took Kaiser by the arm, soothing him with, "Now, Mr. Kaiser, I didn't mean that. Won't you please sit down?" The threatened condemnation never materialized.[7]

Throughout the early 1950s Kaiser's tendency to speak for the program increased. In January 1952 he unilaterally hired Richard Bullis, a physician prominent in medical society affairs in Los Angeles County, commissioning him to improve relationships with medical societies and make the program respectable, a task he later assigned to Keene in 1954. On June 20, 1953, the *Saturday Evening Post* ran an article on prepaid group medical practice. While physicians spoke for the Health Insurance Plan of greater New York, Kaiser was the only one quoted on behalf of the Kaiser-Permanente program. Producing architectural drawings, Kaiser told *Post* writer Lester Velie, "Look, here's my $3,000,000 baby we're building in San Francisco. Here's my $1,500,000 baby we're building at Walnut Creek near Oakland."

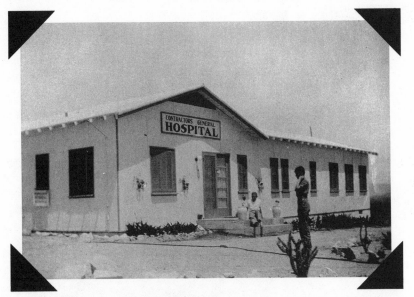

Some time in the mid-1930s, Sidney Garfield relaxes on the steps of the air-conditioned Contractors General Hospital at Desert City.

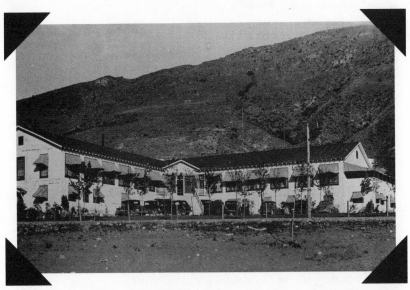

The hospital at Mason City, Washington, served Grand Coulee workers and their families with a program of prepaid comprehensive care.

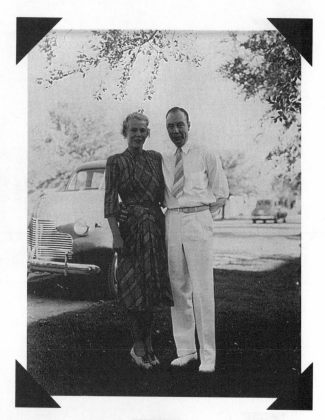

Millie and Cecil Cutting at Grand Coulee around 1940. In later years, many Permanente pioneers remembered the Grand Coulee experience as one of the happiest times in their lives.

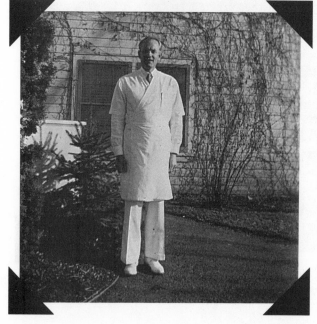

Between 1938 and 1941 Dr. J. Wallace Neighbor served as medical director of the Mason City Hospital at Grand Coulee.

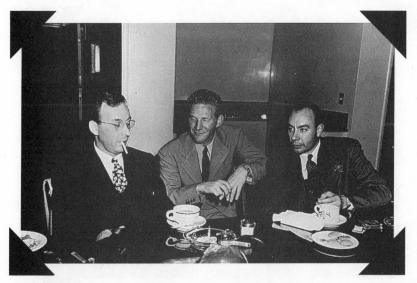

As the Grand Coulee project winds down in 1940, Edgar Kaiser, Sidney Garfield, and Cecil Cutting reflect on their accomplishments and dream of the future.

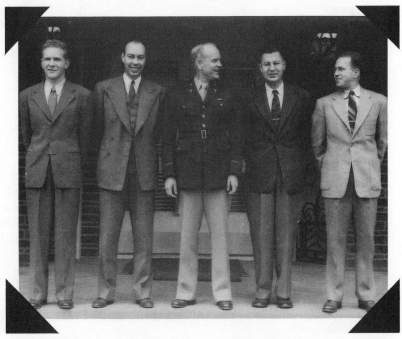

By 1941 the Grand Coulee program was over. J. Wallace Neighbor (center) was already in uniform as Garfield (left) posed for a farewell photograph with (left to right) Cecil Cutting, Neighbor, Ray Gillette, and Eugene Wiley.

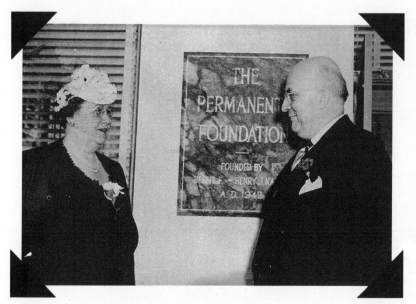

Henry J. and Bess F. Kaiser celebrate the establishment of the Permanente Foundation in 1942.

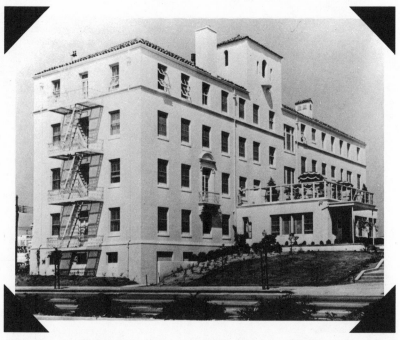

With a line of credit from A. P. Giannini, the Fabiola Hospital on Broadway at MacArthur in Oakland was renovated in 1942 as the first major hospital of the newly established Permanente Foundation.

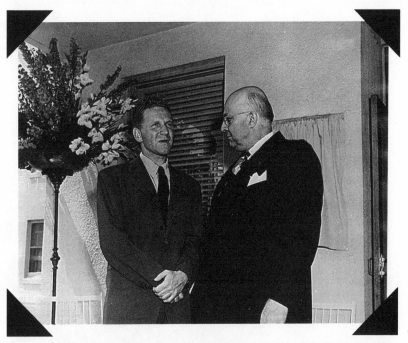

Sidney Garfield and Henry J. Kaiser chat together at the dedication of the Permanente Hospital in September 1942. Kaiser seems characteristically intense.

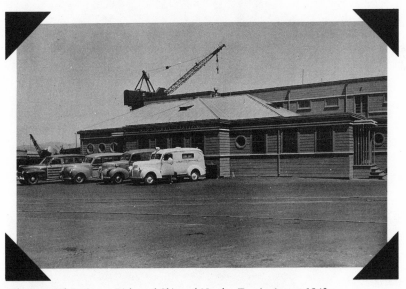

The First Aid Station at Richmond Shipyard Number Two in August 1943.

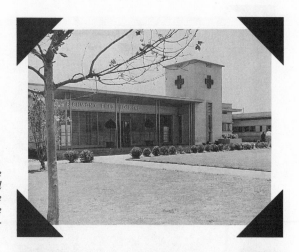

Shown here in 1943, the Richmond Field Hospital was the first in a long line of regional Permanente clinics and medical offices.

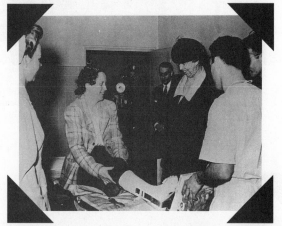

Edgar Kaiser, at the door, escorts Mrs. Franklin Delano Roosevelt on a tour of the Richmond Field Hospital some time in late 1942.

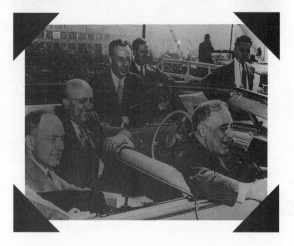

President Roosevelt visited the Richmond Shipyards as well, escorted by a beaming Henry J. and Edgar Kaiser.

PERMANENTE FOUNDATION HOSPITALS

SIDNEY R. GARFIELD, M.D., & ASSOCIATES
C.C. CUTTING, M.D., CHIEF OF STAFF
RICHARD MOORE, M.D., ASST. CHIEF OF STAFF

DERMATOLOGY

BROOKS PRINGLE, M.D., DIRECTOR
GEORGE B. ANDERSON, M.D.

EAR NOSE & THROAT

I. H. WIESENFELD, M.D., DIRECTOR
JAMES H. MC CLELLAND, M.D.
LENA ENGST THIRIOT, M.D.
BENJAMIN THOMAS, M.D.

EYE

THOMAS G. SCHNOOR, M.D., DIRECTOR
F. B. MC DONALD, M.D.
ARTHUR LAYTON, D. OPT.

INTERNAL MEDICINE

MORRIS F. COLLEN, M.D., DIRECTOR
EUGENE B. LEVINE, M.D., ASST. DIRECTOR
DONALD W. ASH, M.D.
FREDERICK BURT, M.D.
THURMAN DANNENBERG, M.D.
J.F. DIDDLE, M.D.
FRANZ R. GOETZL, M.D.
ERIC C. KAST, M.D.
GEORGE O'BRIEN, M.D.
EDWARD PHILLIPS, M.D.
PHILLIP J. RAIMONDI, M.D.
WILLIAM RICE, M.D.
ALVIN L. SELLERS, M.D.
MARGARET STUART, M.D.
ALEXANDER WITKOW, M.D.

NEUROLOGY

J.P. FITZGIBBON, M.D., DIRECTOR

OBSTETRICS & GYNECOLOGY

WILSON FOOTER, M.D., DIRECTOR
LAWRENCE ALLRED, M.D.
HANNAH PETERS, M.D.
MARY H. REHM, M.D.
ELSE ROSS, M.D.
O. D. WILLIAMS, M.D.

ORTHOPEDICS

C. C. CUTTING, M.D., DIRECTOR
PETER J. BARONE, M.D.
JOHN P. EVANS, M.D.
LLOYD D. FISHER, M.D.
THOS. FLINT, JR., M.D.
E. E. FRANKLIN, M.D.
A. BERNARD GRAY, M.D.
WILLIAM HATTEROTH, M.D.
N. MEADOFF, M.D.
RICHARD MOORE, M.D.
H. C. PEDERSON, M.D.

PATHOLOGY

STANLEY L. REA, M.D., DIRECTOR

PEDIATRICS

ALEXANDER HATOFF, M.D., DIRECTOR
DAVID BRUSER, M.D.
MOLLIE CHOLFIN, M.D.
POOI TUEN (BEATRICE) LEI, M.D.
DELPHINE PALM, M.D.

PUBLIC HEALTH

CLIFFORD KUH, M.D., DIRECTOR

RADIOLOGY

OTTO HATSCHEK, M.D., DIRECTOR

SURGERY

R. BRUCE HENLEY, M.D., DIRECTOR
A. LA MONT BARITELL, M.D.
JAMES A. BASYE, M.D.
JOHN BLEMER, M.D.
DAVID G. BORDEN, M.D.
WILLIAM F. BOYER, M.D.
H. DONALD GRANT, M.D.
NORMAN L. HAUGEN, M.D.
ROBERT A. MENDLE, M.D.
DON C. MUSSER, M.D.
LEO D. NANNINI, M.D.

UROLOGY

MILTON Z. LONDON, M.D., DIRECTOR
C. LESLIE COLLINS, M.D.

GENERAL

WILLIAMS BARNES, M.D.
ISABELLA CLINTON, M.D.
DARRELL HAWLEY, M.D.
DAVID HIBBS, M.D.
SAMUEL JAFFEE, M.D.
ROBERT JONES, M.D.
HAROLD MORRISON, M.D.
WILLIAM REINHARDT, M.D.
FREDERICK SHERWOOD, M.D.
R. A. WEILERSTEIN, M.D.

HOUSE OFFICERS

FREDERICK BECKERT, M.D.
ARTHUR A. CIVELLO, M.D.
FRANK HOLT, M.D.
EDMUND D. JUNG, M.D.
S. J. KARSANT, M.D.
E. A. KIBRICK, M.D.
CHARLES LENERT, M.D.
E. P. LISTON, M.D.
WILLIAM THOMAS, M.D.

Sidney R. Garfield & Associates represented the beginnings of a medical group that would eventually enroll thousands of physicians and professional support staff.

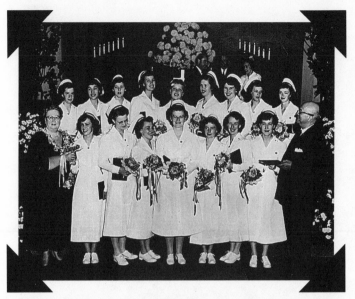

Mr. and Mrs. Henry J. Kaiser award diplomas to graduates of Permanente Foundation School of Nursing. Director Dorothea Daniels is in the rear, near the candelabra on the right.

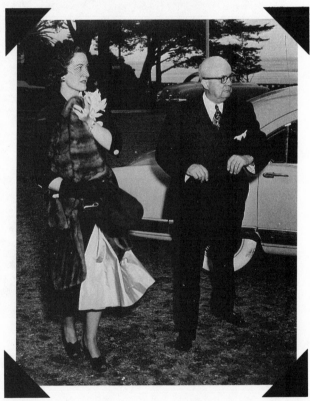

Alyce Chester and Henry J. Kaiser alight from a Kaiser Manhattan automobile for their wedding at the Santa Barbara Biltmore Hotel on June 10, 1951. (Photo by Hal Boucher.)

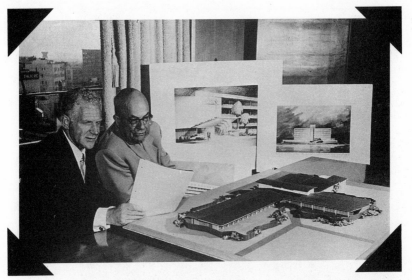

In 1952 Sidney Garfield and Henry J. Kaiser review a model of the proposed Kaiser Foundation Hospital at Walnut Creek, together with renderings of the hospitals planned for Los Angeles and San Francisco.

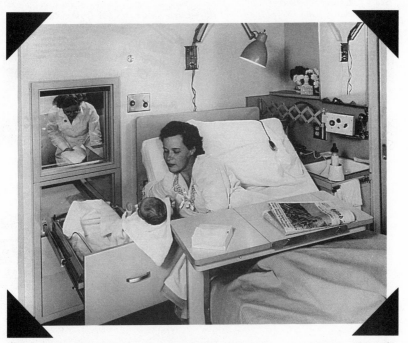

Many of Sidney Garfield's innovative proposals for maternity care were incorporated into the Walnut Creek, Los Angeles, and San Francisco hospitals.

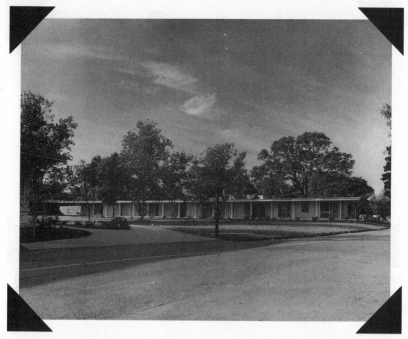

Henry J. Kaiser's insistence that a showplace hospital be constructed in Walnut Creek ahead of other priorities underscored a growing rift between Kaiser and The Permanente Medical Group. The tension was somewhat resolved by the Tahoe Agreement of July 1955.

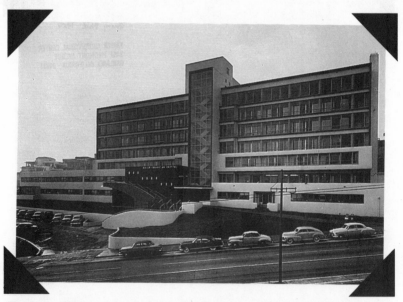

Opening in 1954, the Kaiser Foundation Hospital on Geary Street in San Francisco served the growing West Bay membership of the Kaiser Permanente medical care program.

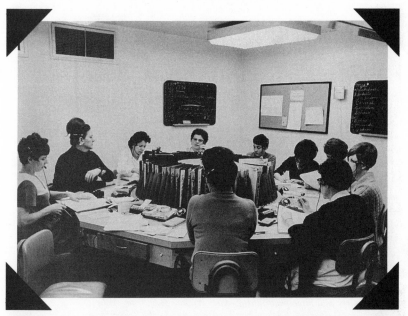

Before the advent of the computer, appointments were kept in files which were rotated from operator to operator on a lazy susan, such as depicted in this scene from Walnut Creek in 1956.

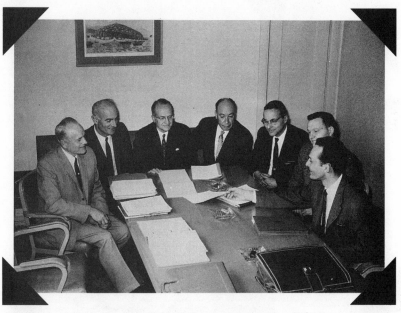

Shown at a working session in early 1950, the executive committee of The Permanente Medical Group established policies for an increasingly complex organization. From left to right: Wallace Neighbor, A. LaMonte Baritell, Morris Collen, Cecil Cutting, David Steinhardt, Paul Stange, and Joseph Sender.

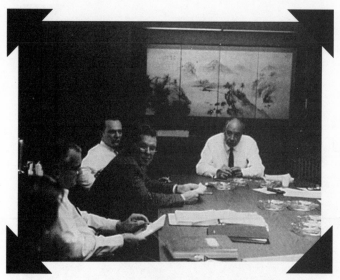

The executive director of The Permanente Medical Group, Cecil Cutting (on the right), confers with three physicians-in-chief: Wallace Cook from Walnut Creek (foreground), John Smillie from San Francisco, and Joseph Sender from Oakland.

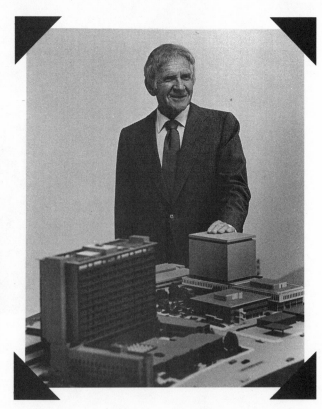

Sidney Garfield enjoyed designing Kaiser Foundation hospitals. Here he stands behind a model of the Oakland Kaiser Foundation Hospital at Broadway and MacArthur after a 12-story addition was completed in 1972. Garfield's hand rests on a model of the historically important and renovated Fabiola Hospital, which he purchased in 1942.

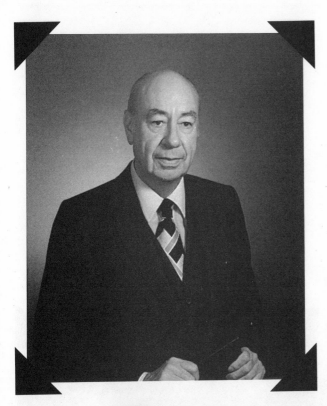

Cecil Cutting, MD, who started with his experience at Grand Coulee, eventually became the first executive director of The Permanente Medical Group. He served in that capacity from 1957 to 1976. (Photo by Allen Studios.)

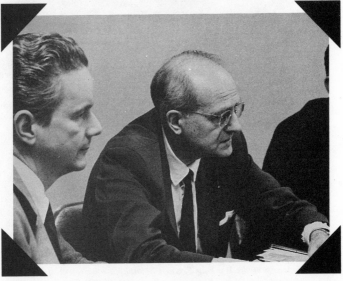

Long-time chairperson of the executive committee, Morris F. Collen (center), presides over a working session of the committee. To Collen's left is Bernard Rhodes, then serving as physician-in-chief at Hayward and the first long-term member of the executive committee.

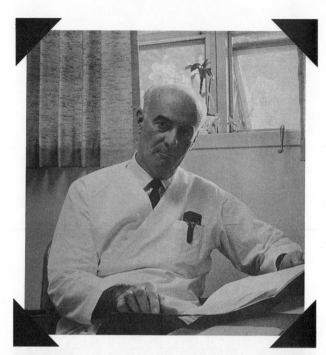

A. LaMonte Baritell, MD, a long-time member of the executive committee, played a major role in the 1950s in helping preserve the autonomy of The Permanente Medical Group.

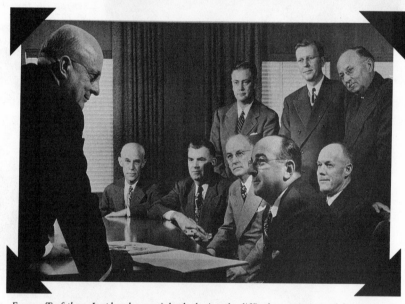

Eugene Trefethen, Jr. played a crucial role during the difficult negotiations of the 1950s. As chairman of the Working Council he brought an element of harmony between Permanente Medical Groups and Kaiser Foundation Health Plan at the Lake Tahoe meeting. Trefethen is shown here in foreground among Kaiser executives talking with Henry J. Kaiser. Mr. Kaiser's first employee, A. B. Ordway, is seated in the rear near the projection screen. (The Bancroft Library.)

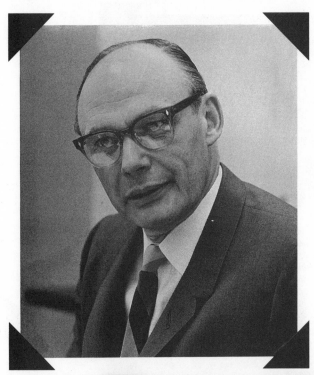

During the tumultuous 1950s, Clifford Keene, MD, served as a liaison between the Kaiser organization and The Permanente Medical Group. In the 1960s Keene became vice president and general manager of the Kaiser Foundation Hospitals and Health Plan and a member of the board of directors.

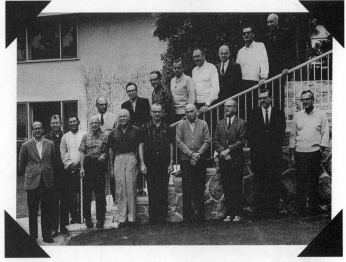

In 1967 the Kaiser Permanente Committee gathered at the Del Monte Lodge in Monterey. After two decades of evolution, experimentation, and frequent stress, the top management had created a way for physicians and administrators to share responsibilities and authority. Left to right, bottom row: Dan Wagster, Robert Erickson, Philip Chu, MD, Ray Kay, MD, Sid Garfield, MD, Walt Palmer, Art Weissman, Bill Price, Irv Bolton, Andrew Gensey. On the stairs, left to right: Clifford Keene, MD, Ernest Saward, MD, Scott Fleming, Jim Vohs, Sam Hufford, William Hughes, MD, Karl Steil, Cecil Cutting, MD.

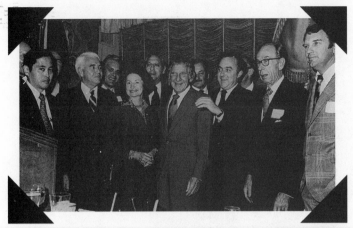

On October 27, 1977, The Kaiser Permanente Medical Care Program became qualified as an HMO. In New York City to celebrate both this event and Sidney Garfield's acceptance of the Lyndon Baines Johnson Award for Humanitarian Service were Ladybird Johnson, HEW Secretary Joseph Califano, and Edgar Kaiser, together with William Dung, MD, medical director of Hawaii (far left), and Max Brown, regional manager for Texas (far right).

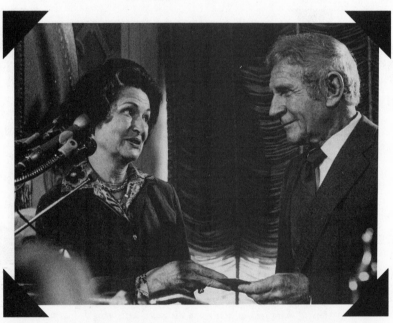

Mrs. Lyndon "Ladybird" Johnson presents the Lyndon Baines Johnson Award for Humanitarian Service to Dr. Sidney Garfield on October 27, 1977, in New York City.

In the course of the same interview Kaiser advocated that American insurance companies set aside a billion dollars for loans to medical partnerships similar to Permanente. "This could build 1000 medical centers across the country," Kaiser claimed, "and give low cost care to 30,000,000 people."[8]

The following year a bill came before the House of Representatives introduced by Representative Charles A. Wolverton of New Jersey establishing a federal government loan insurance program similar to FHA insurance for home building for the private financing of medical care facilities. On January 11, 1954, Kaiser testified in Washington before the Interstate and Foreign Commerce Committee of the House of Representatives on behalf of the Wolverton bill. His 16-page testimony, "A Private Enterprise Solution to Medical Care by the Doctors of this Country," constituted a passionate, detailed, finely reasoned, and eloquently presented argument. From internal evidence of style and phraseology, it is arguable that Sidney Garfield played a major role in the development of this statement.

"This 'New Economics of Medical Care' that we envision as coming rapidly and nationwide," Kaiser told the representatives, "is a free enterprise solution that can be accomplished by groups of doctors throughout the United States. It will make government socialized medicine absolutely unnecessary. In every section of the country, groups of doctors can carry out their own independent adaptations of the pattern of voluntary medical service prepayment plan that has been developed on the Pacific Coast over a period of twenty years."[9]

Kaiser then related a brief history of the Kaiser-Permanente program, noting that it did not start out with preconceived ideas or ideology but developed by adaptation and evolution. The plan worked, Kaiser noted, because it adhered to its four basic principles: prepayment, group practice, well-planned integrated facilities, and preventive medical care. Serving 400,000 members in three West Coast states at a monthly dues rate of $3.25 for a single subscriber, $6.95 for a subscriber and two or more family dependents, the Kaiser Foundation Health Plan showed the nation what could be done in the private sector.

If the Wolverton bill became law, Kaiser urged, 30,000 American physicians could participate in a program financed by $1 billion of federally guaranteed private loans. Lending institutions would provide up to 60 percent of the necessary capital, with medical groups providing the rest. Institutional lenders would be insured for loans covering up to 90 percent of construction costs for new facilities. In a very short time, some 30 million Americans could be fully covered in their health-care needs through the private sector.

In the course of his remarks, Kaiser went out of his way to emphasize physicians' prerogatives in both the Kaiser-Permanente program and any future proposals. "The heart of the medical care program," he noted, "is the partnerships of doctors who supply their services to the members.... The doctors are in complete charge of all medical care, without lay or corporate control over their services to patients."[10]

This statement angered the Executive Committee of The Permanente Medical Group. Not only was Kaiser, a layperson, speaking on behalf of the program, he had the temerity to say that laypeople exercised no control over the Permanente physicians and their medical services. The very fact that it was Kaiser and not Garfield testifying before the House Committee should have spoken for itself. In any event, the Executive Committee determined its intent to inform both Garfield and Kaiser "that testimony before the Wolverton Committee did not correspond to the facts in Northern California."[11] Two weeks later the Executive Committee forwarded contrary information to Representative Wolverton. So bitter had the conflict become, the Permanente physicians seemed willing to endanger the Wolverton bill just so that the record regarding lay interference in northern California might be set straight. Opposed by organized medicine, the Wolverton bill died in committee.

It rankled many Permanente physicians to have Kaiser become the embodiment of their program in the mind of the public. George Duscheck's four-part series in *The San Francisco News* appearing between October 29 and November 1, 1957, underscored in its headline ("Henry Kaiser's Big Medicine") this continuing perception. Not only was Kaiser speaking for the program, he was actively attempting to break up the Northern California Permanente Medical Group into several smaller competing groups in Walnut Creek, Oakland, San Francisco, Vallejo, and elsewhere. Kaiser argued that smaller groups would be competitive with each other and thereby improve service to the public. Kaiser did not mention, obviously, that such a divide-and-conquer strategy would enable him to dominate the physicians. Even Clifford Keene was appalled at the idea of fomenting the breakup of The Permanente Medical Group. "I was distraught when I heard that," Keene later stated. "That's something that I thought would be pretty dumb to do."[12]

Kaiser and his top staffers sincerely believed that they knew what was best for the entire program, the Medical Group included. Cecil Cutting remembers being invited with Morris Collen and A. LaMonte Baritell to a dinner at the Claremont Country Club with Eugene Trefethen, Joe Reis, and Edgar Kaiser. "We had a good dinner," Cutting remembers, "and after dinner they got each of us separate, individually, and were talking to us and patting our shoulders, and telling us what a good job we were doing, but really, we ought to spend our efforts in taking care of the patients in the office and they would run the business. They were the businessmen. We had sense enough to feel that this wasn't quite right. Providing medical care was itself a business, and it was a little different from running cement and steel."[13]

4

Resistance to such dominance over the northern California Permanente physicians naturally centered in the Executive Committee—in Cecil Cutting, A. LaMonte Baritell, and Morris Collen. Quiet by temperament, personally close to Garfield, Cutting pursued a role of internal diplomacy, smoothing out conflicts among Collen, Baritell, and Garfield, on internal issues. Collen and Baritell had specific differences on the allocation of financial resources to research, which Collen favored. In time, Cutting's slow, patient work of internal leadership would result in his being chosen the first executive director of the Medical Group.

Ray Kay of Los Angeles, by contrast, was an outspoken opponent of any intrusion by the Kaiser organization into what he considered the prerogatives of the Permanente Medical Group of Southern California, which had been separately established in 1950. Dealing with Ray Kay, Clifford Keene later remembered, was like standing next to a bonfire with a stick of dynamite in your hand. One noon over lunch at the Brown Derby in Los Angeles, Kay and Keene got into an argument that soon became, in Kay's recollection, part of the floor show. Behind Ray Kay's explosive emotionalism, however, was a well-formulated set of principles. Kay realized that the doctors could not play a dual role in the Health Plan, a nonprofit organization, and the Medical Groups, organizations formed to make a profit; but he was also worried about having the physicians boxed totally into the Medical Groups, with no representation or influence in the Foundation, the Health Plan, or the Hospitals. This effectively reduced them to the status of managed employees. Kay was also concerned about the security of Permanente physicians. "I have to have security for my doctors," Kay told the Kaiser organization. "In ten years when our salaries get higher, you could come in and get a competing group of young guys for much less. We've got to have the security that you can't contract with anyone else in our area."[14]

Neurologist Paul Fitzgibbon, the former football player who had functioned as regional medical director in northern California from 1946 until 1952, also exercised important influence among the resistors as one of the founding partners and a member of the Executive Committee until June 1953, when he resigned from the Medical Group. Some believed that Fitzgibbon resigned because he was experiencing family difficulties. Cecil Cutting tells another story. "He got worried that Mr. Kaiser was going to take over," Cecil Cutting later recalled. "I remember walking clear around the block with him one noon, talking about it, when he was deciding to leave. He said he didn't think much good could come out of it if Mr. Kaiser was going to get involved and take over."[15]

Five months later, in October 1953, the Medical Group was rocked by the resignation (temporary, it turned out) of another founding figure, August LaMonte Baritell, chief of surgery at Oakland. Unlike Paul Fitzgibbon, Baritell did not go gently into the good night. On the contrary, he issued a statement, which was picked up by the Oakland *Tribune*, criticizing the program for failing to pursue excellence. Baritell upbraided the Kaiser organization for not being honest and forthright with the Permanente physicians. He accused Garfield of mismanaging the cash resources of the program. "He thought we ought to spend more money on equipment maybe than Dr. Garfield thought we had money to spend," was how Cecil Cutting remembered it. "Perhaps [he] wanted more doctors, more nurses, things of that sort."[16]

Baritell's stinging criticisms received extensive coverage in Bay Area newspapers. Sensing perhaps that many Permanente physicians agreed with Baritell, Garfield met with The Permanente Medical Group Executive Committee in a special session to discuss the substance of Baritell's complaints. Garfield assured the Executive Committee that it would have a full voice in the enrollment of new groups and that it would share in all financial data regarding the operation of the program. Garfield also stated that his personal desire to be helpful and provide advice had been perhaps misinterpreted by Baritell and others as an attempt at control. After Garfield left the meeting, the Executive Committee drafted a statement affirming its adherence to the principles and ideals of the Kaiser Foundation Medical Care Program. "Recent events," the statement cautioned, "have brought to the surface some crucial problems which are existent between The Permanente Medical Group and the Kaiser Foundation." A masterly piece of understatement!

To effect more satisfactory relations between all associated entities, the Executive Committee recommended a number of reforms. The Permanente Medical Group, first of all, should sign a formal agreement with Sidney Garfield and the Board of Trustees of the Kaiser Foundation reaffirming the principle that the Medical Group was a separate and independent entity. The Group should be reorganized to establish more solidly this separate and equal status. The Executive Committee should appoint an administrator and controller for the Medical Group. It should also set up a nonprofit trust to rent or purchase clinical facilities and equipment and to build up a reserve fund. All hospital services under the direction of physicians — such as laboratory, X-ray, anesthesiology, and physiotherapy — should be under the jurisdiction of the Medical Group. Staff relationships in the Kaiser Hospitals should parallel those of community hospitals. The medical director should become chief of staff. With a competent hospital administrator, a salaried medical director would not be necessary. The board of directors of the Health Plan and the Hospitals should be a policy-forming group and not a managing or administrative entity. The Board of Directors should not interfere in the internal affairs of the Medical Group, either directly or indirectly. Sidney Garfield, finally, should be retained by the Medical Group as a special consultant.

Aside from this first series of internal reforms, the Executive Committee had three other major recommendations. Contracts between the Health Plan and the enrolled membership should be made subject to the approval of the Medical Group, since the physicians were to be held responsible for the services that were being contracted. Medical and administrative representatives from the Medical Group should be present at each meeting of the Kaiser Foundation Board of Trustees to advise and be advised on matters concerning the Medical Group, the Foundation, the Hospitals, and the Health Plan. There should be no major expansion of membership without a corresponding increase in doctors, staff, and facilities.

Two days after this emergency meeting, Baritell informed the Executive Committee at its regular meeting that he considered these recommendations to be the partial answers to his protest and suggested that he might reconsider his resignation. All in all, Baritell remained outside the Group for a little over 4 months. "I remember at the time he scoured the state of California, perhaps the whole West Coast, looking for a proper opportunity for himself," Wally Cook later recalled. "And he told me at the time — I don't remember his exact words — that it was a jungle out there, and he didn't really want any part of it. He did not return with his tail between his legs because everyone wanted him back."[17] In February 1954 Baritell was reinstated in the partnership to the position of physician-in-chief at Oakland and to his membership in the Executive Committee.

At the same October 1953 meeting at which it received Baritell's offer of reconciliation, the Executive Committee also considered the draft of a document submitted by the Health Plan entitled "Statement of Fundamental Policies and Responsibilities of the Various Organizations Associated to Provide the Services of Kaiser Health Plan." Four days later, at yet another meeting, the Executive Committee approved this document, which further delineated administrative structures and responsibilities for the rapidly growing, increasingly complex Kaiser-Permanente program. On October 31, 1953, the trustees of the Kaiser Foundation Health Plan also ratified the document. In theory at least, agreement had been reached that each of the entities had its structures, rights, and responsibilities, and of particular importance to the Medical Group, that the physicians were to be consulted on any action directly or indirectly affecting medical service.

The Executive Committee, meanwhile, busied itself in implementing as many as possible of the reforms called for when Baritell resigned. On October 26, 1953, the Executive Committee established the position of Medical Group administrator, filling it 2 weeks later with the appointment of Daniel Brown. The Executive Committee also met with Hal Babbitt, manager of the Health Plan, and his staff to work out a methodology for securing Medical Group approval of contracts with member groups. The Health Plan agreed to review all contracts with the Medical Group before they were renewed. It was suggested that statistics be kept to determine if different charges should be assessed against groups with different risks. This suggestion was not adopted. In subsequent meetings with the Health Plan staff, a number of other controversial issues were reviewed: coverage for noncontagious tuberculosis, dental X-rays, a flat fee for pregnancies effective the date of enrollment, the termination of troublesome and uncooperative patients, and coverage for emergency out-of-plan medical care. The Health Plan agreed to provide a 24-hour service that would authenticate the eligibility of a patient as a Health Plan beneficiary. Charges for house calls were increased, and the issue of whether it was better to have total prepayment or nominal copayment charges was brought up for continuing discussion. The Executive Committee also secured approval rights for all equipment purchases over $25.

Members of the Executive Committee and Medical Group administrator Daniel Brown met with the labor relations department of the Kaiser Companies to discuss labor relations within the various Kaiser-Permanente entities. It was agreed that labor unions continued to be the core membership of the Health Plan; hence Permanente Medical Group employees would most likely be unionized. In terms of dealing with such unions, the Medical Group and Hospitals would be perceived as one entity and should bargain with the same unions.

A crucial source of intelligence and guidance in all these negotiations came from Morris Collen, the research-oriented internist who had himself resigned as medical director of the West San Francisco Bay Region in December 1953 in protest over the unilateral appointment of a hospital director, Felix Day, by Kaiser Hospitals. Unlike Fitzgibbon and Baritell, Collen did not leave the partnership. Instead, he remained on the Executive Committee as chief strategist of the resistance and an architect of the forthcoming reform. In 1952 when Collen was scheduled to take over as chief of staff in the San Francisco hospital, he had called on his old friend, Gene Trefethen, then serving as vice president of the Foundation Hospitals. If he wanted to be an executive and a medical director, Trefethen cautioned Collen, he would have to learn to put up with a lot of petty harassment. When Collen discovered that a significant percentage of the hassle was coming from the Kaiser organization, climaxed by the imposition of a hospital administrator without consulting the doctors, he resigned his nominal post as West Bay Medical Director and devoted some of his considerable energies to resisting the Kaiser dominance of the organization of which he was a pioneer.

5

Most eyewitnesses to Sidney Garfield's decline from power—Ray Kay, Cecil Cutting, Wally Cook, even Garfield himself—date its beginnings to Kaiser's unilateral decision in 1952 to build the showplace hospital in Walnut Creek. Garfield later admitted that the program really did not need a hospital in the Walnut Creek area at the time. "But I thought it might be a good way to get Mr. Kaiser really interested in the medical operations. With his energy and influence, we could get financing more easily, expand to new communities, improve service. The doctors, Cecil [Cutting], Wally [Neighbor], and the others were skeptical, but I talked them into it. Gene Trefethen and Edgar [Kaiser] opposed Walnut Creek, but the Boss with my backing pushed it through."[18]

Pushing Walnut Creek through, however, had its consequences. In the doctors' minds, Garfield became increasingly identified with Henry Kaiser, especially after becoming his brother-in-law and next-door neighbor. It was Garfield, after all, who first devised the name "Boss" for Kaiser, a sobriquet which Kaiser relished. "Boss" became his preferred designation among the inner circle. The Kaiser-Garfield relationship has frequently been characterized as that of a father to a son. If so, it must be remembered that Henry J. Kaiser could be, as he was to his own two sons, a very demanding father. As a father figure, Kaiser brought much that was positive to the relationship. He respected Garfield as his brother-in-law and personal physician. He admired Garfield's visionary entrepreneurial streak, which he himself possessed. Affectionate in an almost childlike way, Kaiser stuck by those whom he brought into his inner circle, and few were brought more closely into the inner circle than his brother-in-law Garfield. On the other hand, Kaiser had a tendency to dominate even his intimates.

"On various occasions," Clifford Keene remembers, "I saw Mr. Kaiser take on Sidney in the most humiliating circumstances. If a man had spoken to me like that I'd want to fight with him physically. It was most demeaning and I felt sorry for Sidney. Then I guess after Mr. Kaiser cooled down, he would have feelings of remorse. Always there was the awareness of that family relationship, the Kaiser-Garfield cocktail hour, the two women and Henry and Sidney."[19]

Kaiser became especially furious with Garfield when Garfield reminded him that the Permanente physicians did not want to be managed like employees. Kaiser considered the Permanente physicians highly paid producers of services to be managed like a collective bargaining unit. Garfield also opposed Kaiser's plan to divide The Permanente Medical Group into smaller competing entities. "We were great friends," said Garfield of their relationship. "We lived together. I took care of him until he died. But that didn't mean that he had to agree with me or I had to agree with him. He had his great strengths and his great weaknesses like everybody has. There are no gods."[20]

Garfield's identification with Kaiser made it difficult for Garfield to keep the complete confidence of the Medical Group as he tried to play the intermediary. The same held true for Kaiser. Kaiser and the Permanente physicians each perceived Garfield, the would-be intermediary, as the agent of the other side. Garfield also lost credibility in regard to his managerial abilities. The question of finance provides a primary example. Kaiser believed that control of the program by the Kaiser executives on the Foundation Board of Trustees was necessary to ensure major loans from the Bank of America and other lending institutions. Garfield's highly personalized, semi-autonomous management of financial resources thus constituted an anachronism in an organization with a large indebtedness. Some Foundation trustees were troubled that lenders would doubt the financial stability of the program, should they become aware of what they would certainly regard as disorganized management. Meeting infrequently between 1946 and 1952, Health Plan trustees had limited their considerations largely to personnel matters and the ratification of budgets that Garfield presented them. In 1952 the trustees began to request detailed information from Garfield about such matters as the providing of Kaiser automobiles to the physicians through the partnership, leasehold improvements in southern California, the differences in dues and operating expenses between the southern California and the northern California regions, the provision of capital medical equipment for doctors, and the use of the retention fund. All this implied a more systematic level of financial management and accounting than had previously been in effect. "Sid ran a very parsimonious organization," Ernest Saward remembered, "and a great deal of the bookkeeping, I think — not that he didn't have bookkeepers — was in his head. When you go to a bank, the bank wants a very orthodox kind of layout of the finances and how you expect to do it. And I don't think Sid was anymore orthodox in that than in anything else he did."[21]

Organizations require different styles of leadership at different phases of development. It was becoming evident to many that Sidney Garfield's management style belonged to an earlier era. To Saward's way of thinking, Garfield was a born entrepreneur. After the war, in addition to his duties with the program, Garfield was also managing a whole string of apartment houses in Los Angeles, which he owned. Garfield, Saward recalled, was a man of ideas, some good, some terrible. In this he resembled Kaiser himself, whose fecundity of ideas were filtered through the pragmatic realism of Trefethen and other executives. Kaiser's personal assistant and general factotum Lambreth Hancock put it this way: "Sid could only handle something up to the size of where he could control it personally. When it started getting bigger than that, he was not able to delegate."[22]

The Permanente Medical Group Executive Committee resented Garfield's retention of capital for the construction of new facilities as opposed to the improvement of existing facilities, salary increases for physicians, and support of research and education to attract high-quality MDs. Even Garfield's symbolic economies, such as his refusal to allow Scotch tape in the offices or his demand that a pencil stub be turned in before a new pencil was issued, began to rankle and even to be subverted. "Everybody would draw a pencil out of supply," Lambreth Hancock recalled, "break it into three pieces, sharpen the points down to the point where they looked like they had been used up, and turn in three, and get three full pencils back again. And all of a sudden they discovered they were using more pencils than before when he didn't make them turn in their pencil stubs to get the other. This was a form of rebellion on the part of the employees."[23]

This does not imply that the Permanente physicians supported Clifford Keene, who had been brought to California by Henry Kaiser without consultation. Far from it: Permanente opposition to Kaiser dominance focused on Keene throughout the 1950s. For both Keene and Garfield, the situation eventually became intolerable.

Keene, for his part, was expected both to monitor Garfield and to report to him. "I would have lunch with him and dinner with him," Keene remembered, "and spend much of the time going over all that had happened, in great detail."[24] In any other circumstances, Keene later recalled, he would have become friends with Garfield, and with Collen, Kay, and Cutting. They were all, after all, highly competent physicians committed to a philosophy of prepaid group medical practice in which he also believed; but in the circumstances in which Keene, Garfield, and the Permanente physicians found themselves, friendship was out of the question. In a very real sense, the Permanente physicians were wanting it both ways: wanting, that is, to resist Keene as a Kaiser agent, while at the same time agreeing that Garfield's management style had become obsolete. Keene himself believed that he had walked into a mess. The program could no longer afford Garfield's style of running the organization out of his hip pocket, problem by problem.

Keene was especially disturbed by Garfield's highly personalized handling of finances. Garfield, for instance, paid top employees, especially women, according to what he thought they needed to live on, not according to the salaries of people in comparable positions. When Dorothea Daniels, the Los Angeles Hospital administrator with a doctorate in education, discovered that Garfield was paying her less than the going rate on the theory that she was a single woman and did not need much income, she caused an uproar.

Almost immediately upon his arrival, Keene became the person the Foundation trustees sent to the bank when it came time to negotiate loans. Ernest Saward believed that this ability to create the proper image with bankers was Keene's most significant early contribution. "Maybe he wasn't as free-flowing and entrepreneurial as what had gone on in the past," Saward later said of Keene. "But his orthodoxy...was an asset. What would be to some of the physicians a stuffed shirt, to the banks was what they should have seen all along."[25]

Not that any of this endeared Keene to The Permanente Medical Group. Keene might be doing some of the things they wanted done, but he was still the enemy. It was one thing for Garfield's long-time colleagues to oppose him; it was another matter for a non-Permanente physician, responsible only to the Kaiser-controlled Foundation board of trustees, to oppose Garfield in a similar manner. Ambivalent about opposing their founder Garfield, whose entrepreneurial genius had made the program work in its first era, the Permanente physicians alleviated their anxieties by battling Keene, who was, ironically, doing his best to reform the program according to many of the criteria being advocated by the Medical Group.

"The fact that somebody was running the [Kaiser medical care] organization who was a physician bothered them," said Ernest Saward of the Permanente physicians' personalized opposition to Clifford Keene. "And it wasn't that Dr. Keene was doing wrongful things, to them or to the program, not at all. I think he was very helpful. I think even the current management today gives Dr. Keene less credit for what he really did than he deserves. That's my opinion."[26]

"You talk about controversy or disagreement," Wally Cook later concurred, "the Med Group in general never accepted Dr. Keene. They didn't go so far as to call him Mr. Keene, but they didn't accept any management by this doctor from outside the Med Group. He wasn't one of our own. He wasn't from the Med Group."[27]

Cook correctly underscored the growing perception of Keene as a loyal Kaiser executive. Keene worked closely with Eugene Trefethen in the Foundation. In the late 1950s Keene set up industrial health-care programs in Brazil, Argentina, Australia, India, and various countries of Africa as the Kaiser Companies established operations abroad. "No Kaiser boss ever was away from a telephone," Keene later recalled. "You've seen those surrealistic paintings of telephones on a man's ears. That's the way it was. No matter where I was or whatever I was doing, regardless of the time of the day, night, Christmas, New Year's, whatever, I had to be near that telephone. And that was true of Edgar, true of Gene, and true of everybody else that was running a company."[28]

Clifford Keene believed he could make a difference in the Kaiser Permanente Medical Care Program. He was disheartened by the Permanente physicians' reception of him but was willing to endure their resentment because he believed in himself and the job he was doing. At times, he was tempted to quit; but he regarded quitting as failure, and Clifford Keene, a seasoned surgeon, a veteran of fierce campaigning in the South Pacific, did not like to fail.

In psychological and organizational terms, the program was in deep trouble by 1955. The current impasse could not continue without serious damage to the program. If 1955 was the nadir year in terms of dissension, it also contained within itself the dynamics of its own correction. Both sides, after all, were growing weary of the conflict. It was fast becoming time for both sides to negotiate their differences and get on with the business of pioneering a new and very much needed program of health care delivery.

8

The Tahoe Agreement

Problems between the Permanente doctors and the Kaiser organization finally came to a head in 1955. During World War II Kaiser was a purchaser of services from Garfield. He established the Permanente Foundation at Dr. Garfield's request in order to own tax-exempt hospitals, but these hospitals were leased and operated by Garfield. Even after the war, Kaiser functioned as a benign sponsor and supporter of Garfield's medical care program. Until 1952, the Permanente Foundation Health Plan Board of Trustees met infrequently and allowed Garfield to do as he pleased. After 1952, with the building of Walnut Creek Hospital and the change of name of Health Plan and Hospitals from Permanente to Kaiser, Henry J. Kaiser declared that the Kaiser organization ran anything in which it was involved. The doctors rejected this concept, maintaining that medical care was entirely different from ships, dams, steel companies, and cement plants. Medical care, they argued, was best left to the management of the physicians. The doctors felt that they should decide the sites and sizes of medical facilities (the Walnut Creek issue), select management personnel (the Keene issue), and oversee the operations of the Health Plan and Hospitals. The knowledge that Kaiser wanted to break up The Permanente Medical Group into small partnerships posed a constant threat to their sense of security and self-esteem.

Money, of course, was also an issue. The doctors were not certain of a sound base of compensation nor was any retirement program in effect. Moreover, physicians expressed concern that someone from the Kaiser organization might ask to scrutinize The Permanente Medical Group's internal finances, including the pay of individual doctors. During the financially shaky period after the war, the doctors had contributed a share of their own earnings to a Retention Fund. This fund was to be used to cover contractual health benefits for Plan members in the event of financial failure. What would happen to it now?

The Kaiser organization saw matters differently. First of all, there was the indebtedness of $14 million guaranteed by the Kaiser Industrial Companies for the medical care program. Second, and directly related to the debt issue, was Sidney Garfield's off-the-cuff style of management. Kaiser was concerned how the lenders would evaluate an organization managed in the Garfield manner. Kaiser people also insisted on being dominant in management of the enterprise. It was a business, after all, and should be run by businesspeople. Physicians should take care of patients.

Efforts were made to avoid confrontation. In 1953 an administrative council had been established as an advisory and liaison body concerned with the problems resulting from the interactions of the Health Plan, Hospitals, and medical groups. Aside from suggesting that eventually power and responsibility would have to be shared and structured in the growing organization, the administrative council proved to be ineffective in reducing conflict.

In March 1954, upon the recommendation of Clifford Keene, the trustees of the Kaiser Foundation Health Plan established a more sophisticated administrative structure for the Kaiser components of the program. Health Plan was assigned its own president, who reported to the Board of Trustees. There was also an overall executive director for the three regions—southern California, northern California, and Oregon-Washington—covered by Kaiser-Permanente physicians. Each region would have a regional director, vice president, secretary and assistant secretaries, and a controller. Thus each of the regions was given its own localized administrative structure, intended to promote flexibility and responsiveness.

At the same meeting the board of trustees agreed to release the Retention Fund. By March 1954, the Retention Fund had grown to $750,000. Citing the demonstrated success of the program and its present economic base, the board of trustees voted to disestablish the Fund, dispersing half of it through the Hospitals and half of it to The Permanente Medical Group. On the other hand, the trustees continued to demand return-on-investment information from all hospitals, clinics, and medical programs. Such information, while financial in nature, could not be divorced from its medical context;

hence, the Medical Group continued to regard such scrutiny as intrusions into its prerogatives.

During this period, the first half of 1954, some of the most far-reaching organizational thinking was carried on by the Executive Committee and subcommittees of The Permanente Medical Group. Three possible alternatives resulted from these discussions. First of all, the physicians could become employees of the Health Plan. Or separate partnerships could be organized at each facility, a plan Henry J. Kaiser strongly favored. Third, the partnership could stay intact but with a new emphasis on each of the medical centers in the region. Each of the three alternatives was considered according to the following criteria: adequacy or availability of professional services, quality of professional services, patient satisfaction, Health Plan member satisfaction, physician satisfaction, and economics. In June of 1954 the legal committee appointed by the Executive Committee, consisting of Neighbor, Baritell, Cook, and Melvin Friedman, made its report in favor of the medical partnership staying intact. "The partnership has weathered a stormy period," the legal subcommittee reported, "and seems to be reaching a state of stability. This would be no time to instigate, let alone institute, radical departures from a single partnership."[1] The Executive Committee accepted this recommendation.

Thus, embryonically, an eventual solution asserted itself even in these troubled years. The Health Plan and Hospitals remained under central control but were also diversified into regional administrative units. These regional administrations offered points of local contact with the Medical Group that would eventually work against the conviction on the part of the physicians that they were being directed by a remote board of laypeople using its power over finances as a way of controlling medical policy. When Garfield's physician employees had trifurcated themselves into southern California, northern California, and Oregon-Washington partnerships, localization within a controlling central framework had been enhanced and intensified among the physicians, as it was among lay administrators with the creation of regions. Ahead lay the challenge of making this confederation, at once centralized and localized, work in a way that satisfied trustees, administrators, and physicians alike.

By April 1955, despite some administrative advances, dissension among the various components of the Kaiser-Permanente community induced in the organization a virtual state of paralysis. "Expansion was stopped," Cecil Cutting later remembered, "membership was stopped, spending of money was stopped, everything ground to a halt."[2]

On April 21, 1955, the medical groups of each region suggested in a joint letter to Eugene Trefethen the formation of a working council to deal with the impasse. "We consider the basic problems," the letter stated, "to be the obtaining of a mutually satisfactory integration of all management activities, mutually satisfactory representation at policy-making levels, mutually satisfactory methods of monetary distribution and control, and mutually satisfactory methods of selection of all key personnel." In the letter the medical groups recommended establishment of a working council composed of Henry J. Kaiser, Sr., Edgar Kaiser, Trefethen, and attorney George Link, all these representing the board of trustees, representatives from each of the three medical groups, and Sidney Garfield. The working council should meet on a semimonthly basis for 6 months and assess the organizational arrangements of every aspect of the program. During this period, the entire organization would remain on a status quo basis, pending the recommendation of the working council. "During this series of conferences it should be possible to develop an understanding which, it is hoped, will lead to a mutually acceptable solution that will enable us to continue our medical care program together."[3]

The working council met for the first time on May 12, 1955, at the Kaiser Building, 1924 Broadway, in Oakland. Baritell, Collen, Cutting, and Neighbor represented The Permanente Medical Group in northern California. Kay and Weiner represented the Southern California Permanente Medical Group; and Saward and Frink represented the Permanente Clinic in Oregon-Washington. Henry J. Kaiser could not attend this meeting, but Edgar Kaiser, Eugene Trefethen, and George Link were on hand to represent the trustees. Sidney Garfield was also on hand, as was Clifford Keene. Before Keene could be seated as a member of the working council, however, there was some maneuvering and discussion. As ever, Keene, a physician in the employ of the Kaiser organization, served as a red flag to Permanente physicians. Trefethen, by contrast, a skilled organizational leader, a sympathetic layperson, posed no threat and was easily chosen as chair.

The meeting got under way with a reading by Dr. Baritell of a memorandum prepared by the medical groups. The memorandum rehearsed the growth and development of the various components of the Kaiser-Permanente program. In each stage of development and reorganization, the physicians "were told and sincerely believed that all these changes would maintain adequate policy representation and would not destroy our basic concept of an integrated operation of clinics, hospitals, and Health Plan under physician management." It was this very concept of physician management that had enabled the organization to recruit well-qualified physicians and grow to its present size.

Beginning in 1952, a change began to become apparent in the attitude of the trustees. The board began to ignore Sidney Garfield and to intervene unilaterally in administrative decisions. With the board's encouragement, the Health Plan and the Hospitals became increasingly autonomous from the recommendations of the Medical Group. "These events culminated in a movement of defense by the doctors," the memorandum argued, "which developed an autonomy of its own in an effort to strengthen and maintain its remaining integrity. We are now convinced that the continuance of these policies of separation would result in the destruction of everything we have achieved together." Only by returning to the principle of physician management, the doctors concluded, could the organization save itself. "We urge a return to these fundamental principles, not only for our benefit, but for that of our successors, and our imitators, and for what all of us believe to be an ideal of medical practice worth maintaining."[4]

With this strong unilateral declaration, the first session of the working council commenced in an atmosphere of challenge and confrontation. Taking up the gauntlet, Edgar Kaiser suggested that George Link prepare a legal evaluation of the doctors' statement. Lines were thus immediately drawn. In an effort to keep the meeting productive, Trefethen then suggested that rather than lay down challenges to each other, the members of the working council should deal with the announced agenda: the evolution of a satisfactory structure of representation at all policy making levels. Trefethen suggested that a permanent advisory committee be established of representatives from each of the three medical groups, together with Garfield, Keene, Edgar Kaiser, and himself. This advisory committee would review and recommend all matters scheduled to go before the boards of the Health Plan and Hospitals. The advisory committee would have the authority to initiate matters for presentation to these boards. The boards of the Health Plan and Hospitals, however, and the governing bodies of the medical groups would retain final authority on all matters brought before them. The medical groups caucused over Trefethen's proposal, then requested more time to consider it. Trefethen adjourned the meeting until the following day.

The next day, May 13, Baritell restated the positions affirmed in the previous meeting, then reasserted the doctors' message in even stronger terms. In his remarks, Baritell took strong exception to a statement made in the previous session by Clifford Keene that the original idea for the program and its successful development (160,000 members by

1952) was due primarily to the lay board of trustees and not to the physicians. "Contrary to your statement yesterday," Baritell rebuked Keene, "the original idea and its successful development was principally the product of physicians, not a lay board."[5]

Despite Baritell's reassertion of this hard-line position and his face-to-face rebuke of Keene, this second session of the working council did not, as might have been expected, end in deadlock. On the contrary, once Baritell had stated this most uncompromising view of things, the Medical Group representatives put five major options on the table. The medical groups could take over the entire operation of the Health Plan, or the medical groups could take over the entire operation of both the Health Plan and the Hospitals. In another scenario, the medical groups could be given equal representation on the boards of trustees of the Health Plan or the Hospitals or both. As a fourth option, the differences could be resolved by contractual arrangements between the medical groups and the Health Plan. As a fifth option, matters might be allowed to remain as they already were. The trustees, that is, would continue to be responsible for the management of the Health Plan and the Hospitals, while the medical groups remained responsible for medical care.

As bold as the medical groups' first two proposals sounded, there was little likelihood that the physicians would ever be in a position to buy out the Hospitals and the Health Plan. The third option, Medical Group representation on the boards of trustees of the Health Plan and the Hospitals, had some possibilities of resolving conflicts, although this proposal made no provisions for the day-to-day points of contact in an intricate medical care delivery system. Nor did the fifth option, leaving things as they were, offer much of a solution. The status quo, after all, had created an atmosphere of mistrust and paralysis.

Option four, contractual agreements between the medical groups and the Health Plan, contained the possibilities of a long-range solution. This way out of the impasse through contractual agreements did not at this point strongly impress the working council, which merely directed attorney George Link to consider the tax and other administrative consequences of all five proposals. With this, the working council adjourned on the second day of its first working session, agreeing to meet on the same agenda once Link had prepared his analysis.

In the memorandum he prepared for the working council, Link clearly joined the various issues. Although there were no insurmountable legal obstacles to having the medical groups take over the Health Plan and the Hospitals, Link reported, there were some legal and financial difficulties—and some rather formidable ethical problems as well. Owning the Health Plan, Link pointed out, would put the doctors in the position of being responsible for the solicitation of patients, which was clearly unethical. Should the medical groups merely operate the Health Plan while not owning it, the physicians would still be in the position of dominating terms of contract with the Hospitals, even though the Hospitals would continue to remain under the control of its own board of directors. Such a drastic change, moreover, would have to be approved by the Bank of America, which had loaned the Kaiser Foundation substantial amounts of money on the understanding that the Foundation, the Hospitals, and the Health Plan would be operated under Kaiser management with the moral responsibility of the Kaiser organization, including the Kaiser industrial companies, to repay the debt.

Link then went on to list a number of staggering tax consequences arising from the various proposals that the physicians take over the program. The Kaiser Foundation Hospitals were tax-exempt community hospitals. Any adjustments in their ownership and/or governance endangered the tax-exempt status, which had been so carefully worked out. If the medical groups assumed control of the Hospitals, and the Hospitals thus lost their nonprofit status, the Hospitals would have to pay additional property, payroll, rental, and income taxes from its operation. Link calculated that these taxes for the period January 1, 1955, to December 31, 1959, would total an estimated $4,339,600.

If the component organizations remained under Kaiser ownership, on the other hand, but the doctors were allowed equal representation on all boards, the tax-exempt status of the Foundation and the Hospitals would also be jeopardized. Should the Foundation and Hospitals lose their tax-exempt status, a retroactive deficiency demand for back taxes would exceed $2 million plus interest. Such a lump-sum obligation, Link stated, would bankrupt the Kaiser Foundation itself and the Kaiser Foundation Hospitals. Supplementing Link's financial observations, Trefethen noted in an appended memorandum that should the medical groups choose to purchase the Kaiser Foundation Hospitals, their book value as of December 1954 was $15,416,000, with mortgages totaling $6,225,000. A prospective purchaser would need approximately $9.2 million in cash.

Such financial considerations grounded all further discussion in reality. Whatever their objections to lay control might be, the physicians had to recognize that the present set-up had allowed a significant portion of the program tax-exempt status. Without such tax exemptions, the Kaiser-Permanente program—and hence the physicians' personal incomes—could not have flourished. The physicians could not have it both ways. If they chose to own and operate the program, or even to serve on the boards of trustees, they would have to assume the financial consequences.

Significantly, Link considered the fourth proposal by the medical groups, that of contractual agreements, to be the most feasible. Actually, Link pointed out, the contractual agreements already in effect gave the medical groups the authority to approve or disapprove Health Plan contracts with new groups and individual members and to determine the scope of benefits. The physicians took Link's statement with a grain of salt. Just recently the Health Plan had unilaterally agreed to provide the ILWU dual-choice coverage at the same rate it charged for 100 percent enrollment—but had not bothered to consult the physicians. When Link, on the other hand, pointed out that the present contracts made no provision for the long-term security of the Permanente Medical Groups, he struck a deep chord. Under current agreements, the Health Plan was theoretically free to contract with competing groups of physicians. Clearly, this difficulty would have to be resolved in any further contractual arrangements. The reassertion of option four, contractual agreements, ended the first session of the working council on a relatively optimistic note. Through a glass darkly, a resolution was glimpsed.

2

Meeting on June 7, 1955, at the Kaiser Building in Oakland, the second session of the working council was not as productive. Henry J. Kaiser was personally present. Also on hand were Henry J. Kaiser, Jr., the formidable A. B. Ordway, Todd Inch, and Robert Elliot. Henry J. Kaiser opened the meeting with a threat. Some members of the medical groups, Kaiser said, felt they no longer needed the Health Plan and Hospitals in their present format. Very well, he was working on a program in which the trustees would withdraw entirely and permit the doctors to manage the enterprise through small independent groups. Given the financial consequences of such action already outlined by Link and Trefethen, it was difficult to make sense of this proposal by Henry J. Kaiser. Kaiser was going over old ground. Contractual agreements, and not any other formula, offered the only solution. Everyone knew this.

Even before this second session of the working council, Kaiser had been debating with Ray Kay of the Southern California Permanente Medical Group. Meeting with Kay at the Bel Air Hotel, Kaiser kept Kay up until 3 in the morning discussing the prospects of selling the Hospitals to the Medical Group. "I knew he was bluffing," Kay later stated. "I knew he wasn't going to sell it to us. But I thought it was worth exploring." Interestingly enough, the Southern California Medical Group was less hardline than its northern California counterparts in the matter of lay participation in program management. "The Southern Group," Ray Kay later wrote, "agreed that the Medical Care entities should be under physician control and that Dr. Garfield should continue to play an important role as the key advisor to all entities; however, we also felt that the Kaiser organization had a great deal to contribute and that we must find a way to work together."[6]

Henry J. Kaiser did not contribute to the possibilities of cooperation with his opening gambit at the first meeting of the second session of the working council. Understandably, the minutes record that "a great deal of discussion" followed Kaiser's opening statement. A lot of points previously considered were heatedly rehashed. As with any committee meeting finding itself in a floundering condition, it was agreed to form a subcommittee to study Kaiser's proposal that the trustees withdraw from responsibility and turn the program over to smaller partnerships. Trefethen appointed Collen and Baritell to represent the physicians on this subcommittee, together with Paul Steil, the regional manager in southern California, Joe Reis, and George Link to represent the trustees. Meeting on June 20, 1955, the subcommittee accomplished only one piece of business, the election of Morris Collen as chair. After some discussion, the subcommittee unanimously agreed to seek clarification of their assignment. Clearly, Kaiser's proposal, even if it were to be taken seriously, was getting nowhere.

Henry J. Kaiser was unable to attend the third session of the working council, which met on the afternoon of June 21, 1955. Some progress was made on these deliberations—but not immediately. While physically absent, Henry J. Kaiser continued to dominate the proceedings. The first day's meeting was wasted in a fruitless discussion of Kaiser's proposal to sell the Plan and the Hospitals to smaller medical partnerships. The next day's meeting on the morning of June 22 opened with Trefethen's announcement that he had discussed with Kaiser moving a portion of the hospital located at the Kaiser steel mill to the town of Fontana. The doctors were disconcerted. It had been agreed that there would be no changes or expansions of facilities as long as these talks were occurring. Kaiser, however, had approved the Fontana move because it was advantageous to the steel company. Trefethen soothed the doctors' ire with the promise that the Fontana decision did not involve a precedent.

Trefethen then returned to a question left on the table from the discussions of the previous day: whether the subcommittee appointed at the end of the first session was mandated to find methods by which the medical groups could purchase facilities on a cash basis — or whether the subcommittee could also pursue other reasonable methods of resolving the impasse in governance. Trefethen stated that any solution could be explored as long as it did not encumber the Kaiser Foundation. The working council then expended more time discussing possible methods of financing a buyout by the physicians before Trefethen requested that they return to the matter of seeking satisfactory structures of representation at policy-making levels. Trefethen reminded the working council that he had already proposed a permanently established advisory committee with members from the Medical Group, the Health Plan, and the Hospitals, which would screen and initiate policy matters coming before the boards of trustees. Trefethen now added another role to this proposed advisory committee: to serve as a coordinating body for matters arising between the Kaiser boards and the medical groups. As in the case of the medical groups' suggestion of specified contracts, Trefethen's proposal constituted a form of mediation welcome to both sides, and so, despite the distrust in the meeting, it was tentatively approved. If these crucial sessions of the working council had a hero, it was Trefethen, ever searching for the common ground.

At this point, discussions continued in a positive vein. The working council attacked the problem of finding a satisfactory method to select all key personnel. The physicians were anxious to have some input into the appointment of hospital administrators and regional managers. A draft statement was presented, discussed, revised, and also tentatively approved. It stated that the cooperation between the physicians and the other entities was necessary because it was "believed desirable to have key personnel acceptable to all entities." To achieve this common objective, "it is understood that the appointment or removal of individuals in key positions should be reviewed by the Advisory Committee before action is taken, so that the views of each of the several entities be known. The right of final action was vested in the entity involved."[7]

Here was an important compromise. The physicians would be consulted on nonphysician appointments, but the prerogative to appoint would remain with the Health Plan and Hospitals. On the other hand — and this represented an important concession by the physicians—the physicians also agreed to check their own medical group appointments with the Health Plan and Hospitals, while retaining a comparable authority. How exactly such a mutual consultation would be worked out on a practical day-to-day level was left unstated; but this commitment to mutual consultation constituted an important step in the direction of an eventual solution.

It then came time for the medical groups and the representatives of the other entities to read statements of objectives and goals to each other, as had been promised in the first session. Attorney George Link read into the record that these statements should not be interpreted to purport to state all the objectives of either group. With this caution, the physicians read their statement. Despite the opening salvo fired by the physicians at the first session, in which they argued for physician control of every entity, they now backed off from that position. They, too, were searching for common ground.

The first objective of the medical groups regarding the Health Plan, the statement read, was "to cooperate with the trustees of the Health Plan to achieve necessary teamwork between Medical Groups, Hospitals, and Health Plan, and to assure the attainment of the objective of the program, which is high quality medical care for the people at the most reasonable cost." Having made this concession, the medical groups then went on to assert their objectives, which they believed to be rights as well. Medical groups had the right to approve contracts with persons and groups of new Health Plan members, together with all contract terms and conditions. The Health Plan could not unilaterally enroll new member groups. The medical groups also wanted the right to review and approve all methods used by Health Plan representatives in dealing with Health Plan members and the general public. The medical groups also called for the proper distribution of monies so as to assure (1) high-quality medical care at a reasonable cost, (2) amortization on the debt of all present and future facilities, and (3) funds for research, education, and charity. The medical groups, finally, wanted to develop policies that would stimulate its physicians to provide the highest quality possible medical services.

It was now time for the Kaiser side to respond. Their statement, "Proposed Objectives of the Board of Trustees of Kaiser Foundation Health Plan" likewise began on a note of cooperation. The Health Plan, the statement began, sought "to cooperate with the Medical Groups to maintain the Kaiser Foundation Health Plan as the agency which assures the attainment of the objective of the program, which is high quality care for the people at the most reasonable cost." The Health Plan also sought to conduct its operations so as to prevent charges of solicitation against the medical groups.

The Health Plan sought a fair and equitable allocation of Kaiser Foundation Health Plan revenues among the medical groups, Kaiser Foundation Hospitals, and itself. The Health Plan would also continue to utilize the Kaiser Foundation Hospitals in a manner consistent with commitments to banks and other creditors.

On the level of formal objectives, neither of these statements contradicted each other; on the contrary, each side was struggling to establish common ground. With this encouragement, Trefethen then moved the proceedings to consider a third and most difficult area of discussion: the satisfactory integration of the management activities of the Health Plan, Hospitals, and medical groups. It was here, after all, in the pragmatic world of day-by-day administration, that authority and responsibility had to be shared between the physicians and administrators. To start off this difficult discussion, Trefethen suggested that the word "teamwork" be substituted for the word "integration." Everyone agreed. It was much easier to cite a spirit of teamwork than to wrestle with the administrative intricacies of integration. Seizing the initiative, Trefethen suggested that a committee be appointed to work out the teamwork approach in the northern California region. Ray Kay asked for a similar committee for southern California. The committees were appointed and charged with reporting on proposals at the next meeting, scheduled for July 12, 1955. Citing the time they were losing from medical practice, the physicians requested that this July 12 meeting constitute the final session of the working council. It was agreed that the session would continue for as many days as were reasonably necessary to accomplish the major goals. The second meeting of the second session adjourned with every hope of resolving the conflicts between the physicians and the trustees and administrators which had brought the Kaiser-Permanente health-care program to such an impasse.[8]

Henry J. Kaiser alone persisted in pursuing the matter of smaller partnerships. On a more positive note, Kaiser offered the use of his Lake Tahoe estate for the final session of the working council in July 1955.

3

Like everything associated with Henry J. Kaiser, his Tahoe estate was larger than life. Called *Fleur de Lac*, Flower of the Lake, the sprawling complex occupied a mile of Lake Tahoe waterfront. *Fleur de Lac* consisted of a great stone lodge surrounded by a network of guest cottages, each of them the size of the average summer home. Kaiser liked to bring guests en masse to *Fleur de Lac* for action-filled days, barbecues, water skiing, and motorboat racing, which constituted Kaiser's only form of outdoor activity other than barbecuing steaks and hamburgers. Celebrities were frequently on hand—such Kaiser cronies as screen actor Robert Cummings, radio personality Art Linkletter, Howard Hughes, and Ava Gardner on another occasion—together with scores of Kaiser executives and their families, invited up to this Sierra lake to bask in the Boss's favor for a job well done. Never one to forget business, Kaiser used these summer weekends as a way of bonding key executives to the organization, which meant to himself, and reviewing or setting in motion lines of activities in his far-flung empire.

"It's not that it wasn't fun," remembers Wally Cook, who as a young physician in charge of Walnut Creek was frequently a guest at these Tahoe gatherings, "and that it wasn't a constant party, but whenever you were with Henry you weren't talking about baseball or travel or anything—you were talking about business. He was building a new beach at that time, and he had the bulldozers in....I can't estimate how much sand he brought in. It turned Tahoe into Waikiki. Of course, the sand all washed away later, but, anyway, that was the kind of thing he did."[9]

Kaiser maintained a fleet of power boats on the lake, including the hydroplanes in which he was at the time seeking the world's speedboat record. One Fourth of July, Wally Cook remembers, Kaiser packed his guests onto a 160-square-foot raft, then towed it out to a vantage point on the lake where the guests could enjoy the hydroplane races. Protected by a railing that ran around the raft, the guests sat on deck chairs, sipping daiquiris, and viewing the competition.

The Permanente physicians and Kaiser organization staff who assembled at Tahoe on July 12, 1955, however, were not at *Fleur de Lac* on a holiday. They were there to conduct the third and final session (albeit the fourth actual meeting) of the working council, assembling under a self-imposed mandate to deal in some way with the issues that divided the physicians from the rest of the organization. Subsequent memory has made of this Tahoe Conference and the Tahoe Agreement that resulted from it a legendary encounter. Very soon, the Tahoe Conference became, justifiably, a watershed in the history of the organization.

At Tahoe, first of all, the founder, Sidney Garfield, for so long caught between his brother-in-law Henry J. Kaiser and the Permanente physicians, was eased out of the line of authority with the consent of both parties. Here also, Henry J. Kaiser and his executives encountered, perhaps for the first time as far as their personal conviction was concerned, the steely, resistant will of the Permanente doctors refusing to become employees in the Kaiser organization. On the other hand, it also dawned on many of these very same Permanente physicians at Tahoe that the talk of their going it alone, of buying the Hospitals and themselves running the Health Plan, was impractical.

Surprisingly, no minutes were kept at the Tahoe Conference. Subsequent recollections by participants, however, describe scenes of heated debate, adversarial posturing, demands and counterdemands, with both sides taking time out to caucus. Eugene Trefethen, the point person in countless negotiations on behalf of Kaiser Industries, later described the Tahoe Conference as the toughest negotiating session he had ever experienced. It might have been tougher for Trefethen had Henry J. Kaiser been more active in the negotiations, but the evidence suggests that Kaiser attended only 1 day of the 3-day session.

"You're challenging me," Kaiser exploded at one point to Ray Kay, the feisty head of the Southern California Medical Group. "You're challenging me, and I won't stand for it."[10]

At this meeting, Ray Kay purposely talked very little, and he did not feel that Henry J. Kaiser's exasperation was legitimate. However, Ray Kay's *bete noir* and *idée fixe* was Clifford Keene. Kay internalized as a personal insult the notion that Kaiser wanted to place Keene, an outsider, over the Permanente Medical Groups. The fact that Keene was also a loyal Kaiser executive and a board-qualified surgeon with a distinguished military career and medical record only served to rub further salt into these wounds. In this resistance Kay was joined by Morris Collen, the leader of the northern Californian forces. Like Kay, Collen was an instinctive leader. Whereas Kay argued in the open, Collen worked in close and up front, countering his opponents with stiletto thrusts. Of all the physicians, Kaiser attorney George Link later recalled, "Morrie Collen was one of the persons who was particularly adamant on the concept that it was their Health Plan and they really didn't need the kind of management they were getting from the Kaiser people."[11]

Heading the Kaiser side of the negotiations from the vantage point of being the chair was Eugene Trefethen, who stood as close to Henry J. Kaiser as anyone. A close fraternity friend of Edgar Kaiser's at U.C. Berkeley, Trefethen had joined Kaiser as a young man out of the Harvard Business School. By the mid-1950s Trefethen had become the de facto prime minister of Kaiser Industries. Loyal to his friend Edgar

Kaiser, Trefethen nevertheless enjoyed a unique relationship with Mr. Kaiser. It was Trefethen who had told Cecil Cutting that whatever Kaiser people were involved in, they ran; and yet, it was Trefethen also who had guided the first two sessions of the working council to whatever levels of reconciliation had been achieved. In the long run, it was Trefethen who in many ways saved the program and facilitated its necessary realignment of power and responsibility.

Henry J. Kaiser had said that he wanted his brother-in-law Sidney Garfield removed from all administrative responsibilities, whether in the Health Plan, the Hospitals, or the medical groups. The day before the Tahoe Conference convened, Kaiser had sat Garfield down in his home office in Lafayette and asked him to resign. Lambreth Hancock, who was there, remembers Garfield fighting back like a tiger. "He didn't want it taken away from him," Hancock recalled. "And this is with people who loved him very dearly, starting with Mr. Kaiser, his brother-in-law. But it had to be done. It finally came to a point where Mr. Kaiser finally had to say, 'Sidney, whether you want it or not, it's got to be done'."[12]

Believing that he would be backed at Tahoe by the medical groups, a shaken Garfield agreed to resign—but only if the medical groups approved. "I didn't think they would," Garfield admitted. "When [Kaiser] met with them the next day, they accepted it immediately. I felt let down. They tacked onto it that they would not accept Cliff Keene in that position. After that, my job was planning and building facilities."[13]

From the perspective of attorney George Link, Henry J. Kaiser was justified in, as Hancock described it, defrocking Sidney. "Management had to be clarified," Link believed, "and as long as Sidney was there, it was going to be a mishmash. Sidney never did get out completely, but the responsibilities began to really get divided at Tahoe." Even after this defrocking, however, Garfield worked as an advisor to the Permanente Medical Groups which had acquiesced in his removal. "He was in there constantly talking to them and advising them," George Link remembered, "...on a kind of *sub rosa* basis."[14]

"I made two big mistakes," Garfield later admitted. "I turned over control of the Hospitals to the Board of Trustees with complete faith that we could continue to run it the way we wanted to. I turned over control of the Partnership to the partners with complete faith that they would let me work with them and continue as I had been. I learned my lessons."[15]

Garfield left Tahoe as executive vice president of facilities and planning. Clifford Keene, however, was not promoted as Garfield's replacement. Kaiser and his executives had bargained away Clifford Keene's position, agreeing that Keene would not be given a top management position but would remain a liaison between the Hospitals, the Health Plan, and the Kaiser organization. Not until June 1960, seven years after he had come out from Willow Run, was Clifford Keene made vice president and general manager of the Kaiser Foundation Hospitals and Health Plan. By that time, the power struggles of the mid-1950s were over. "While no one sent me several dozen American Beauty roses to put on my desk," Keene said of his long-deferred promotion, "no one threw any bricks either."[16]

4

After 3 days of continuing and frequently stormy discussion, the Tahoe Conference resulted in a document entitled "Decisions of Working Council," subsequently known as the Tahoe Agreement. Dated July 19, 1955, and prepared by George Link, the working council secretary, the Tahoe Agreement contained six major provisions.

First and most importantly, there was an expression of commitment from all parties that the medical care program had to be preserved and that all entities within Kaiser-Permanente must seek to find a working relationship among themselves. To that end, an advisory council, composed of key representatives of the Health Plan, the Hospitals, and the various medical groups would be permanently established. There would also be the creation of regional management teams that would integrate at the level of staff authority the regional Health Plan manager, the Hospital manager, and the key physician administrators of each region. All major problem areas were to be covered by the contract. Such problem areas would include the approval of Health Plan contracts, the question of advertisement and/or solicitation, the establishment of continuity of contract with the Health Plan, and the assurance that the Health Plan would not develop competitive groups in the regions. Fifthly, financial arrangements were established and agreed upon in which both the Hospitals and the Permanente Medical Groups would be supported in their basic needs. Excess revenue would be equally distributed. Finally, Permanente Services, to be jointly owned by the Hospitals and the Medical Groups, would be established as a service organization supporting all entities.

Each side gained, and each side gave up something. The physicians had secured the right to review and approve the individuals and the groups who were to be enrolled in the Health Plan. They could now monitor the delicate area of how the Health Plan contacted prospective members, an activity that the medical societies monitored with watchdog surveillance as they hunted for instances of unethical solicitation. The medical groups also could now formulate and approve the terms and conditions of proposed contracts with Health Plan members and had the responsibility for handling all medically related claims and complaints. In this way, physicians would not have to be evaluated on medical matters by lay administrators. In one sense these were minor gains in that they were prerogatives that the physicians had always been exercising; but now they were formalized by agreement. More importantly, the medical groups gained a measure of psychological security in the promise of the Health Plan not to contract with other medical groups within the various service areas as long as a high standard of medical care continued to be provided. Thus the medical groups countered Henry J. Kaiser's constantly reiterated preference for smaller, competing medical groups. This exclusivity represented a major gain.

On the other hand, the medical groups surrendered all claims to ownership and control of the Health Plan and the Hospitals. In return, the physicians gained the right to participate at the policy-making level on the advisory council. The physicians thus theoretically reestablished themselves in the management of the organization, for the advisory council would supervise all administrative and operational functions. The advisory council would serve as the sole channel between the regional management teams, the trustees and directors, and the executive committees of the medical groups. The advisory council was empowered to initiate matters on its own volition and to review for recommendation all matters scheduled to go before the trustees and the directors. Theoretically at least, the physicians would no longer be the recipients of the unilateral decisions of Kaiser executives. In the matter of personnel, especially in the sensitive appointments of regional managers and hospital administrators, the advisory council was empowered to review all appointments and removals in key positions before action could be taken: another major gain by the medical groups.

All these powers assigned to the advisory council were ultimately advisory in nature. The advisory council possessed no absolute authority. Each entity, including the medical groups, retained full authority to disregard the recommendations of the advisory council and to take such actions as it felt necessary and proper. Despite this purely advisory role, the advisory council did represent a convergence of medical and lay responsibilities. While adhering to a clear distinction between medical and nonmedical lines of authority, the advisory council brought physicians and lay administrators into a dialogue that contained within itself the elements of an ultimate solution.

The advisory council was set up to include a medical group representative for each 100,000 members of the Health Plan. Baritell, Collen, Cutting, and Neighbor represented The Permanente Medical Group in northern California. Kay, Frederick H. Scharles, and Herman Weiner represented the Southern California Permanente Medical Group. Ernest Saward was appointed to represent the Permanente Clinic in Oregon. Henry J. Kaiser, Edgar F. Kaiser, E. E. Trefethen, Jr., and George Link represented the trustees. Two other physicians, Sidney Garfield and Clifford Keene, also came on as trustee representatives. Thus the advisory council had 10 physicians and 4 laypeople, a very favorable ratio of MDs. The physicians had effectively lobbied their case at the Tahoe Conference.

The Tahoe Agreement also established a framework for interentity cooperation at the regional and unit levels. Regional management teams were created in northern and southern California. These regional management teams were established to maintain a medical care program in the region of high quality at reasonable cost; to review matters scheduled to go before the advisory council and to serve as a direct channel between regional personnel and the advisory council; and to coordinate and review all activities within the region of the Health Plan, the Hospitals, and Permanente Services. These regional management teams were not intended to supersede existing administrative structures. Each of the regional entities in the Health Plan, the Hospitals, and the medical groups retained its basic authority and responsibilities.

From the start, the regional management teams differed from each other. No regional management team, for instance, was established in Oregon-Washington. Without any objections being voiced by the trustees at the Tahoe Conference, Ernest Saward, MD, the medical director of the Permanente Clinic in Oregon became the de facto chief executive officer for the Health Plan and the Hospitals. In northern California, a complete regional management team was appointed, with Collen and Cutting representing The Permanente Medical Group, Baritell representing Permanente Services, Hal Babbitt representing the Health Plan, and Felix Day representing the Hospitals. A doctor rotated as chairperson every 6 months. In southern California, by contrast, Ray Kay became the permanent chair. Nor were places on the regional management team necessarily attached to specific constituencies among the various Kaiser-Permanente entities.

The Tahoe Conference also created a third level of administration called area management teams. These area management teams consisted of the physician-in-chief or associate medical director of each area and the local hospital administrator. At Tahoe it was agreed that neither the physician-in-chief nor the hospital administrator could, without prior mutual consultation, take any action that might affect the other. In northern California—but not in southern California—this consultation had to be evidenced in writing. In both this and the matter of the more informal method of selection to the regional management team, southern California seems to have been a more trusting place.

The Tahoe Agreement failed to create a precise plan for the distribution of money. It did, however, spell out the principles to be followed in paying the costs of the Hospitals and medical groups. Joseph Reis was designated to develop the necessary financial information to determine contract prices. Hospitals would receive a portion of Health Plan revenues sufficient to pay the costs of operations, research, charitable and educational activities, and the amortization of loans, together with a fixed percentage of hospital assets to be used either for expansion or for the amortization of loans in areas that did not produce sufficient income. The medical groups, the Health Plan, and the Hospitals would receive a share of income sufficient to cover their base needs. Any excess above this base would be shared between the Hospitals and medical groups on a negotiated percentage basis. The medical groups might use this excess revenue at their own discretion for the improvement of medical services. The Hospitals would use the excess at the discretion of the trustees for additional research, charitable care, construction of facilities, or other activities consistent with the role of hospitals.

"Lake Tahoe was a traumatic period," Cecil Cutting reminisced with typical understatement. "We had the feeling that we would either come back with some sort of compromise, or we'd have no program."[17]

The Tahoe Agreement did not end all controversy, but for all its weaknesses, which would soon appear, the Tahoe Agreement did delineate the compromise that Cutting correctly believed to be necessary. The Kaiser-Permanente medical program had over the 20-plus previous years developed as an activity that encompassed the profession of medicine, the profession of management, and the social responsibilities belonging to both management and medicine. Whatever its sketchiness, the Tahoe Agreement acknowledged that while the practice of medicine was the responsibility of physicians, experienced managers had much to add to the operation of medical systems. Nowhere was this more apparent than in finance. After Tahoe, the doctor-patient relationship stood reaffirmed, but there also emerged a new respect between medicine and management in the service of patients. It would take a few more tumultuous years for this newly asserted mutuality of respect to solidify itself as a permanent feature of the Kaiser-Permanente corporate culture. Perceived in retrospect as a watershed, as a near-legendary battle of giants, the Tahoe Conference and the subsequent agreement set the stage for the more viable solutions and the more lasting agreements that were to come.

5

The advisory council established by the Tahoe agreement was intended as an administrative solution to the problem of sharing authority between the physicians and the Kaiser organization. In point of fact, the advisory council became a continuation of the Tahoe deliberations. The advisory council met seven times between August 1955 and June 1956. There were no meetings between February 16–17 and June 21, 1956, which means that the advisory council held most of its deliberations in the 5 months following the Tahoe Conference. In addition to its appointed representatives, the advisory council was assisted by a small staff, which included Joseph F. Reis, a senior Kaiser financial officer, Scott Fleming, later the senior vice president and manager of the Oregon region, and Arthur Weissman, a medical economist. Also attending advisory council sessions and acting as resources were Karl Steil, southern California Health Plan manager; his brother Paul, a regional manager for southern California; Sam Hufford, Oregon-Washington regional manager; Karl Palmaer, a financial advisor; L. E. Bullis, an accountant; Hal Babbitt, northern California Health Plan manager; William Price, northern California comptroller; and E. B. Dodds, the representative for properties. The inner staff, Reis, Fleming, and Weissman, reported directly to Eugene Trefethen and devoted its full energies to working on the problems of the Kaiser-Permanente program. Dealing with these problems became the fundamental business of these 6 months of intense advisory council sessions.

"In retrospect," Scott Fleming later wrote, "I see this as a period of necessary preparation for a fundamental restructuring of the program in which a synthesis of essential elements from contradictory positions created a mutually acceptable and constructive outcome."[18]

Since Fleming served as secretary to the advisory council and took extensive notes, it is easy to see that this synthesis was achieved only after intense conflict. The climate of emotional antagonism that preceded the Tahoe conference did not disappear with the signing of the Tahoe agreement. The removal of Sidney Garfield had been a traumatic event, putting long-established friendships and associations under severe strain. Whatever his faults, Sidney Garfield, the founder, had also served as a liaison between the Kaiser camp and the doctors. In his idiosyncratic way, Sidney Garfield had kept the program together. The Kaiser executives and the Permanente physicians now faced each other without his mediating influence. To complicate matters, the regional management teams established at Tahoe did not work out as they were intended. The teams tended to polarize along the familiar lines of physicians versus Kaiser management. In northern California, management by committee proved especially cumbersome. The regional hospital administrator, for example, purchased a large order of manual typewriters just as electric typewriters were becoming available. The regional management team spent several meetings trying to decide which secretaries would get electric typewriters and who would end up with manual models.

To review Scott Fleming's minutes of the advisory council meetings is to encounter debates and confrontations that represent a continuation of the Tahoe sessions. The first meeting, held on August 2, 1955, in Oakland, was concerned mainly with administrative matters. Officially, Garfield's forced resignation as executive director of the Kaiser Foundation Health Plan and Hospitals was accepted. The position of executive director was itself eliminated. Keene resigned as medical director of the Health Plan and Hospitals. That position was also eliminated. When the Kaiser Foundation transferred its assets to Kaiser Foundation Hospitals on June 30, 1955, Clifford Keene was appointed program coordinator, in charge of the charitable, educational, and research activities of both the Kaiser Foundation and the Kaiser Foundation Hospitals.

From these initial minutes and from the minutes of the subsequent meetings of the advisory council, it is apparent that the central authority in the program had become Eugene Trefethen, Jr., executive vice president of the Kaiser Foundation Health Plan and Hospitals, the job that Clifford Keene had been promised but would have to wait until 1960 to attain.

Throughout his career in the Kaiser organization, Trefethen functioned as an alter ego for Henry J. Kaiser and a close personal friend and associate of Edgar Kaiser's. Henry J. Kaiser respected Trefethen enormously. When Trefethen spoke, Kaiser listened. During the Tahoe period, Trefethen bore the major responsibility for orchestrating the discussions. Having long since grown reluctant to face directly the physicians he could not control, Kaiser had delegated to Trefethen major responsibilities, not only to serve as executive vice president of the Health Plan and the Hospitals, but to negotiate with the medical groups. Ironically, the medical groups were willing to accept Trefethen in such a leadership role in a way that they would never accept Clifford Keene. "Trefethen was the main guy," Ray Kay later remembered. "Edgar [Kaiser] was a sweet lovely guy. When we'd have the fights, we'd go to Edgar. But Edgar would agree with everybody, and he was a sweet guy. Trefethen was the guy we had to fight with, and Trefethen was the guy you really had to work out a problem with. He was the one that counted."[19]

At the second meeting of the advisory council, held on August 8, 1955, the debate on personnel appointments surfaced immediately. At Tahoe it had been agreed that the doctors, operating through the advisory council and the regional management teams, would have review and recommendation rights regarding key administrators. But then a Kaiser executive by the name of Fred Tennant, who had not even come out of the Foundation, the Health Plan, or the Hospitals, was made regional manager for northern California. The Permanente physicians were furious that a Kaiser Industries executive should be unilaterally appointed to such a major position. Requesting an executive session of the advisory council, Ray Kay read a strong statement protesting the bypassing of the advisory council in personnel matters, contrary to the Tahoe Agreement. Kay also protested the fact that in organizational charts Keene, now a program coordinator with the Health Plan and Hospitals, was shown as being in a line capacity between the executive vice president and the operating level of management.

Trefethen disagreed. Hospital administrators and comparable managers, he argued, must have line responsibility to the board of directors. The concept of such line authority was part of the Tahoe understandings. Line responsibility extended from the operating management levels to the executive vice president, who represented the directors of the entire program and its entities. The executive vice president – meaning himself, Trefethen – or someone in his place would continue to have line authority and responsibility. Finally, Trefethen pointed out, both the advisory council and regional management teams were advisory bodies only. Edgar Kaiser attempted to soften Trefethen's hard-line position, emphasizing the powers of review that had been granted to the advisory council. Morris Collen argued that the regional management teams and the advisory council possessed an importance and dignity at least equal to direct management authority. Edgar Kaiser then suggested that the executive vice president, Trefethen, also had heavy responsibilities for other Kaiser Company enterprises. He needed an assistant, and Clifford Keene should fill that position. The medical groups agreed with the need for assistance but as usual objected to any line authority being granted Clifford Keene. They preferred that Keene should work as a staff assistant to Trefethen. Not wishing to push the point, Trefethen agreed. Obviously, some new organizational chart was needed for the Kaiser-Permanente program. A subcommittee of Trefethen, Collen, and Cutting was appointed to draw up such an organizational chart. The task was never completed.

The third meeting of the advisory council, held 4 weeks later on September 8, 1955, centered on another perennial problem, money. The Tahoe Agreement, Trefethen pointed out, provided for the establishment of the base needs of the Health Plan, the Hospitals, and the medical groups. Any excess over these base needs was to be shared by the medical groups and the Hospitals on the basis of a negotiated percentage. This agreement, Trefethen argued, could be interpreted in two ways. Contracts could be drawn up providing a percentage division of total revenue in which all parties would bear all risks and enjoy all benefits. Or there could be contracts that fixed only the percentage of excess revenues to be shared by the medical groups and the Hospitals. Trefethen stated that he had understood the Tahoe Agreement to mean the first alternative, namely, that all entities would bear all risks and enjoy all benefits. Collen indicated that he had understood the second alternative, namely, that the medical groups and the Hospitals were entitled to a fixed percentage of excess revenues without their being a commitment to financial liability for the entire program. Both Trefethen and Collen, however, agreed that the language of the Tahoe Agreement could bear either interpretation. Scott Fleming was commissioned to draft a restatement of this section of the Tahoe Agreement.

In October 1955, the advisory council met twice, on October 5 and 6, and again on October 26 and 27. At the first meeting, Fleming submitted a redraft of the revenue-sharing statement, and Trefethen suggested that ultimately this matter would have to be settled by a contract. At the second meeting, Trefethen introduced a list of further areas to be covered by future contractual arrangements between the Kaiser Foundation Health Plan and the medical groups. The advisory council unanimously agreed to this solution of problems through contractual agreements. Again, as in the past, contractual agreements served as sign posts to future solutions. Not that these October meetings were unanimous–they were not. At the second October session, the medical groups asserted that no person or entity outside the medical groups had any standing in determining the compensation payable to an individual doctor. The medical groups also expressed their belief that all interim financial arrangements between themselves and the other entities contained an overly rigid commitment to fixed-price contracts. There had to be more flexibility.

The remaining four meetings of the advisory council accomplished little, if anything. By the last meeting, June 21, 1956, it was apparent to everyone that the advisory council would not continue as a permanent part of the Kaiser-Permanente administrative structure. All was not lost, however. Contractual solutions to problems had emerged in the most fruitful of the sessions. Trefethen was keeping his staff busy developing a series of contract proposals between the Kaiser Foundation Health Plan and the Permanente Medical Groups. These contract proposals eventually came to be known as the Medical Service Agreements, and they were to take the program into a new era.

Another development in evidence was the emergence of a well-staffed central office. In the first era, Sidney Garfield constituted the central office. In 1951 Henry J. Kaiser hired Arthur Weissman of the U.S. Public Health Service to gather statistical information for the program. In the fall of 1952, Scott Fleming, a young attorney in the Kaiser legal department, was detailed to work with the medical care program. In 1954 Clifford Keene arrived. Keene formed a close working relationship with Fleming and Weissman, whom he considered one of the most brilliant people he had ever met. By the end of 1955 the central office staff consisted of Sidney Garfield, Clifford Keene, Joseph Reis, Arthur Weissman, Karl Palmaer, and Scott Fleming. Having attended all sessions of the advisory council, these administrators were thoroughly familiar with the concerns of the Permanente physicians. It was this group, then, working with the medical groups, that set about developing the Medical Service Agreements. The central office had replaced Sidney Garfield as the buffer zone.

In the field, meanwhile, at the operating level, smooth working relationships between physicians and lay administrators were also being established. In 1950, when the Permanente program moved to southern California, Paul Steil was hired from the Justin Dart Industry. Steil and Garfield became close friends. When Garfield was divorced from his first wife Virginia, he depended upon Steil as a source of moral support for both him and his former wife. Paul Steil watched over the care of Virginia Garfield during her final illness. Although Steil later quarreled with Ray Kay and left Kaiser-Permanente, he introduced his brother Karl to the program. In 1956 Trefethen recommended Karl Steil as regional manager in southern California, and the Southern California Permanente Medical Group concurred. An instinctive diplomat committed to working with the physicians, Karl Steil did much to soothe the tensions of this era. Such successful working associations at critical administrative staff levels created a counterforce to the confrontations of this period. It was already apparent that the Kaiser-Permanente medical program, so comprehensive, so intricate, ever-growing, needed many types of talent to flourish.

_____ **6** _____

In November 1955 Eugene Trefethen convened a meeting at the Kaiser headquarters in Oakland of the top central office staff, which was by then reporting directly to him. The advisory council, Trefethen told the staff, was not working. Where should the program go next? A freewheeling discussion ensued. At its conclusion, Trefethen summarized the proceedings. There were, he stated, five priorities that could satisfactorily restructure the program.

First of all, there needed to be a specific proposal for a method of contracting between the Health Plan and the medical groups. Second, an organizational structure had to be devised that would integrate the medical and the administrative components. Third, management by committee would never work and should be abandoned. The fourth and fifth priorities dealt with finance. Fourth, there was a need to develop some kind of incentive system to provide the Permanente physicians a financial stake in the effective operation of the program. Fifth, the physicians needed a retirement plan. Trefethen charged his staff to develop these proposals within all applicable legal, ethical, and financial constraints. Relieved from their advisory council activities, the staff went to work through the remaining weeks of 1955 and on into the spring of 1956. The staff developed proposals centered upon eight avenues of concern and solution. Each of these eight policy areas became an important building block of the Medical Service Agreements, which saved the program and should thus be itemized and listed separately.

Per capita method of contracting. Previously, contracts between the Health Plan and the medical groups had been based primarily on a percentage of prepaid dues. The staff proposed that the payment system now be based on a mutually agreed upon per capita rate. This way, revenue was closely tied to actual operating experience.

Minimum capital generation requirement. The minimum requirement for the financial stability of the Health Plan and Hospitals could best be met by a straight-line depreciation plus 4 percent per year of the historical cost of the land, buildings, and equipment utilized in the program. A base line was now established. The program must generate revenues to meet its basic per capita costs and depreciation plus 4 percent. Such obligations constituted the minimum consistent with long-term financial self-sufficiency.

Incentive compensation. Once the formula for minimum capital generation had been established, the question of excess revenues reasserted itself. These additional earnings were to be divided equally between the medical groups and the Hospitals as a financial embodiment of the partnership concept, as a financial incentive for the physicians, and as a means to increase Hospital earnings from the minimum to adequate levels.

The program revenue concept. Revenue from all sources should be combined into a single total of revenue available to support all operations of the program. Because of legal and ethical concerns, only revenue from house calls was exempted. House call revenue belonged exclusively to the medical groups.

Regional financial autonomy. Each region should be considered financially autonomous in terms of revenue and accountability.

Simplified organizational structure. The Kaiser Foundation should no longer function as an ownership or holding entity. The Foundation had already made a donation of all facilities to Kaiser Foundation Hospitals. It should now cancel the balance due on the promissory note. From now on there should be three major entities in the program: the Health Plan, the Hospitals, and the medical groups.

The joint management concept. The regional management teams were not working and should be abandoned. The partnership concept, however, must be kept intact. There should therefore be a joint medical director–regional manager concept. The medical director would be the chief executive of the medical group. The regional manager would be the chief executive of the hospitals and Health Plan in the region. Each of them would be responsible for the functioning of their respective organizations, and they would be jointly responsible for the effective functioning of the total program in the region. The joint management concept also implied the right of review and concurrence in the matter of key personnel appointments.

Physicians' retirement plan. Since the program was now nearly 15 years into its formal operation, it was necessary to explore the best possibilities for a retirement plan for the Permanente physicians. There should be a wholesale review of all legal and financial options.[20]

In his directives to his staff at the November 1955 meeting, Trefethen had urged them to emphasize the southern California region in their planning. At an advisory council meeting in February 1956, in fact, Trefethen had already sketched out possible solutions and had met with a favorable response from the southern California representatives. Despite the confrontational style of Ray Kay, relations between the physicians, the Health Plan, and the Hospitals in southern California were actually functioning more cordially than in the north. Ray Kay and Karl Steil were already working out a de facto joint management structure. Southern California was also in a period of major growth and was hence doubly anxious to achieve arrangements that would allow it to get on with the business of providing prepaid comprehensive health care to the rapidly expanding southland.

In the late spring of 1956, the Trefethen proposals were presented to the Southern California Permanente Medical Group. These proposals included the concepts of regional autonomy, per capita payment to the medical group on a per member per month basis, and an incentive compensation system that established a contingency fund of 30 cents per member per month. This fund could be increased by favorable operating results or decreased by unfavorable operating results in the region. Hospitals would receive 50 percent of this incentive fund for capital generation. The Medical Group would receive the other 50 percent as an incentive to provide good service, which would increase enrollment, and avoid any unnecessary utilization of resources. With some modifications, the Southern California Medical Group accepted the Trefethen proposals on a trial basis. This first Medical Service Agreement went into effect on January 1, 1957.

The Permanente Clinic in Oregon, by contrast, preferred to continue under the existing arrangements. Ernest Saward dominated the decision-making process in the Oregon region. The primary issue to Saward's way of thinking was not governance but the financing of a hospital on the Portland side of the Columbia River since few Portlanders wished to enroll in a program based in Vancouver, Washington.

It would take almost 2 years for The Permanente Medical Group in northern California to accept the Medical Service Agreement. Negotiations began in late July 1956 when The Permanente Medical Group received the proposed contract. The Health Plan and Hospitals were represented by Fred W. Tennant, recently named regional manager for northern California. The main point of contention was the insistence by the Health Plan that ancillary revenue belonged to the Health Plan. The Medical Group insisted that all ancillary revenue should belong to the Medical Group. In the discussions, the Medical Group pointed out that in the Southern California Agreement, private (nonmember), industrial, and house call fees were collected by the Southern California Medical Group. Morris Collen, as chair of the Executive Committee of the Medical Group, played a major role in these negotiations. Again and again Collen emphasized that the prime producer in the Kaiser-Permanente Medical Program was the individual physician. That meant that the individual physician had to be competitive in terms of his or her personal practice of medicine. It also meant that the individual physician was entitled to incentives for extra work or for an outstanding performance. That is why the question of ancillary revenue was so important. It provided an incentive to the physicians to competitive excellence.

On the other hand, Gardiner Johnson, legal counsel to the Medical Group, cautioned that there could be some legal and/or ethical difficulties in thus mixing a prepaid program within the framework of the nonprofit Health Plan and a system of competitive financial incentives. In October 1956 the executive committee informed the Health Plan that the question of ancillary revenue presented so many difficulties that discussions would have to continue. Eight months later, in May 1957, Collen reported to the partnership that negotiations were continuing in an encouraging fashion.

That same month, the executive committee created the position of executive director of The Permanente Medical Group. Collen was especially insistent that such a position was necessary now that each region had a regional manager representing the Health Plan and the Hospitals. As chair of the executive committee, Collen was a leading candidate for this position, as were Cecil Cutting and Monte Baritell. Each candidate had much to recommend him. Personable and articulate, Baritell had served as treasurer and chair of the finance committee and had an excellent understanding of the financial affairs of the program. Baritell had also played an important role in preparing medical group positions for working council and advisory council meetings before and after the Tahoe Conference. As chair of the executive committee, Morris Collen was already de facto leader of the medical group. For more than a decade Collen had been a key leader in the partnership. Both Baritell and Collen, however, were as controversial as they were effective. Having operated for so long at the center of resistance, they had made enemies in the Kaiser organization. The choice, then, revolved to the more conciliatory figure of Cecil Cutting.

With the organization since Grand Coulee, Cutting had remained a close personal friend of Sidney Garfield. After Garfield, Cutting was the senior physician active in the organization. Although Cutting could be firm in negotiation and debate, he was also by temperament and developed skill a patient listener whose even-handed approach to problems had earned him wide respect among his colleagues. On May 23, 1957, a majority of partners voting approved the appointment of Cecil Cutting as executive director of the medical group. "I think both Dr. Collen and Dr. Baritell were brighter," Cutting later stated with characteristic modesty. "They were more dynamic people than I, but I did seem to have the ability to calm things down a little bit."[21]

As executive director, Cutting represented the executive committee of the medical group in all management, coordination, and supervisory activities. At a later meeting, the executive committee granted the executive director all management functions that had been assigned the standing committees, which were discontinued. The executive committee also relinquished some of its long-held authority over expenditures, allowing the executive director to approve purchases of up to $1000.

After 6 years of struggle between the physicians and the Kaiser organization, the entire Kaiser-Permanente community had grown weary of infighting. With Cecil Cutting as negotiator, progress was made regarding the Medical Service Agreement. On March 27, 1958, the executive committee at long last approved the proposed contract, which was then discussed at a meeting of the partnership. A majority of the partners present also approved. The Medical Service Agreement of 1958 established a framework—a Mayflower Compact, if you will, a Constitution, and a Bill of Rights—between the Kaiser Foundation Health Plan and The Permanente Medical Group which has lasted to this day. With clarity and simplicity, major points of contention fell quietly into place after long struggle and debate.

Several introductory sections of the agreement described the nature
and functions of the Health Plan and the Medical Group and the relationships these entities had to each other. While these sections made
clear that the Health Plan and the Medical Group were separate and
autonomous organizations, it was also stated that the Health Plan would
contract exclusively with The Permanente Medical Group so long as the
group would satisfactorily serve the needs of the Health Plan and the
membership. Similarly, the Medical Group would contract exclusively
with the Health Plan and not render professional services to any other
prepayment plan in the area. A list of specific medical and hospital services for which the Medical Group was responsible in the Health Plan's
contracts with members was spelled out. Excluded were psychiatric
care, cosmetic surgery, fertility studies, intentionally self-inflicted injuries, alcoholism, and a long list of communicable diseases. Some of these
excluded categories would later be included in Health Plan coverage.

Most significantly, the Health Plan no longer threatened to divide
The Permanente Medical Group into smaller partnerships. The Medical Group, moreover, retained the right to review all terms of all contracts with members as well as review the addition of new enrollees. The
Health Plan, for its part, was prohibited from advertising or soliciting
for a medical practice. The physicians thus protected themselves against
charges of solicitation, an unethical practice by the standards of the
time.

A major part of the Medical Service Agreement dealt with financial
matters. The Health Plan assumed responsibility for collecting revenue
and providing facilities and equipment. Responsibility for handling
claims was divided. The Medical Group was responsible for handling
claims primarily related to medical services. The Health Plan retained
responsibility for claims over disputed benefits and enrollee contract
provisions.

Ending one major point of contention in advisory council meetings, a
definition of net Health Plan revenue was agreed upon. Specifically,
funds generated for and contributed to capital—including depreciation
plus 4 percent of the historical cost of land, buildings, and equipment—
were not considered as part of the net Health Plan revenue. The definition of Health Plan revenue also clarified the long dispute over the
issue of ancillary revenues collected at the point of service—registration
fees, for example, supplemental charges for laboratory and X-ray procedures, and co-payments for obstetrical care. Such revenues belonged
to the Health Plan. Fees for medical services rendered by Permanente
physicians to nonmembers, however, fees for industrial care, witness

fees, fees for rendering medical reports, and income from the sale of medical equipment were excluded from Health Plan revenue and could be collected and retained by the Medical Group.

The base compensation to the Medical Group was explicitly stated. Instead of a negotiated percentage of dues, it became a capitation contract based on a per member per month compensation. A refreshingly simple formula established incentive compensation. The Health Plan agreed to pay the Medical Group 50 percent of the net Health Plan revenue, if any. The Hospitals received the other fifty percent of net revenue, if any, to be used in community service activities or in the generation of capital. The agreement specified the method by which net revenue would be calculated, together with the frequency of payment of net revenue to the Medical Group. The Medical Group retained sole responsibility for establishing a method of distribution to individuals within the Medical Group. This allowed the physicians the freedom and flexibility in establishing incentives for both performance and recruitment.

In the matter of retirement, the Medical Service Agreement provided for the payment of 12 cents per Health Plan member per month to a Bank of America trust fund for a retirement program for physicians of the Medical Group. The Medical Group was assured that the Internal Revenue Service would approve this plan; subsequently, however, the IRS ruled that these funds represented current and taxable earnings by the Permanente physicians.

With the signing of the Medical Service Agreement nearly 3 years after the Tahoe Agreement, a threat to the survival of the Kaiser-Permanente program was successfully resolved. Cecil Cutting, who would lead the Northern California Permanente Medical Group into the era of expansive cooperation that was to follow, gave much of the credit for this successful resolution to Eugene Trefethen, who had assumed responsibility for solving the crisis.

"I think the thing that broke the road block," Cutting later stated, "was Mr. Trefethen's coming up with the specific contractual relationship."[22]

Said Trefethen, "The relationship and the arrangement passed all the tests because all parties believed in what we were doing in our approach to meeting health care needs."[23]

9

Progress, Evolution, and Continuing Challenges— 1957–1961

––––––––––––––––––– 1 –––––––––––––––––––

Throughout the mid-1950s, the Kaiser-Permanente Health Plan continued to grow. At the end of 1955, the year of the Tahoe Agreement, Health Plan membership in northern California stood at slightly more than 301,000. Over the next 5 years, 98,000 new members were enrolled. This rapid expansion focused the attention of the Medical Group upon the critical area of physician recruitment. The Medical Group calculated that it needed one new physician for every thousand new Health Plan enrollees. This meant the recruitment of more than 98 physicians between 1955 and 1960. Not only did physicians have to be recruited, the entire cadre of physicians had to be allocated correctly throughout the northern California region.

Demographics was a nascent science in the mid-1950s; hence it was difficult to predict exactly how or where membership would be developing in the northern California region. It was also difficult to predict which medical departments would incur the greatest volume of patients. The recruitment of new physicians and the assignment of the entire complement of physicians in the Medical Group depended upon such information. Already, some departments were short of personnel while others were adequately staffed.

The Executive Committee had learned to depend upon the chiefs of departments as the key to successful medical operations both in terms of forecasting and ongoing medical care. The burden of balancing quality of care and economics rested squarely on the shoulders of these department chiefs, which further reinforced Morris Collen's constantly reiterated point that in the Kaiser-Permanente program, the individual physician was the profit center. A procedure evolved in which the department chief, perceiving backed-up demand, initiated a request for an additional physician. If the physician-in-chief concurred, he obtained the approval of the executive director, Cecil Cutting. It was up to the department chief to recruit and negotiate with candidates. The additional physician was not hired, however, until the Executive Committee reviewed and approved his or her qualifications. By the late 1950s, starting salaries for Permanente physicians ranged from $800 to $1000 per month.

Not only did new physicians have to be recruited to keep up with growth, replacements had to be hired for physicians leaving the Medical Group. Most physicians leaving the group were salaried employees, not partners. Some left voluntarily, seeking other opportunities; others were encouraged to leave for a variety of reasons, including unfavorable reviews of their medical practice with the group. Each new physician was expected to serve 3 years as a full-time salaried employee before becoming eligible for election to partnership. During the third year, the physician employee was classified as a "participant" and received a modest bonus. New participants and partners were elected each July.

The question of compensation remained a matter for internal discussion in the Medical Group. In the late autumn of 1956, the Health Plan provided the funds to increase physician compensation by an overall 5 percent. The Executive Committee proposed a uniform across-the-board increase of 5 percent for each Permanente physician. At a partnership meeting before Christmas 1956, several partners protested this across-the-board increase because it did not reward excellence in medical practice and other positive contributions to the success of the group. They dubbed this across-the-board increase a reward for mediocrity. The partners nevertheless ratified the Executive Committee's proposal. An across-the-board increase, however, was never repeated. Subsequent adjustments of salary or drawing account were considered merit increases.

The Medical Group was acutely aware that both poor-quality medical care and underservice cost money, and all such costs mitigated against incentive earnings within the Medical Group. A patient, for example, who suffered medical complications as a result of inappropriate diagnosis or treatment could require additional expensive hospitalization and physician care. If such a patient had to go outside the Kaiser-Permanente system to receive such follow-up care, the Hospitals paid all outside hospital expenses, and the Medical Group paid outside physician claims. These outside expenses, so many of them unnecessary in the first place, cost the partnership and the program money. Even when subsequent corrective care was provided within the Kaiser-Permanente system, it represented an additional drain on physician and hospital resources.

To ensure quality control, an informal but strong peer review system was generated. Second opinions on all diagnoses and treatment were readily available. The medical records of each patient were seen by each physician concerned with that patient. Physicians who created more than their share of unnecessary expenses through the poor quality of their treatment were encouraged to leave the Medical Group.

However, despite all such precautions, organized medical societies continued to voice their disfavor. The Solano County Medical Society denied membership to the Permanent physicians in Vallejo. The San Francisco Medical Society admitted only a few Permanente physicians. A meeting was arranged between the leaders of the San Francisco Medical Society and the chiefs of departments of The Permanente Medical Group based in San Francisco. This dialogue eventually brought forth many beneficial results as a growing number of Permanente physicians applied to the San Francisco Medical Society and were accepted. In Oakland, Richmond, and Walnut Creek, Permanente physicians began increasingly to be regarded as part of the professional community. Permanente physicians served on committees of the Alameda–Contra Costa Medical Society and participated regularly in its affairs. Even members of these nondiscriminatory medical societies, however, continued to counsel physicians against joining The Permanente Medical Group. This hurt.

"I know it has bothered you," Sidney Garfield remarked of this continuing opposition in his fifteenth anniversary speech, "and it may have disturbed your wives. I can speak with authority on this subject because I am a battle-scarred veteran of opposition. The appearances I have made before councils, committees, and so on, would fill a book. Almost invariably, when I have come out of one of those meetings, I have felt good. Most of the opposition was based on misinformation and lack of real knowledge of our objectives and Plan. When I had an opportunity to tell the doctors about us, as I did in those instances, they liked what they heard."[1]

Garfield's optimism restrained the response of the Medical Group to what it considered unfair resistance and discrimination. For instance, the Medical Group could have obtained relief through the courts, had it elected to do so. Already, there were several powerful precedents. In Washington, DC, the District of Columbia Medical Society and the AMA were found to be in violation of the Sherman Act by denying membership to physicians associated with the Group Health association, a consumer-owned and sponsored prepaid group-practice plan. The Supreme Court upheld this decision, and similar decisions were handed down in Seattle and San Diego.

The Permanente Medical Group in northern California, however, chose not to force the issue through litigation. The Executive Committee established a standing committee on professional relations under the leadership of Dr. Robert King, which was charged with continuing the dialogue with organized medicine while remaining vigilant as to the rights of individual Permanente physicians. Such opposition, of course, could have been disastrous had not the Kaiser-Permanente program maintained its own hospitals. Since Permanente physicians could admit and care for Health Plan patients in Kaiser Foundation Hospitals, organized medicine could not prevent them from practicing their profession. In the matter of professional self-esteem, however, this persistent opposition continued to prove disquieting.

In January 1959, a thorn long in the side of prepaid group practice was extracted. Ever since 1953, the Kaiser-Permanente program had existed under the threat that the AMA might eventually declare all forms of prepaid group practice unethical, as advocated in the worrisome Resolution 16 brought up before the 1953 AMA convention but tabled for further study. In January 1959 the AMA Commission on Medical Care Plans chaired by Dr. Leonard Larson made its report. The Commission supported the tradition of freedom of choice of physician by the patient. It went on to acknowledge that such freedom included the right of the patient to choose a system of medical care or health plan. The very principle that threatened to be used against Kaiser-Permanente, freedom of choice, was now invoked in its defense. Commenting on the AMA report, the *San Francisco Chronicle* published an editorial cartoon showing a patient labeled as Prepaid Group Practice getting out of a hospital bed and asking his doctor, who was labeled the American Medical Association, "Now that I'm well, Doctor, what was wrong with me?"

Meanwhile, tensions in northern California continued between the Permanente physicians and the managers of the Health Plan and Hospitals, regardless of the Medical Service Agreement signed in 1958. The Permanente physicians resented the fact that they had not been consulted regarding the appointment of Fred Tennant as regional manager in April 1957, nor had they been consulted when Arthur Reinhart was appointed Health Plan manager during the same period. The doctors especially resented Tennant because he did not have a background in health-care administration but came, rather, from the Industrial Relations Department of the Kaiser Companies. Felix Day, by contrast, the regional administrator of the Kaiser Foundation Hospitals, had been with the program since Grand Coulee. Yet even Felix Day, with his long association with the Permanente program, came into conflict with some physicians when he appointed a hospital administrator who did not have the support of the medical center physician-in-chief. The physicians were not totally opposed to lay administrators. The Medical Group itself appointed Gerald C. Stewart as general administrator of the Medical Group on July 1, 1957, thereby implanting an element of lay administration at the core of the partnership.

In an effort to improve relations between the physicians and the administrators, a series of conferences was held between 1958 and 1960. The first conference, convened in the autumn of 1958, was considered a disaster by those who attended. The Executive Committee, physicians-in-chief, chiefs of major departments, and key managers from the Hospitals and the Health Plan met together at the Feather River Inn, a remote lodge 200 miles from Oakland. Jack Chapman, a member of Tennant's staff, arranged to have three professors on hand—one from Berkeley, another from Stanford, and the third from UCLA—with expertise in group dynamics. On the first day of the conference, the group assembled without an agenda. Two of the faculty facilitators arrived late and went to the front of the room. They sat quietly staring at the participants for about 10 minutes, saying nothing, smoking cigarettes, waiting for the confrontation to begin. The participants waited for the faculty to start talking about group dynamics. The minutes passed; the silence continued; the tension mounted.

Finally, one of the faculty facilitators broke the silence, saying, "We're here to talk about your problems."

From somewhere in the room, a Health Plan official offered loudly, "We don't have any problems."

At that, a Permanente physician retorted, "What do you mean we don't have any problems? We have a board of directors that is trying to control the doctors!"

A disorderly and acrimonious discussion ensued, angry invectives being hurled even during coffee breaks and meals. The academic advisors never succeeded in directing the conference into positive channels. When the participants rode by bus back to Oakland on Sunday afternoon, the atmosphere was subdued.

Two follow-up conferences for middle management personnel were held in 1959 in Santa Rosa. While not as acrimonious as the Feather River Inn Conference, these Santa Rosa meetings accomplished little. In May 1960 the first interregional management conference was held at the Mark Thomas Inn in Monterey. Sponsored by the central office, this conference brought together the key operating managers from Oregon-Washington, northern California, and southern California and had as its theme forecasting and planning for the decade 1960 to 1970. The dominant topic addressed by this Monterey conference was whether or not the program should continue to build new Kaiser Hospitals or to use community hospitals. Although membership in the Northern California Health Plan had increased to 365,000, no new Kaiser Foundation Hospitals had been constructed in this region since the completion of the facilities in Walnut Creek and San Francisco. A 50-bed hospital had been purchased in south San Francisco, however, and additional satellite clinics had been opened in Martinez, San Rafael, and Sunnyvale. Noting the construction of new hospitals in the other regions, the Permanente physicians in northern California grew progressively more dissatisfied. A shortage of hospital beds in northern California frequently made it difficult to admit patients.

The Monterey Conference, however, did successfully encourage long-range planning. Arthur Weissman of the central office predicted that the Kaiser-Permanente program was generating experiences, procedures, statistics, and other associated data that would eventually prove of great value to American medicine. Sidney Garfield, who the month previously had been appointed to the board of directors of the Health Plan as the best way to keep him active on the policy level after he had been stripped of his management role, urged the Kaiser-Permanente community to realign its interests toward the prevention of illness and the maintenance of health. The Kaiser-Permanente program, Garfield argued, should not be a sick plan but a health plan in the full sense of the term: an ongoing commitment to the maintenance of health in the membership. Garfield's appointment to the board of directors returned the physician-founder to the core of Health Plan power and authority, thereby returning Garfield to formal influence and bringing a Permanente-oriented physician into the core of the decision-making process in the Health Plan. As a director of the Health Plan, Garfield was in a key position to ease tensions between lay administrators and physicians. Placed beyond the fray, Garfield tended to become, increasingly, "Sid," the wise uncle to whom the family might come to help adjudicate differences.

The greatest strain placed on the Kaiser-Permanente program during the late 1950s resulted from Henry J. Kaiser's decision to establish a fourth region in Hawaii. Kaiser had first visited Hawaii with Bess and had fallen in love with the Islands. In the home Kaiser built for his second wife Alyce in Lafayette, he had the architect incorporate Hawaiian motifs. In 1954, Alyce and Henry Kaiser vacationed in Hawaii. Finding hotel accommodations scarce on Waikiki Beach, they rented a house near Diamond Head. In 1956, Henry J. Kaiser, then in his midseventies, retired from the active direction of the Kaiser Companies and moved to Hawaii with Alyce. For the first 6 months of his retirement, Henry J. Kaiser tried to relax.

A lifetime of vigorous activity, however, could not be brought to a halt so abruptly. As a young photographer, Kaiser had witnessed the rise of Miami as a tourist and convention city. Honolulu, he decided, possessed the same potential—if it were properly developed; and Kaiser, then 75, decided that he would be that developer. Spending $3 million for a beach site bordering on Waikiki, he began the Hawaiian Village Hotel complex, which included a 100-room hotel, 70 adjacent thatched-roof cottages, a 1000-seat convention auditorium, and a 14-story residential tower. By October 1960, when *Time* magazine profiled Kaiser's Hawaiian empire, he had completed 1600 hotel rooms, together with massive convention facilities. To support this frenzy of construction, Kaiser opened a Permanente Cement plant with an annual capacity of 1.7 million barrels. He also entered radio and television broadcasting, the tour boat business, and residential development at Hawaii Kai, a city unto itself. Among the homes he built was his own million dollar mansion on Mauna Loa Bay, which featured a competition-sized swimming pool, a restaurant-sized kitchen, and a Hollywood-style screening room.

Hawaii was offering Henry J. Kaiser a way of starting over in his midseventies. He awoke each morning at 5 and spent a good part of each day at construction sites, supervising every detail. Hawaii was providing Kaiser one last chance to play social planner. Hawaii Kai was in one sense a quasi-utopian community in shocking pink concrete (Kaiser's favorite color), in which every facility and detail would bear the unmistakable imprint of Henry J. Kaiser.

Kaiser also determined to create in Hawaii a health plan that he would run directly. As in the case of Walnut Creek, Kaiser plunged immediately into the construction of a hospital. A previous study by the Stanford Research Institute had indicated that Honolulu did not need another hospital. The local medical insurance plan, moreover, called the Hawaiian Medical Service Organization, was adequately meeting local needs. In January 1958, however, Kaiser began building a hospital on Waikiki Beach a few hundred yards from the Hawaiian Village hotel. He financed this effort with a $2.5 million grant from the Henry J. Kaiser Family Foundation. Concrete was poured before Kaiser had secured final approval from the Honolulu authorities. Among other disputed points, Kaiser had determined to surface the hospital in layers of lava rock, which the city building code forbade because it created crawl spaces for rats. Kaiser had the first two floors of the hospital sheathed in lava sheets before the planning authorities had an opportunity to protest.

During construction, Kaiser would visit the site as often as six times a day, urging a faster schedule. He would call Clifford Keene daily across the time zone, usually getting Keene on the phone by 7 in the morning Pacific Standard Time. "I am not a religious man," Keene later remarked of these early morning calls from Mr. Kaiser, "but when I woke each morning, I prayed for the end of the world before 7 A.M."[2] Midway through construction, Kaiser decided to use a $250,000 contingency reserve to add another story. Within 10 months, the hospital was completed.

During this extraordinary activity, Kaiser not only built a hospital, but he also personally recruited a medical staff. Upon moving permanently to the Islands, Kaiser and his wife began socializing with three socially prominent Honolulu physicians in fee-for-service practice. These physicians were not in partnership but were sharing office space. With typical persuasiveness, Kaiser prevailed upon the three to form a medical partnership that would then establish the medical program at the hospital under construction. Upon the advice of Eugene Trefethen, who warned that a Caucasian-only partnership would not succeed in multiracial Hawaii, Kaiser recruited two other prominent physicians, one of Chinese and the other of Japanese ancestry, to join the three Caucasian physicians in the original partnership.

Kaiser called on only one member of The Permanente Medical Group, Fred Pellegrin (whose luncheon steak Kaiser had once appropriated back in Lafayette) for assistance in establishing the Pacific Medical Associates, as the Hawaii partnership called itself. Clifford Keene and Scott Fleming from the central office were flown over to conduct a crash program in prepaid group medical practice for the newly recruited medical partners. In the summer of 1958, Keene and Fleming embarked upon a 2-week intensive seminar at the Hawaii Kai Hotel on the medical and economic aspects of prepaid group practice. Kaiser himself attended most of these sessions and did not hesitate to enter the discussions. His enthusiasm tended to sweep away any discussion of the special challenges and difficulties inherent in prepaid group medical practice. When the seminar was over, Kaiser bundled Keene and Fleming back on the plane to California. Keene had fully expected to be asked to stay on as an advisor, perhaps even medical director, in the early stages of the program; but Kaiser wanted to run this show himself.

Kaiser made only two appointments from the Health Plan on the mainland. Robert Jack, who had been business manager for the Southern California Permanente Medical Group, was appointed Medical Center administrator; and Fred Carroll, an experienced Health Plan representative from southern California, was made enrollment director. For his regional manager, Kaiser appointed Lambreth Hancock, a public relations aide-de-camp with no previous background in medical administration. Prior to this, Hancock served Kaiser as a construction and hotel manager at the Hawaiian Village, also without previous experience. Hancock assumed his new duties with the breezy self-confidence that was absolutely necessary for anyone having such a close working relationship with Henry J. Kaiser. "Fortunately," he later remembered, "the hotels helped me in getting going with the hospital, because hospital operations are basically the same as hotels. You have house guests, who are your patients, instead of the tourists. You have your prima donnas, which then would be the showpeople in hotels, Alfred Apaka and the orchestra and all that. At the hospital your prima donnas are your doctors. You have the same business problems of income and expenses. You have your same housekeeping problems. So hospitals and hotels are very similar. You don't have any bars to worry about, but you do have a pharmacy. So, you know, it was not that much of a shock as when I first tried to take over the Hawaiian Village."[4]

As Kaiser's Honolulu Medical Center neared completion in late 1958, Kaiser called Keene and asked for a list of supplies and equipment. Working at the accustomed fast-track Kaiser pace, Keene complied. Shortly after the Honolulu Medical Center opened on the last day of 1958, its shortcomings became obvious. The central elevators were too small to contain a hospital gurney, hence all interfloor transfer of patients had to be by service elevators only. The halls were not air-conditioned and the kitchen soon proved inadequate. The consulting architects had incorporated many of Sidney Garfield's innovative ideas on hospital design, including the outside access to patient rooms. Unfortunately, the severe tropical storms of Hawaii battered against these glass-enclosed outside corridors with telling effect. Flooding was frequent, and at the least, great drafts of air surged through the building during tropical storms. In 1986 the Honolulu Medical Center, constructed in 10 months in 1958, was dynamited to rubble after 28 years of use.

Health Plan enrollment also proved a disappointment. Actuarily, between 15,000 and 16,000 Health Plan members were necessary to start the program off on a sound fiscal basis. The Honolulu Medical Center opened with only 5000 enrollees. The Asian communities of the Honolulu area had strong personal attachments to their own fee-for-service physicians, many of them associated with the Hawaiian Medical Service Organization insurance plan. Recruitment from the Asian community proved difficult. With the exception of the ILWU and the Hotel and Restaurant Workers' Union, the Honolulu area did not support an extensive union community; hence recruitment in this area, a traditional source of Kaiser-Permanente enrollment on the mainland, proved a disappointment. After 18 months, enrollment had grown to 35,000; but this was still not enough to pay the costs of the Honolulu Medical Center and the 33 employee physicians under contract to Pacific Medical Associates.

By this time, the original five partners of Pacific Medical Associates were becoming increasingly disgruntled. In recruiting these physicians, Henry J. Kaiser had stressed financial incentives. When enrollment proved insufficient to generate surplus income, these incentives were not forthcoming. Furthermore, the partners found themselves in the position of exacting increasingly larger amounts of work from the physician employees in order to meet costs; hence the relationship between the partners and the employee physicians degenerated. In order to remain cost effective, moreover, group medical practice demands that each physician work daily on a consistent basis. When partners and employee physicians took unscheduled days off, as was possible in fee-for-service practice, the system, dependent as it was upon the advance scheduling of patients and medical services, suffered.

Under their agreement with Kaiser, the partners of Pacific Medical Associates were entitled to continue fee-for-service practice, thus violating a basic tenet of prepaid group-practice medical care. Complaints were soon forthcoming that fee-for-service patients at the Honolulu Medical Center, many of them wealthy tourists from the mainland, were receiving the red carpet while prepaid Health Plan patients were receiving second-tier treatment. Nor were the partners and many of the employee physicians accustomed to the consistent economies that prepaid practice demanded. In fee-for-service practice such costs — such as multiple tests and X-rays — can be passed on to patients. In prepaid practice they have to be absorbed by the health plan. The absorption of costs at the Honolulu Medical Center had not been correctly calculated and continued to prove troublesome.

Nor were the physicians and their wives prepared for the professional and social ostracism they soon experienced. This was especially difficult for the wives of a number of the founding partners, who prior to joining Kaiser had enjoyed social prominence in Honolulu. Suddenly, the physicians found themselves cold-shouldered by the local medical society. Physicians and wives alike found themselves increasingly excluded from the social life of the fee-for-service medical community. "They ostracized them to the point that they were just blackballed," recalls Lambreth Hancock. "From everything. Their wives, who had always been very close to one another — played bridge, played golf, all that sort of thing, in each other's homes all the time for dinner — whoosh, one wife wouldn't speak to the other wife. I mean, it was just a cold-blooded freeze-out."[5]

Many of the problems could be laid at the door of the hasty inauguration of the program. The partners entered the program without a full understanding of the implications of prepaid group practice. Not surprisingly, they began to attribute their difficulties to the Kaiser management. Henry J. Kaiser, in turn, disappointed by the lagging enrollments, the complaints about service, the cost overruns, and the other difficulties, began to blame the Pacific Medical Associates.

Swallowing his pride, Kaiser began to call on the mainland for assistance. Sidney Garfield was already on hand, having come over to help in the architectural design of the Honolulu Medical Center. But Kaiser had deliberately kept Garfield out of all medical and administrative matters, having blamed Garfield — so Garfield believed — for the confrontations that began with the expansion of the program to Walnut Creek. "I stayed out of it," Garfield later recalled of these difficulties between Kaiser and the Pacific Medical Associates, "but every once in a while he'd bring me into it. When he was having trouble with those five doctors, he asked me to intervene and see if I could help him. I would talk to the doctors and get them to agree to certain things, then I would leave and come back here [to the mainland] and it would all blow up again! But, I got no direct responsibilities — that was fine with me."[6]

Sometime in mid-1959, regional manager Lambreth Hancock began keeping a confidential chronology of events. It detailed a progressively deteriorating situation, pitting the Pacific Medical Associates against the Kaiser organization in a manner all too familiar to the mainland. Kaiser's visionary concept of a system superior to that operating on the mainland disintegrated.

At Kaiser's request, Clifford Keene began to make frequent trips to Honolulu to monitor the situation. At the request of Trefethen and Keene, Ernest Saward, the director of the Kaiser-Permanente program in Portland, spent the month of April 1960 as, ostensibly, a visiting practitioner at the Honolulu Medical Center. Saward's real mission was to observe the situation there and report back to Trefethen as to what was happening. Aware of Saward's mission, many of the employed physicians engaged him in private conversation. They complained of how the partners of the Pacific Medical Associates were exploiting them in a difficult situation. Saward also formed his own judgments as to the individual competence of the Honolulu Medical Center physicians, employees and partners alike.

In the early summer of 1960, the five partners, despite the fact that a firm contract existed for the entire year, demanded immediate increases in their compensation. The problems in the Hawaii operation, they argued, were being caused by the Kaiser organization, not themselves. The Health Plan, or even Henry J. Kaiser personally, must continue to subsidize the program and must meet the demands of the Pacific Medical Associates for a midyear increase in compensation — "or else."

It was the "or else" that gave the central office its opportunity. Clifford Keene later took personal responsibility for the decision that followed, but he also checked it through with Trefethen and Edgar Kaiser before taking any definite steps. No sooner had Keene discussed the matter with Trefethen and Kaiser than he heard from Henry J. Kaiser himself on the telephone. "Clifford," Keene later remembers Kaiser saying to him, "you're all on your own. If you come a cropper on this, you're just out the back door. You'll lose everything."[7]

On Saturday, August 20, 1960, Keene fired the Pacific Medical Associates, serving them with a written notice to vacate the premises by 5:00 P.M. of the day following the receipt of the "or else" ultimatum. The remaining 33 employed physicians were assembled and invited to continue practice as a medical group. All but two elected to stay. Keene phoned Saward, then attending a postgraduate course at Cornell University, and asked him to fly to Honolulu to help manage the situation.

Saward left the next morning and assumed the role of acting medical director. The Pacific Medical Associates, meanwhile, had called their lawyers, and were threatening lawsuits. Keene, Saward, and other Kaiser staffers, Arthur Weissman and Scott Fleming, who flew to the scene, had simultaneously to deal with the fired partners and to reorganize the medical group.

Appointing himself regional manager over Hancock, who was glad to have someone from the Health Plan in charge, Keene assumed overall control of the reorganization. Saward, meanwhile, concentrated his energies on forming the new medical group. Keene had chosen Saward for this task because the Permanente Group in Oregon had a strong director model, as opposed to the shared authority of the southern California and northern California groups. In the course of the reorganization, the Southern California Medical Group sent physicians to Hawaii as advisors. The Permanente Medical Group in northern California, however, was not approached directly for assistance, although Pellegrin and Baritell went over as individuals.

Keene and Saward chose Philip Chu, a Chinese-American surgeon on the Honolulu Medical Center staff, to be the director of the reorganized Hawaii Permanente Medical Group. Saward spent considerable time in personally coaching Chu in the management of prepaid group practice. As in the case of the Oregon region, Hawaii developed as a strong one-person directorship, with Chu exercising central authority. Saward felt himself at some risk during this period since he did not have a medical license in Hawaii; however, no complications resulted from his sojourn as temporary medical director.

In the immediate aftermath of being fired by Keene, the partners of the Pacific Medical Associates waged war against Henry J. Kaiser through a series of indignant press releases. Kaiser, however, owned a television and radio station and controlled a public relations apparatus within his own organization that outgunned the embattled partners. On or about the fifth day of this exchange of press releases, the fired partners requested and received an agreement to discontinue fighting the battle in the newspapers. The partners then took the battle to court, claiming major damages for breach of contract. The Kaiser Foundation Health Plan eventually agreed to a token out-of-court settlement.

According to Trefethen, it took 5 years to put the Hawaii Kaiser-Permanente program on its feet. In 1969 the Hawaii region expanded its services to the island of Maui. Whatever mistakes were made, Trefethen later argued, the Kaiser-Permanente program was eventually established in Hawaii, and that constituted a major plus for prepaid group medical practice in the United States. From Sidney Garfield's perspective, the entire Hawaii experience reemphasized the fact that not just any physician, however competent, could make the transition into prepaid group medical practice. After Hawaii, great care was taken in selecting the core cadre for any new medical group.

From Clifford Keene's perspective, Hawaii conclusively proved — at first negatively and then positively during the reorganization — the necessity for close cooperation and a community of sentiment between the Health Plan–Hospitals and the physicians. Hawaii was difficult, Keene later admitted, but in the long run it strengthened the entire program. "It took a few years off my life, straightening that one out."[8]

3

In January 1961, executive director Cecil Cutting made an optimistic annual report to The Permanente Medical Group. Revenue for the Medical Group had exceeded expenses by $450,000. The contingent incentive payment from the Health Plan was averaging $300,000 per quarter, reflecting solid growth. Health Plan membership had increased to 398,500. One-third of all eligible federal employees in the region had subscribed to the Kaiser Foundation Health Plan by the end of 1960. Health Plan enrollment had grown so rapidly, in fact, that it was necessary to close enrollment of new groups and individuals in San Francisco, San Mateo, and Marin Counties until hospital and clinical facilities could be expanded. Twenty-eight new partners were welcomed that year, giving The Permanente Medical Group in Northern California a total of 226 partners. After a long discussion, a retirement program had been instituted. The Medical Group now had its own headquarters at 1924 Broadway in Oakland, formerly the headquarters of Kaiser Industries.

In spite of all this solid achievement, however, the leadership of The Permanente Medical Group of Northern California was still uncomfortable sharing "their" program with the Health Plan. "The Medical Group felt that it was the primary agent in the health care program," Collen later remembered, "and that Hospital and Health Plan were of secondary importance. In order to demonstrate that, the Medical Group decided to set up its own program, completely proprietary, under Medical Group governance."[9] As a growing city without a competing prepaid medical care program, San Diego soon emerged in Medical Group discussions as the best place to establish a physician-owned and physician-managed program that would at once be profitable and show the Kaiser organization that MDs could run their own enterprise. Before proceeding any further, The Permanente Medical Group in Northern California sought and received the approval of the Southern California Permanente Medical Group for the venture. Between April 3 and 7, 1961, four members of the Executive Committee, Baritell, Collen, Cutting, and Neighbor, visited San Diego to examine two hospital properties available for purchase. On April 13, 1961, the Executive Committee unanimously approved a motion to purchase the 46-bed Lake Murray Hospital in San Diego for an amount not to exceed $475,000 and to initiate there "a medical care program under the ownership, control, and operation of The Permanente Medical Group."

At the next regular partnership meeting 4 days later, 95 out of 116 partners present voted to authorize the Executive Committee to proceed with the San Diego venture. Since this was not an absolute majority of all partners eligible to vote, a mail ballot was sent out the following day, April 18, 1961. The final vote was 182 partners in favor of the San Diego project, 26 opposed, a clear majority. The operations reserve of The Permanente Medical Group that had been contributed by each partner on election to partnership status since 1948 was used to start the San Diego venture. Morris Collen was given leave of absence from his duties as physician-in-chief at the medical center in San Francisco to direct the San Diego venture. Collen began to look for a home for his family in the San Diego area.

The Kaiser Foundation Health Plan Board reacted promptly to this new development. The board was concerned principally about conflict of interest. How could The Permanente Medical Group set up a health plan that was in competition for resources with the Health Plan it was already serving? Edgar Kaiser made a verbal proposal "to work with the Medical Group in the attempt to resolve some fundamental differences between the two parties involving problems at both the operational and policy levels." He proposed that the Health Plan cooperate with the Medical Group in a dual control capacity in San Diego.[10] The Health Plan and the Medical Group began discussions of a Moratorium Agreement. It would include four major provisions. First of all, the Health Plan would join the Medical Group as a partner in the prepaid health plan in San Diego. Second, the Medical Group would continue with plans for the acquisition of the San Diego property. Third, the Medical Group would table plans for operation of the plan while the moratorium was in effect. Finally, the Health Plan would reimburse the Medical group for "stand-by" expenses as long as the moratorium held. The

Executive Committee was eager for the execution of the Moratorium Agreement to be followed by negotiations to include improvement of operations under the Medical Service Agreement in the Bay Area.

While this was being considered, The Permanente Medical Group established a nonprofit charitable trust, the trustees of which were six members of the Executive Committee. With funds authorized and advanced by the Executive Committee, the trustees purchased the first and second deeds of trust to the Lake Murray Hospital. The trustees later assigned their interest in these deeds and in certain items of property at Lake Murray Hospital to The Permanente Medical Group. The actual acquisition of the Lake Murray Hospital occurred July 11, 1961, at a public bankruptcy sale on the sidewalk in front of the San Diego Courthouse.

"When Henry Kaiser heard about it," recalled Wally Cook, "there was a mushroom cloud over his Honolulu headquarters. He was really upset that these upstarts would dare to venture down to San Diego and start up a competitive Health Plan."[11] Kaiser's ire was compounded by the fact that the Medical Group was also using the San Diego venture as a way of negotiating further adjustments to the Medical Service Agreement. San Diego, in other words, was not just a way of proving that physicians could run their own program. The San Diego venture now became an instrument of leverage against the existing Medical Service Agreement.

At this point, the board of directors of the Kaiser Foundation Health Plan withdrew from the possibility of participating as a partner in the San Diego venture. Edgar Kaiser informed Cecil Cutting that the directors were now concerned that the San Diego expansion would destabilize arrangements in northern California. It was agreed, however, to continue discussions between the Executive Committee of The Permanente Medical Group and representatives of the Health Plan, including Edgar Kaiser, Eugene Trefethen, Fred Tennant, Felix Day, and Clifford Keene. The first meeting of this group was held on the morning after it was first suggested. A note of caution is clearly evident in the refusal of the Health Plan to oppose directly the San Diego expansion. The Health Plan representatives, in other words, clearly understood the negotiating leverage now possessed by the Medical Group. At a discussion held on July 14, 1961, representatives of the Health Plan board of trustees assured Baritell, Collen, Cutting, and King that no antagonism existed with respect to the San Diego expansion. The Health Plan did request, however, that the Medical Group avoid recruiting Health Plan personnel for San Diego and that the resources of Permanente Services,

Inc., not be used in the expansion effort. Trefethen stressed that the board considered the Health Plan and Hospitals to be its responsibility, but that the Health Plan was nevertheless willing to work out even further levels of partnership between the Health Plan and the Medical Group in northern California. A new series of meetings was organized between Cecil Cutting, representing the Executive Committee of the Medical Group and Fred Tennant, Felix Day, Frank Jones, the new Health Plan manager, and Carlos Efferson of Kaiser Services to study ways to further improve the organization in northern California.

In southern California, meanwhile, Ray Kay objected to the use of either the name Permanente or Kaiser for the San Diego program. If these names were to be used, Kay wanted representation on the board from both the Southern California Permanente Medical Group and the Kaiser Foundation Health Plan. To avoid this conflict, The Permanente Medical Group chose the name Pan-Medical, Inc., for the San Diego venture. All members of the Executive Committee signed the articles of incorporation and became the board of directors of the new health plan organization. A medical, surgical, and hospital services agreement and a subscriber plan contract were drafted and approved. An administrator for both the hospital and the medical group was appointed, together with a health plan manager, and a marketing brochure was drafted. Pan-Medical, Inc., seemed an inevitability.

At this point, Ray Kay, increasingly concerned that another program would block expansion of his operation in southern California, requested a meeting with Henry J. Kaiser in Honolulu. Kaiser agreed to a meeting after Labor Day, provided that Edgar Kaiser come along as well. "I can't see any hope of me being helpful," Kaiser telegrammed Ray Kay on August 31, 1961, "when you and Edgar, Gene and I have gotten absolutely nowhere on the fundamental principles and dangers at stake. Both of you must feel as I do that it is impossible to believe or much less understand that the same persons now contracting with the Health Plan, who have been working with the same principles in the Health Plan for more than twenty years, would suddenly start a competing Health Plan, competing with themselves, their doctor friends, and the Health Plan and would not even, as I'm advised, notify the Health Plan principals that such action was contemplated until decision already had been taken. How can such actions be anything but clear disloyalty? Therefore, where disloyalty and disregard of the threatened consequences which you express concern over are involved, it is difficult for me to understand how further fruitless discussions are either merited or could be constructive. I will look forward to seeing you."[12]

After Labor Day, Ray Kay and Edgar Kaiser flew to Hawaii to discuss the entire matter with Henry J. Kaiser. Kaiser continued to declare his unequivocable opposition. If the Medical Group persisted in its plan to establish Pan-Medical, Inc., in San Diego, Henry J. Kaiser asserted, it would jeopardize the existing contract between the Health Plan and The Permanente Medical Group in northern California. This was the same tactic that Clifford Keene had used in dismissing the Pacific Medical Associates from the Honolulu Medical Center. Henry J. Kaiser, in other words, was threatening to fire the Northern California Permanente Medical Group if it expanded into San Diego.

Kaiser flew to the mainland to handle the matter personally. A meeting was arranged between Kaiser and Cecil Cutting. Kaiser stood looking out at Lake Merritt from the top floor of the Kaiser building. Cutting approached him, but Kaiser refused to turn around, not even to a physician who had lived in his house for months during Bess Kaiser's final illness 10 years earlier. Kaiser kept on looking out the window and remained silent. The silence continued until Cecil Cutting spoke.

"Mr. Kaiser," Cecil Cutting asked, "would you really destroy this plan because of San Diego?"

Kaiser replied that yes, indeed, he would.

"In that case, Mr. Kaiser," Cutting responded, "I will assure you that the Medical Group will not go through with its plans."

At this, Kaiser turned and faced his old friend. "Can you do that, Cecil?" he asked.

Cutting said that he could and that he would.[13]

Cutting kept his word. On September 18, 1961, the partnership authorized the Executive Committee—85 in favor, 34 opposed—to sell Lake Murray Hospital in San Diego. The hospital was eventually sold for $650,000, which represented a net capital gain of $203,895. This profit was distributed to the partners on June 30, 1962, in proportion to their capital contributions to the Medical Group. As a real estate venture, San Diego proved a success.

It also improved relations between the Health Plan and the Medical Group. In his October 1961 report, Cecil Cutting noted an improved organizational atmosphere after the settlement of the San Diego dispute. This point was repeated in the minutes of subsequent meetings of the Executive Committee. From the viewpoint of the doctors, the San Diego dispute had resulted in a growing consciousness of partnership between The Permanente Medical Group and the Health Plan in the Kaiser-Permanente enterprise. No longer would the doctors be taken for granted. Fred Tennant resigned as regional manager for the Health

Plan and for the Hospitals in northern California in December 1962. Karl Steil, the regional manager in southern California, assumed the position of regional manager for both California regions. In northern California, Steil—noted for his smooth working relationships with physicians—was assisted by Martin Drobac, Edgar Kaiser's son-in-law. In southern California, Steil's assistant was James Vohs, another rising Health Plan executive.

In the long run, the Hawaii and San Diego crises proved watersheds. With their resolutions, the conflicts of the 1950s passed, and an era of good feeling ensued. As the Kaiser-Permanente program entered its third decade it would encounter scores of new challenges, but after a decade of controversy it would meet these challenges with one central premise established. For the Kaiser-Permanente program to work properly, there had to be partnership and trust between the physicians and the executives and directors of the Health Plan. That trusting partnership had now been forged in controversy and compromise, which was fortunate, for the growth and social turmoil of the 1960s would require unity and resolve among all participants and groups in the Kaiser-Permanente community.

10

Forging a New Health Plan—Growth and Transformation Through the Mid-1960s

<hr>

1

In September 1962 the physicians of Permanente and the Kaiser Foundation Health Plan, Inc., had corroborated in the strongest possible terms in a profile in *Time* magazine, that their program had come of age. Appearing on September 14, 1962, twenty years after the inauguration of the program in the Richmond shipyards, the *Time* article profiled what had by then become the single largest private group-practice health plan in the United States. All in all, the Health Plan—with its propensity for neologisms, *Time* called it "Medikaiser"—encompassed 12 hospitals, including the just-opened facility at Panorama City and 38 clinics serving 337,000 subscribers (911,000 family members) in California, Oregon, and Hawaii. In its program, the Health Plan stood unique; its closest runner-up, the Health Insurance Plan of Greater New York, did not provide or pay for hospital care.

In the article, *Time* focused in on The Permanente Medical Group of northern California, then at 278 partners and 142 employed physicians. The article allowed both Sidney Garfield and Cecil Cutting to explain the program. Cutting's remarks virtually exuded an audible sigh of relief that the great battles for control of the program of the 1950s had at long last been resolved through the Medical Service Agreements.

"Organized medicine has a legitimate worry that prepaid care could open up medicine to lay control," Cutting told *Time*. "We are the proof that this need not be so. We physicians in these groups run our own show."[1]

Cutting thus unofficially opened up a new level of dialogue with organized medicine that would continue through the 1960s. Having admitted the dangers of lay control and having successfully confronted them in the 1950s, the Permanente physicians were now willing to take their case to the nation. Which is exactly what Sidney Garfield was allowed to do in the *Time* article: make a most dramatic defense of the entire prepaid concept. A little more than a decade earlier, Garfield had been threatened with loss of his license for advocating the prepaid group-practice concept; and now, in 1962, he was emerging as the founding father and continuing spokesperson for a concept of medical care that over the next 20 years would alter the structure of American medicine.

The 1960s was a period of unprecedented growth. By the end of 1965 the Health Plan in northern California counted 646,000 enrollees, a net growth of 61.9 percent in 5 years. The 1960s would also witness the exporting of the Health Plan out of the west coast. It would be characterized by new levels of financial complexity. It would bring a new generation of physicians into the Permanente partnerships. The 1960s would also see a growing involvement of government in medicine. The year 1942 saw the program established in its first lasting form. The year 1952 witnessed it growing but embattled. The year 1962 found the program thriving as the largest prepaid group-practice health plan in the nation. Between 1962 and 1972 a series of internal adjustments were made and gains consolidated. By the early 1970s, the Kaiser Foundation Health Plan would be an accepted paradigm for the future organization of American medicine (footnote in *Time*, September 12, 1962).

But first, some unfinished business. Henry J. Kaiser had favored the proliferation of smaller medical groups as opposed to the all-encompassing four Permanente partnerships in Oregon, California, and Hawaii. Only one such smaller group, the Eden Medical Group of San Leandro, 8 miles south of Oakland, managed to become established. It began in October 1953 under the direction of John Mott, a Permanente physician, and continued until September 1962. "John was a pioneer in spirit," Cecil Cutting later observed of Mott. "He was a little restless within the confines of the partnership of Oakland, which seemed to be a little bit too bureaucratic. He, and David de Kruif, Leonard Rubin, George Eckhart, and a pediatrician, Edna Schrick—she later went to Hawaii—decided to start a little clinic in San Leandro."[2]

Cutting's personal friendship with John Mott allowed this deviation from official doctrine to take place. It worked well for a decade because Mott and his staff, despite their independence from The Permanente Medical Group, were fully aligned with the programs and practices of the entire plan. Since the Eden Medical Group operated under a subcontract with The Permanente Medical Group, and not on a direct contract with the Kaiser Foundation Health Plan, and since most of the Eden physicians had been Permanente physicians before the formation of their group or had been resident physicians in the Kaiser Foundation Hospital in Oakland, conflict was kept at a minimum.

The Eden physicians received a base salary, plus a modest fee per office visit. By 1962, however, they were asking for an increase in per visit fees. "Look," Cutting said to Mott, "I can't do this, because this is just getting into a fee-for-service, getting one step away from prepayment. As long as you can keep it at one prepayment level, fine...but I just can't start increasing it. Why don't you come back into the partnership?"[3]

John Mott took a long breath, Cutting recalled, and then agreed to return. In September 1962 the physicians of the Eden Medical Group returned to Permanente. The San Leandro Clinic was phased out and a new Kaiser Permanente Medical Center was established in Hayward. Most of the former Eden physicians were assigned there so as to capitalize on their existing momentum as a team. With the absorption of Eden, a fundamental aspect of the Kaiser Permanente genetic code, unified group medical practice, was restored to its full integrity.

2

One of the forces propelling growth in the Health Plan in the early 1960s was the growing participation of employers in capitation prepayment. During this period, the percentage of members for whom the employer paid some or all of the dues increased from 68 percent to 91 percent. This dramatic growth underscored an important evolution in the traditional compensation and benefits package in the United States. Another relevant dynamic was the enrollment in the Health Plan of federal, state, and local government employees. This was stimulated by the Federal Employees Health Benefits Act of 1960, which became in turn the model for similar legislation by the state of California.

Until 1960, federal employees generally did not have the same kinds of choices of health insurance benefits that were available to many employees in private industry. In seeking to redress this, the Eisenhower administration proposed a nationwide program for federal employees that would use a single indemnity insurance carrier. The proposed program would be limited to coverage of major medical (catastrophic) expenses. It would not cover basic health services. Blue Cross–Blue Shield responded with a proposal for a nationwide account covering federal employees in the event of catastrophic illness. The Blue Cross–Blue Shield proposal, however, would not allow federal employees the option of being covered by prepaid group-practice plans. The Kaiser Foundation Health Plan thus stood in danger of losing one of its largest enrollment groups, federal employees, if they were to be covered either exclusively by a single indemnity insurance company or by a Blue Cross–Blue Shield nationwide account. By 1960, approximately 16 percent of the total health plan membership in northern California, some 65,000 members, were federal employees and they would be forced to disenroll from the Health Plan if the government settled on a single insurance system. The other Kaiser Foundation Health Plan regions in southern California, Hawaii, and Oregon would be similarly affected. Not only would such a disenrollment constitute a disaster to the Health Plan, it would also violate the freedom of choice of those federal employees who were happy in the Kaiser-Permanente system.

It thus became necessary to persuade the federal government that dual choice was both just and workable. Meanwhile, Blue Cross–Blue Shield, together with indemnity insurance companies who had their eye on the nationwide federal contract, were arguing that a dual or multiple choice option for individual federal employees would be totally impractical for a nationwide account. At this critical juncture, an accident of history worked on behalf of Kaiser-Permanente. The chairperson of the senate subcommittee for the Federal Civil Service was Richard Neuberger of Oregon, a member of the Kaiser Foundation Health Plan in Portland. Ernest Saward was his personal physician. When Arthur Weissman and Avram Yedidia of the Health Plan called on Senator Neuberger to persuade him that a system which provided basic coverage was preferable to major medical insurance for federal employees, Neuberger listened. Neuberger also knew from his own experience that dual choice was workable and practical.

From his strategic position, Neuberger refuted the claims of the Eisenhower administration and Blue Cross–Blue Shield that dual choice was unworkable. Refuted by Neuberger, the major national carriers modified their position and accepted the option of several carriers in order to avoid being bypassed in the forthcoming legislation. The Federal Employees Health Benefits Act of 1960 provided basic health services as well as catastrophic coverage and affirmed the principle of dual or multiple choice. Not only would Kaiser-Permanente keep its federal employees as members, the door was opened to further enrollments.

"If somebody from, say, Nebraska had been the chairman of that committee," Ernest Saward later remarked, "it might have proved impossible to get multiple choice into such a program."[4]

The insertion of the principle of dual choice in a program designed for the largest employee group in the United States created an important precedent, establishing a mandate for dual or multiple choice in all subsequent programs, whether publicly or privately sponsored.

The Federal Employees Health Benefits Act stimulated similar legislation in California. In 1962 the California State Employees Retirement Board, through its appointed Medical Advisory Council, requested a presentation by Cutting of the Kaiser-Permanente program. Much of the discussion focused on the quality of medical care. Not only did Kaiser-Permanente wish to be in a position to serve the thousands of state employees in Sacramento, but it also had enrolled many state employees assigned to the Bay Area. When these employees were relocated to Sacramento, as frequently happened, they were faced with a choice of transferring to another carrier or traveling more than 50 miles to the nearest Kaiser-Permanente Medical Center in Vallejo. Further pressure for expansion to Sacramento was added by the California Employees Association itself, which demanded that Kaiser-Permanente establish a Sacramento facility if state employees were to be enrolled in the program.

Throughout the summer of 1964, Cecil Cutting participated in discussions with Health Plan management regarding the Sacramento venture. By the end of 1964 a decision was made to begin operations in Sacramento in June 1965. Between 10,000 and 15,000 members were expected in the initial enrollment, with growth to 30,000 in the first year. Kaiser Foundation Hospitals purchased the Arden Hospital in Sacramento and leased medical offices for 12 physicians. John Mott, previously the head of the Eden Medical Group and the Hayward Medical Center, was appointed physician-in-chief of the new Sacramento Medical Center. "As a pioneering spirit," said Cecil Cutting of John Mott, "[he] was the only guy that was willing to go to Sacramento. He burnt his life out making Sacramento a success."[5]

According to the Medical Service Agreement, expansions such as this to Sacramento, together with the enrollment of new groups in existing facilities, had to be approved by the Executive Committee of The Permanente Medical Group, which it was.

The minutes of the Executive Committee from this period reflect constant attention to problems brought on by growth and expansion. Take the matter of outpatient drug coverage, which was considered at length. In 1963 the Executive Committee agreed to Health Plan coverage of all costs of immunizations. It also agreed to cover half the cost of outpatient drugs, provided that the amount received through prepayment dues was equal to the revenues from cash counter sales. By this decision, the Executive Committee in effect extended the prepayment concept to include outpatient drug coverage, an important, if little noticed at the time, step in the direction of a more comprehensive medical care plan. Each Kaiser Permanente Health Plan member could now purchase drugs on an outpatient basis at half cost, which represented a considerable saving in the years to come as pharmaceutical costs soared.

Then there was the tricky question of alcoholism. Since the earliest era, Permanente physicians had resisted the idea of comprehensive care for alcoholism, self-inflicted wounds, or other self-induced illnesses. There was also continuing debate as to the extent and range of psychiatric care that could be offered. When the Federal Civil Service Commission, representing the largest consumer group contracting with the Kaiser Foundation Health Plan, requested coverage for alcoholism in 1968, this resistance began to crumble. In a cautiously worded statement, the Executive Committee approved "the general concept" of coverage for alcoholism, leaving the details and terms of coverage to later negotiation. The question of alcoholism foreshadowed the then-expanding definition of health care. The 1960s was experiencing a shift in psychological and social consciousness that would soon have a dramatic impact upon what constituted the definition of health, healthfulness, and health care entitlements and which therefore escalated the cost of care.

Meanwhile, growth continued. During the 1960s the net gain in Health Plan enrollment always exceeded the forecast. The Health Plan, for example, informed The Permanente Medical Group in July 1964 to expect a 55.6 percent increase by July 1970, for a net gain of 275,000 members in 6 years. The actual gain as of December 1970 exceeded this forecast by 200,000. Some 477,000 new members were enrolled, representing a growth rate of nearly 100 percent. Within 6½ years, 1964 to 1970, enrollment had doubled.

3

Growth of such dramatic proportions meant that new physicians had to be recruited on an accelerated basis. Between 1961 and 1965, 245 physicians were recruited to Kaiser-Permanente. In 1965, during which the Health Plan grew by 101,000, The Permanente Medical Group alone added 95 physicians, the equivalent of the entire graduating class of a medical school with 400 students. By September 1968 when the Health Plan enrollment stood at 845,000, The Permanente Medical Group had 917 full-time equivalent physicians. This put the physician-member ratio at 1:921, the most favorable ratio in the history of the Medical Group.

This favorable ratio was achieved, despite the competition in the recruitment of new physicians. In the boom years of the late 1950s and early 1960s, a shortage of physicians developed. The pool of physicians interested in group practice was small. A smaller pool existed of physicians interested in prepaid group practice. Moreover, within this smaller pool, an even smaller number of physicians were capable of meeting Medical Group standards. Thus recruitment remained a continuous challenge.

Because resident physicians training in Kaiser Hospitals had already expressed an interest in the program by being there, recruitment of physicians finishing their residency in Kaiser-Permanente became a top priority. Permanente physicians took it on themselves to be on the lookout for prospects among classmates and a wide variety of professional friends. Recruitment also occurred above the entry level. Henry Shinefield, for example, then on the staff of the Cornell Medical School in pediatrics, was recruited directly from Cornell and made chief of pediatrics in San Francisco. Others were recruited from teaching institutions. John Mott was especially active in recruiting physicians for Sacramento when enrollment at that expansion site exceeded all expectations. Mott spent time on the road across the United States interviewing prospective physicians. At times it became necessary to close enrollment in Sacramento because of the physician shortage. Mott reported to the Executive Committee that he and his department chiefs were simply unable to recruit enough physicians to keep up with the rapid growth. Accordingly, in June 1966 the Executive Committee authorized a $500 per month increase in salary for Permanente physicians willing to accept a temporary transfer to Sacramento.

The recruitment of minority physicians began from ground zero. Permanente had been criticized in the 1950s for requiring the assignment of a black intern to only those hospitalized patients willing to accept a black doctor. Not until the 1960s did black physicians, male or female, begin to enter the system in any numbers. Ninety-five black physicians celebrated their association with Permanente at a reception during Black History Month in 1990.

Understandably, the suggestion arose that Kaiser-Permanente should establish its own medical school as a source of recruitment. By this time, the Stanford University School of Medicine had moved from San Francisco to Palo Alto. San Francisco thus had an empty medical school facility just a few blocks away from the Kaiser Hospital. In late 1963 the Kaiser Foundation Health Plan Board of Directors, operating through Edgar Kaiser, began tentative conversations with the Presbyterian Medical Center of San Francisco and the University of the Pacific (UOP) in Stockton regarding the possibility of establishing a Presbyterian-UOP–Kaiser-Permanente medical school in the city. The Foundation was not only interested in this proposed medical school as a source of recruitment, but it was also desirous of the respectability that such an institution would bring to the program. Moreover, the facilities of the Presbyterian Medical Center would also become available to Kaiser-Permanente, thus giving the program a second hospital in the city. At the time, with the removal of the Stanford Medical School to Palo Alto, the Presbyterian Hospital was experiencing a patient shortage. As intriguing as this medical school idea was, however, it never moved beyond the conversation stage. The University of the Pacific did eventually establish a school of dentistry in San Francisco, but an important opportunity to empower the Health Plan and the various Permanente medical groups with its own university-affiliated medical school was lost for want of action at this moment of opportunity.

Meanwhile, The Permanente Medical Group wrestled with the problem of appropriately allocating its physicians, experienced and newly recruited alike. The Executive Committee reviewed new hires, full- or part-time, on a physician-by-physician basis. The minutes from this period reveal a series of argued and reargued questions as the committee continued to grapple with the problem of staffing its rapidly expanding program. Which medical center had the greatest need for an additional doctor? What specialty was understaffed? What starting incomes and benefits were necessary to obtain specialists in anesthesiology, orthopedics, neurosurgery, and radiology?

Once physicians were added—in increasingly larger numbers—they also had to be oriented into the social and psychological milieu of group practice. The culture of The Permanente Medical Group had to be transmitted. Such transmission is always a challenge after passing the first pioneer era. The new physician associates coming into Permanente could not be expected immediately to understand the complex history of the group or the rules and procedures the group had evolved for its survival. The first vehicle for cultural transference was, obviously, the senior physicians of the group: physicians such as Cecil Cutting, J. Wallace Neighbor, Phil Raimondi, Lamont Baritell, H. Donald Grant, Robert King, Norman Haugen, and Morris Collen. Since most of these physicians were on the Executive Committee, this body functioned as a council of elders as well as an administrative committee. As executive director of the Medical Group, Cecil Cutting assumed personal responsibility for orienting new physicians to the program. Cutting's files eventually teemed with the transcripts of talks he gave new physicians. Cutting also spoke to gatherings of physicians' wives, joined by a husband or two as women increasingly joined the medical staff. One of his most ambitious addresses, dealing with the entire history and present and future challenge of the program, was given to the annual luncheon meeting of the Permanente Wives' in San Francisco, held on March 6, 1963, at the Owl and Turtle Restaurant. In this address Cutting prophesied the emergence of the Health Maintenance Organization movement with Kaiser-Permanente as a model. Gradually, after constant repetition, Cecil Cutting developed a finely chiseled, factually rich, and well-delivered set speech, such as that given to a conference of new Permanente physicians in December 1966—which set forth the history, five-part genetic code, and future prospects of the program.

This 1966 conference for new physicians was but one of a series of intensive group orientation meetings held during these years for new physicians. They usually occurred on weekends at hotels away from the daily routine of home, hospital, and office, and constituted at once a vehicle for the transmission of The Permanente Medical Group culture and a way of allowing older Permanente physicians to get in touch with the next Permanente generation. Apparently, these and other programs, together with the more important fact of actual practice in the Kaiser-Permanente program itself, worked. As of 1963, nine out of every 10 doctors who joined the group completed their 3 years of associate employment and entered the partnership.

While new physicians were being recruited, it also became necessary to provide for the eventual retirement of a generation which was then midway through its professional career. The Southern California Permanente Medical Group was first to come to an agreement in 1958 with the Kaiser Foundation Health Plan. This southern California program was discussed and modified by The Permanente Medical Group in northern California over a period of 2 years. A retirement plan for northern California physicians was initiated in 1960. Under terms of the agreement, the Health Plan contributed approximately 12 cents per member per month to a trust fund administered by Aetna Insurance Company. Each participating physician had a tentative account in this trust fund, based partially on length of service, but taking into consideration salary rates as well.

For 2 years, the matter seemed to have been settled; but then the northern California region of the Internal Revenue Service (IRS) ruled that the retirement funds with Aetna, since they were tentatively allocated to individual physicians, were considered taxable current income of each individual physician. By contrast, the IRS in southern California had made an opposite ruling. The northern California IRS also challenged the division of net revenue between the Kaiser Foundation Hospitals and The Permanente Medical Group. Bearing down even further, the IRS in northern California challenged the arrangement which provided hospitals with 4 percent of the historical cost of land, buildings, and equipment for amortization of loans.

Counsel for The Permanente Medical Group argued that the physicians did not realize any income at the time that the Health Plan contributed to the trust fund. The income would be received only after retirement. Ownership of the fund did not vest in individual physicians at the time the Health Plan made its contribution. Physicians who withdrew from the Medical Group, for instance, or who died before retirement, such as David De Kruif, forfeited their benefits.

Adding insult to injury, the IRS proposed to collect back taxes from the individual physicians of The Permanente Medical Group. Since the Medical Group indicated that it would take the matter to court, the IRS agreed to assert deficiencies, for the time being, against only six or fewer physicians so that the matter could be brought to court. The majority of physicians executed waivers to avoid forcing the IRS to assert deficiencies immediately, since the statute of limitations on some of the past monies the IRS considered due had expired. In the event the IRS obtained a favorable decision in court, it could then assert deficiencies against the remaining physicians.

The selected physicians paid their alleged deficiencies and then sued the IRS for a refund. Since James Basye, an obstetrics-gynecology specialist at the Kaiser Permanente Medical Center in Oakland, was the first test case named to be listed alphabetically, the case went into the courts as *The United States vs. Basye.* On November 29, 1968, the U.S. District Court ruled in favor of the Medical Group. The IRS appealed. On November 23, 1971, the Ninth Circuit Court of Appeals affirmed the District Court decision. The United States then obtained a writ of certiorari on April 3, 1972, which took the case to the Supreme Court. *The United States vs. Basye* was argued before the Supreme Court on December 11, 1972. To the disappointment of the Medical Group, the Supreme Court reversed all decisions of the lower courts on February 27, 1973. Justice Powell wrote the majority decision. Only Justice Douglas dissented. The IRS then proceeded to assess deficiencies against all the remaining Permanente Medical Group physicians. Fortunately, the Kaiser Foundation Health Plan utilized its invested trust funds to provide all physicians with the amounts assessed against them by the IRS.

Clearly, an alternative retirement plan was necessary. Such an alternative, in fact, had been under discussion for nearly a decade before the adverse decision of the Supreme Court. Under this new program, known as the Common Plan, the Kaiser Foundation Health Plan assumed the liability to pay the retirement income for all doctors serving Health Plan members in all four regions. Set aside and invested, these funds were recorded as both an asset and a liability of the Kaiser Foundation Health Plan. Unlike most retirement plans, these funds were unprotected from the potential demands of Health Plan creditors. In effect, each physician's claim for retirement income was at risk if the Health Plan were to fail. On the other hand, physicians could now transfer from one Permanente Medical Group to another without forfeiting retirement benefits.

Under the terms of the Common Plan, retirement income was calculated by a formula relating years of service to a percentage of peak earnings. Initially, the Health Plan sought to reduce its obligation by subtracting a physician's expected Social Security benefits. The physicians resisted this decision. This controversy disturbed the harmonious relationship between the Medical Group and the Health Plan that had been established following the San Diego venture. After several years of debate, the Social Security offset was withdrawn. Other benefits were added as well. Life insurance, for instance, was provided, with premiums paid by the Medical Group. The Medical Group also assumed responsibility for keeping the retired physician and his or her family in the Kaiser Foundation Health Plan. For its part, the Health Plan agreed to fund these new Medical Group obligations through an increase in capitation payments. The Health Plan also agreed to increase the face value of life insurance policies, to improve short-term disability benefits for physicians who had used all sick leave compensation, and to establish an improved program of long-term disability insurance. By February 1968, after a decade of discussion, court cases, negotiations, and renegotiations, a satisfactory retirement and benefit program was in effect.

There still remained the question of the retention fund. Between 1948 and 1954, the Health Plan had created a fund that could be used for the care of member patients in need of continuing attention in the event that the Health Plan was dissolved. The retention fund was thus a form of self-insurance. Half of these funds had been withheld from otherwise distributable earnings of the Medical Group. In February 1964, ten years after the last contribution to the retention fund had been made, the Health Plan returned to the Medical Group the portion of the retention fund physicians had contributed. These funds were then distributed to partners of record from the 1948–1954 era who were still active in Permanente. The IRS taxed it as 1964 income.

Meanwhile, the Medical Group revised and updated some of its internal arrangements. Three elected short-term positions were added to the Executive Committee in an effort to make the Executive Committee more responsive to younger physicians. In 1965 it was decided to replace permanent members of the Executive Committee, as they retired, withdrew, or died, with long-term members, elected for a term of 9 years. Thus the Executive Committee became further democratized.

Sadly, it soon became necessary to exercise this option. On July 29, 1965, Dr. Robert King, a founding partner of The Permanente Medical Group and a permanent member of the Executive Committee, died unexpectedly. An outstanding student athlete at Stanford, a gold medalist in the 1928 Olympic Games in the high jump, King had won for himself a reputation as a conscientious and compassionate obstetrician-gynecologist. As chief of obstetrics and gynecology at Oakland, King had established a respected residency program. Many of King's residents stayed on with the Medical Group. In the tumultuous years of the 1950s, King's quiet demeanor and wry sense of humor had contributed a necessary note of dispassionate thoughtfulness to the frequently stormy Executive Committee proceedings. King had also played an important role in bettering relationships between the Medical Group and the Alameda–Contra Costa Medical Society. Under terms of the new arrangements, King was replaced by Bernard Rhodes, physician-in-chief at Hayward, the first long-term member of the Executive Committee.

This smooth transition did not suggest that conflict had absented itself from The Permanente Medical Group. The debate on Article Five, for instance, remained a divisive issue. Article Five of the Partnership Agreement prescribed a work week of 11 half-days per week per full-time physician. Many physicians used the eleventh half-day for educational purposes, making departmental rounds at the University of California or the Stanford Medical Schools. Physicians who chose to work the half-day were compensated a meager 15 dollars per session or 60 dollars per month. Those physicians who made departmental rounds at California or Stanford considered this added income a reward for ignorance. The physicians who worked the extra half-day argued that the value of doing departmental rounds at university hospitals was overestimated. In 1967 Article Five was amended to reduce the work week from 11 to 10 half-days. The work week was now equal for everyone. To compensate for this loss of educational time, the Executive Committee established an intramural staff education program, outside regular clinic hours, coordinated by Leonard Rubin.

By 1966 it had become time to reconsider the staffing of the office of the executive director of The Permanente Medical Group. From 1957 until 1965 Cecil Cutting had functioned as executive director with a staff of one secretary, who was occasionally aided by part-time secretarial assistance. Cutting also managed to continue his surgical practice as well. As the Medical Group grew, however, Cutting found himself in need of a physician executive assistant. In December 1965, Donovan McCune, formerly on the faculty of the College of Physicians and Surgeons at Columbia University, a noted pediatrician and bibliophile, and for some time physician-in-chief at the Vallejo Medical Center, was appointed assistant to the executive director, the first physician, aside from Cutting, to be added to the Medical Group regional staff.

4

At the Monterey Conference in 1960 Sidney Garfield had made three dramatic challenges to the Medical Group. New methods of providing health care as opposed to sick care must be tested. New technology must be used to acquire and store medical information. Nonphysician medical personnel must be brought further into the health-care process, under physician supervision, so as to extend the scope and efficiency of physician treatment. When the San Diego venture collapsed, Morris Collen, scheduled to head the San Diego enterprise, was now free to pursue such studies.

A board-certified internist with research interests and a long list of publications, Collen had a degree in electrical engineering from the University of Minnesota and for some time had taken a special interest in the relationship between the emerging computer technology and medicine. Intellectually, Collen was at home in medicine, medical research, and medical technology. In September 1961 the Executive Committee established a division of Medical Methods Research with Collen as director. The new division was given a broad mandate, in the words of its empowering directive, "to explore and develop to the fullest extent the 'health' aspects of our medical care activities." Thus the Medical Methods Research division oriented its activities to the very challenges Sidney Garfield had made the previous year in Monterey. Significantly, a founding partner, Morris Collen, would now direct this ambitious program.

The Medical Methods Research division program got off to a strong start in 1962 with a grant from the U.S. Public Health Service to the Kaiser Foundation Research Institute for the study of automated multiphasic health testing. Under this program, patients completed a medical history and then were put through several examination stations for testing in blood pressure, weight, eyesight, followed up by X-rays, electrocardiograms (ECG), and other laboratory tests. The results of these tests were then recorded on a punch card to be stored in a large computer for ready access. After each multiphasic examination, the patient had an appointment with an internist who had on hand the printout data pertaining to the individual.

As in the case of most innovation, there was much debate. A number of internists felt they were being burdened with information they did not need, or that false positive tests required time-consuming and expensive validation, together with the need to reassure patients. At a partnership meeting in October 1968, the question was put to the Executive Committee: "What does it cost The Permanente Medical Group to run the automated multiphasic study?" Collen replied that all routine tests—blood pressure, for example, blood count, urinalysis, and other usual aspects of health appraisal—were Kaiser-Permanente expenses. The Public Health Service contract bore the cost of all other laboratory procedures that were being tested for their predictive and cost-effective values. Collen went on to argue that the Medical Group was saving money through automated multiphasic examinations, as opposed to the traditional method in which a single internist would take up to an hour doing an individual examination and medical history, followed up by another appointment.

Once the multiphasic examinations were automated in 1964, long-range studies became possible. In 1979 the comparative results of 15 years of multiphasic examinations were used to determine whether periodic health checkups resulted in reduced morbidity, mortality, and disability in persons between the ages of 25 and 54. By comparing Kaiser-Permanente members who had been through the multiphasic process with those who had not, it was determined that there were significant differences in disability and mortality in middle-aged men between the ages of 45 and 54 primarily due to the early detection and treatment of hypertension and cancer of the colon or rectum. No significant differences were found in younger men, ages 35 to 44, or in women between the ages of 25 and 54. The results of this evaluation received wide coverage in the medical literature. The results also stimulated a more precise focus for the testing program. The complete annual physical checkup for healthy members was replaced with specific tests known to be useful for persons at risk for certain medical conditions on the basis of their medical history, age, gender, or other factors. These specific tests were also scheduled at intervals appropriate for these risks as they related to the life cycle.

In the meantime Kaiser-Permanente's automated multiphasic health testing program did show that such testing was acceptable to patients, an effective method of health surveillance, and speedy and economical in comparison to the traditional 1-hour checkup. The data collected by Kaiser-Permanente from a half million patient examinations in Oakland and San Francisco over the course of 15 years provided valuable information for a variety of spin-off research studies. Some 200 multiphasic programs throughout the world were stimulated by the Kaiser Permanente experiment.

In addition to the automated multiphasic health testing program, the Medical Methods Research division carried out other research projects. The very size of the Kaiser-Permanente program, together with the controls and data-gathering capacities inherent in prepaid group medical practice, made it a magnet for medical research. Throughout the growth years of the 1960s, the Medical Group participated in a number of important national studies. These studies not only contributed to medical knowledge, they also brought to the attention of the national medical establishment the extent and sophistication of the Kaiser-Permanente program. Research had its public relations effect, and by the early 1970s, with the emergence of the HMO movement, Kaiser-Permanente was no longer the pariah or even the exception to the rule, but a model for a valid philosophy and practice of health care.

In 1966 the Medical Methods Research division signed a contract with the Food and Drug Administration to establish a drug reaction monitoring system in San Francisco. In 1968 the National Center for Health Services Research of the Department of Health, Education, and Welfare (HEW) selected the Medical Methods Research division of The Permanente Medical Group as one of its seven national health service centers. It is interesting to note that another of the seven centers was in the Kaiser-Permanente Northwest Region in Portland, under the direction of Merwyn Greenlick, Ph.D.

Once again, the focus was on automation. HEW was interested in computerized medical databases, with which Kaiser-Permanente already possessed extensive experience. In the course of the program at the San Francisco Medical Center, physicians made over 1 million computer-readable clinical entries. Drug data for about 1200 prescriptions per day were entered by the pharmacy. A terminal was placed in the emergency department for physicians to have access within seconds to clinical, pharmaceutical, and laboratory data. Lasting several years, this project helped pioneer the introduction of the computer in health care management.

At the 1960 Monterey Conference, Sidney Garfield had spoken eloquently of health education and preventive medicine. These goals were followed up in the 1960s. In 1967 a Health Center project was financed through Kaiser-Permanente community service funds. The project had two components, health education and preventive medicine. A pioneering health education center was established by the Health Plan in 1969. The center had a theater and a library. It prepared exhibits that toured Kaiser-Permanente facilities. It also established a counseling system for health members and a specialized counseling system for patients in the recovery process. The emphasis of this counseling program was upon personal responsibility. In doing this, Kaiser-Permanente helped pioneer a shift of consciousness that would become fully evident by the 1980s when health was no longer envisioned as something that doctors gave patients, but as something that healthy members maintained for themselves through a healthy lifestyle.

This message of preventive service was also taken to paramedical personnel as well. Under the supervision of Permanente Medical Group physicians, nurse practitioners and physician assistants were trained in the management and maintenance of certain chronic or recurrent conditions, such as arthritis, back pain, diabetes, hypertension, obesity, and the smoking habit. Not only did this program meet Garfield's challenge of preventive health maintenance, but it also responded to his urgings that paramedical personnel be used to extend the range and efficiency of physician services.

In 1977 the National Center for Health Services Research and Development of HEW contracted with Kaiser-Permanente for another project. Interestingly enough, what HEW had in mind also dovetailed with one of Sidney Garfield's contentions: namely, that "the worried well" and the asymptomatic sick posed special challenges to a comprehensive medical care program. How were these two categories of patients, the one well but worried about being sick, the other sick but showing no evident symptoms, to be distinguished from each other and treated? In this second HEW project, Kaiser-Permanente members in Oakland who requested appointments for checkups were assigned to study and control groups and given automated multiphasic examinations. The on-line test results and patients' histories were immediately available to nurse practitioners who performed physical examinations under the direct supervision of an internist. An individualized assessment and disposition was then made. The results usually came in four categories: the well, the worried well, the symptomatic sick, and the asymptomatic sick. Persons determined by this process to be healthy but worried were given supportive counseling, with an emphasis upon the promotion of healthy lifestyles. The persons determined to be symptomatic sick were referred to physicians for follow-up treatment. Some asymptomatic sick were also referred to physicians. Others determined to be asymptomatic sick were put on preventive maintenance regimes. Evaluation of this Medical Care Delivery System (MCDS) showed that 70 percent of physician time and costs could be saved through the process. Sorting out the worried well, the symptomatic sick, and the asymptomatic sick made possible efficient follow-up programs. Once again, valuable data were compiled. Between 1961 and 1975, in fact, so Collen reported in 1976, some 150 articles or chapters in books emerged from these experimental programs.

In addition to the health services research carried on in the 1960s, Permanente physicians were involved in basic and clinical research projects as well. As early as 1943 Sidney Garfield had been seeking money to research new methods for the treatment of syphilis. All in all, Garfield raised some $50,000 for this project. In 1958 the Kaiser

Foundation established a Research Institute headquartered in Richmond. Under the auspices of the Kaiser Foundation Research Institute, a division of Kaiser Foundation Hospitals, a number of full-time basic research projects were supported. These included a laboratory of comparative biology and a laboratory of medical entomology, together with study projects into the epidemiology of cancer and a study into the biological and environmental aspects of child development. While Permanente physicians were seldom principal investigators in these projects, a number of them participated as researchers on their own time.

By contrast, in the case of clinical research, Permanente physicians became more actively involved. The very nature of the Kaiser-Permanente program, with its large enrollments of a cross section of the community, provided a strong demographic credibility to clinical research done within the program. In the 1960s clinical research in cardiovascular disease, cancer, diabetes, allergies, and psychosomatic disorders was pursued by Permanente physicians. In most cases Permanente physicians functioned as the principal investigators. In some instances these clinical research projects were pursued in conjunction with investigators at other institutions. In 1967 the Executive Committee authorized a field study on the safety and effectiveness of a new vaccine for mumps. The pharmaceutical company provided the liability coverage. The Executive Committee also authorized a contraceptive drug study in Walnut Creek, funded by the National Institutes of Health. At the time, the recently introduced contraceptive pill remained a controversy. Many claimed that the pill had adverse side effects. The Walnut Creek study showed that no adverse effects of the pill could be detected in healthy nonsmoking young women. Certain critics attacked this report, however, and the controversy continued.

While the Executive Committee gave its approval of these clinical research projects, it also steadily maintained the point that the primary mission of Permanente physicians was patient care. The financial arrangements and medical protocols of each project were closely scrutinized by a research committee headed by Ben Feingold, chief of allergy in San Francisco. Committed to research programs as a form of physician education and Medical group prestige, Feingold lobbied on behalf of a permanent research facility in San Francisco and was successful. In 1962 the facility opened in a two-story building adjacent to the San Francisco Medical Center. Among the research projects pursued under Feingold's direction was an investigation into the problem of insect bite reactions, a special problem in the flea-ridden San Francisco peninsula, and a later investigation, which received wide national publicity, into the cause-and-effect relationship between certain food additives and hyper-activity in children.

Proponents of research in The Permanente Medical Group argued that these activities helped to attract well-qualified professionals to the group and helped also to maintain a high intellectual level among the Permanente physicians. Continuing education constituted an even more important intellectual activity. Beginning in the early 1960s, The Permanente Medical Group and the Kaiser Foundation Hospitals jointly sponsored an annual symposium open to all physicians dealing with the topic of general medical or scientific interest. More frequent seminars were offered in internal medicine, general surgery, obstetrics-gynecology, and pediatrics. In 1961 alone, some 2000 physicians and scientists from 8 na-tions attended these programs sponsored by Kaiser-Permanente.

The 1960s also witnessed a formalizing of intern and resident programs. Supported by the community service budget of the Kaiser Foundation Hospitals and approved by the American Medical Association and the board of examiners of the various medical specialties involved, intern and resident programs nevertheless remained controversial within the Permanente Medical Group. Some Kaiser Foundation Hospitals, Oakland and San Francisco for example, had intern and resident training pro-grams; others, such as Walnut Creek, Hayward, Vallejo, and Redwood City, did not. Critics of this imbalance argued that the hospitals with resi-dents and interns were able to ease the burden of night and weekend call schedules in a way that was not fair to Permanente physicians at hospitals without such programs. Some argued that the presence of residents and interns interfered with the Permanente philosophy of primary responsibil-ity of the attending physician for health care. It was also argued that resi-dent and intern programs were overly expensive to maintain. Supporters of the teaching programs argued that the presence of bright young minds fresh out of medical schools stimulated good doctors to be better doctors. Far from being shortchanged, Kaiser-Permanente patients actually bene-fited from receiving the latest forms of diagnosis and treatment. Flourish-ing intern and resident programs, furthermore, increased the prestige of the Medical Group, which in turn helped the recruitment and retention of high-quality physicians.

Many of the best young doctors coming into the Medical Group were being recruited from residencies in Kaiser-Permanente hospitals. Such young residents had already worked in prepaid group practice and thus understood its philosophy. They were also committed to northern Cal-ifornia as a place to live. Best of all, their professional skills, manners, and suitability for group practice had been repeatedly evaluated by Permanente physicians and department chiefs during their years of residency; indeed, so close was this scrutiny, up to 6 months' credit toward election to partnership was being granted by the Medical group to physicians who had completed residencies in the Kaiser Foundation Hospitals in northern California.

Defenders of the intern and residency programs also pointed to the gratifying record being compiled by Kaiser-Permanente residents in their certifying examinations. By 1976 Kaiser-Permanente residents taking certifying examinations from the American Board of Internal Medicine were consistently scoring in the top quartile of physicians from 350 training programs in the United States. In certain subspecialty subject areas, in hematology and oncology, for instance, residents from San Francisco Kaiser Foundation Hospital programs were one year ranked second among residents from the top 10 programs in the country. Not surprisingly, with their experience in group practice, Kaiser-Permanente residents scored particularly well in questions dealing with patient management problems and distinguished themselves in dealing with questions of cost effectiveness, having absorbed the Permanente philosophy that the best care is not necessarily the most expensive.

Thus the 1960s in general witnessed the deepening and strengthening of The Permanente Medical Group as a medical organization. By assuming responsibility for research and postgraduate education and training programs, The Permanente Medical Group in northern California committed itself to as complete as possible a practice of medicine, ever seeking high levels of quality. Just a few years earlier, the very competency of Permanente physicians was being questioned by medical societies violently opposed to prepaid group practice. By the end of the 1960s such attacks had become absurd. Not only were Permanente physicians practicing good medicine, but they were also utilizing their unique environment with its demographic inclusiveness, with well-established research protocols and controls, and its vast input of automated data, collected over 15 years, to contribute to both medical science and the socioeconomics of medical care delivery. By 1969, the challenges presented to Kaiser-Permanente by Sidney Garfield at the Monterey Conference had not been completely met. Sidney Garfield, after all, had a way of always operating on the cutting edge of the future. But the challenges had been confronted and in many cases channeled into successful programs, and from this experience there had been consolidated in the Medical Group an even stronger sense of internal identity and a creative, positive relationship to the medical world at large.

11

Construction, Expansion, and Governance— The 1960s

1

In 1967 the founding era receded further into history with the death of Henry J. Kaiser. Even as this era passed, another was emerging. Just as the question of governance dominated the 1950s, the central challenge of the 1960s was coping with growth and expansion. Although some intraorganizational tensions did surface in the 1960s, they were minor. Without the agreements and relationships hammered out in the 1950s, the extraordinary growth and expansion of the 1960s could not have taken place.

The challenges of the 1960s began with the need for new hospitals, which in turn involved new levels of capitalization, and this in turn made necessary the further intensification of a central identity. As a rule of thumb, Kaiser Foundation Hospitals and The Permanente Medical Group worked on a ratio of two hospitals beds per 1000 Health Plan members. By 1960 in northern California there were 1115 licensed beds for 399,000 enrollees, representing a ratio of 2.9 beds per 1000 members. Theoretically, this ratio should have been more than adequate.

But 335 of these available beds were in Vallejo, where many of them were being used for the Rehabilitation Institute. Others were not being staffed because they were not required at the time for the acute care of the Health Plan population in Vallejo. In other areas, by contrast, such as Redwood City and Hayward, the need for acute care beds sometimes exceeded local resources. The question, then, became one of targeted expansion of hospital facilities. At the Santa Clara Medical Center, for instance, with its growing population and Health Plan membership, 159 beds were added by 1964. By then, a new hospital in Hayward was also under construction. All in all, between 1960 and 1965, 282 beds were added in selected locations, bringing the overall bed to patient ratio to 2.16 per 1000 members.

Buying land, building hospitals, clinics, and doctors' offices, equipping and staffing them—all this required millions of dollars of capital. Since 1942 the bank of America had provided Kaiser-Permanente with practically all of its loans. This willingness of the bank to finance the riskiest venture possible, hospitals, proceeded in large part because of the personal relationship between Henry J. Kaiser and A. P. Giannini, founder and chair of the bank, who was willing to extend credit to the Health Plan and Hospitals because of the total assets of Kaiser Industries. Without such assets, Giannini might have balked at extending credit to a medical organization as he had in 1942. Prior to 1962, Eugene Trefethen and George Woods, a Boston banker with strong ties to the Kaisers, had sought unsuccessfully to raise money in New York for the Hospitals and the Health Plan from lending institutions other than the Bank of America. Trefethen and Woods discovered that the major lending institutions did not consider the Kaiser Foundation Health Plan and the Kaiser Foundation Hospitals viable. enterprises in their own right. They were considered, rather, dependent agencies of the overall Kaiser organization; hence, any credit extended to them had to be through the Kaiser Companies channel.

In 1962 a breakthrough occurred: the First National Bank of Portland agreed to extend a line of credit to the Health Plan and Hospitals for its expansion in that area. Not only did the First National Bank of Portland extend this credit, but one of its leaders, Charles Marshall, also persuaded other banks and pension funds in the area to get involved. All in all, Clifford Keene raised $35 million from these new sources. By 1966, the Kaiser-Permanente Medical Care Program was benefiting from a 3-year, $42 million construction program, which included a $6.5 million high-rise hospital tower over the top of the existing Oakland structure, the completion of the Hayward Hospital and Clinic ($4 million), a new Redwood City Medical Center ($7 million), additions and renovations to the San Francisco Hospital ($9.7 million), and purchases of hospitals in San Rafael ($1.6 million) and Sacramento ($9.35 million). In 1968 the Health Plan negotiated another $45 million for facilities in the northern California region. All told, by 1968 Kaiser Foundation Hospitals was able to borrow a total of $268 million from various lenders. Keene and his staff—Irving Bolton, Arthur Weissman, Scott Fleming—became skilled at making sophisticated presentations to bankers and the guardians of pension trusts. Initially turned down in 1962 by Atwood Austin, guardian of the Kaiser Steel Pension Trust, Keene had the pleasure by 1967 of having Atwood go to Trefethen and complain that the Health Plan and Hospitals were borrowing money from every pension plan but those connected with the Kaiser Companies! Satisfied with Kaiser Steel Pension Trust rates, Keene signed for the loan.

Some of this new financial credibility came from the appointment of an outside director to the board of directors of Kaiser Foundation hospitals. This outside director was the very same George S. Woods, chairperson of the board of the First Boston Corporation, who had tried unsuccessfully along with Trefethen to raise money for the Hospitals in the pre-1962 period. As the head of an internationally respected financial institution, George Woods helped bring the needed fiscal credibility to the board of directors of Kaiser Foundation Hospitals, which now included Henry J. Kaiser, Edgar Kaiser, Eugene Trefethen, Clifford Keene, Sidney Garfield, A. B. Ordway, William Marks, George Link, Paul Marrin, and new member George Woods. In 1968, thirty years after the dean of the School of Medicine at Stanford had cautioned Cecil Cutting against jeopardizing his career by joining Sidney Garfield at Grand Coulee, the Vice President for Medical Affairs of Stanford University, Dr. Robert Glaser, became the second outside director of Kaiser Foundation Hospitals. This appointment underscored the growing respectability and national attention the once-embattled Kaiser-Permanente program was now receiving.

In 1961, for instance, the United Steelworkers of America conducted a national survey of medical care programs across the country participated in by their union membership. The survey favorably reported on the Kaiser-Permanente program in the San Francisco Bay Area and at Fontana. That same year, the American Hospital Association invited Cecil Cutting to a national workshop on the organization of hospital inpatient services. The AMA, meanwhile, invited Arthur Weissman of the central office to serve as a special consultant to an AMA commission on the costs of medical care. Then came the favorable coverage in *Time* on September 14, 1962. A year later, Congressmember Chet Holifield of

California read into the *Congressional Record* for February 28, 1963, a laudatory description of Kaiser-Permanente. The following October, Cecil Cutting published a scholarly article, "Medical Care: Its Social and Organizational Aspects, Group Medical Practice and Prepayment," in the prestigious *New England Journal of Medicine.*

In the decade that followed, Cecil Cutting became increasingly active as a writer for medical journals and periodicals and as a spokesperson for prepaid group medical practice in general and the Kaiser-Permanente program in particular. Cutting also became increasingly involved with the activities of the California Medical Association (CMA) and the AMA, a far cry from the standoffish attitude of these two organizations a decade earlier. In early 1965 the Bureau of Research and Planning of the CMA invited Cutting to participate in a discussion of "The Role of Medicine in Society." Later that same year, the AMA specifically invited Cutting to attend a meeting of its Council on Medical Services. Also in 1965 Dean John Snyder of the Harvard School of Public Health personally called upon Clifford Keene in Oakland to invite him to give the annual Milton J. Rosenau Lecture in public health. Keene lectured on "The Social Organization of Medicine." Keene later served on the Visiting Committees of the Harvard School of Medicine, the Harvard School of Dentistry, the Harvard School of Public Health, and a committee of the Harvard Business School dealing with medical economics. He also served on boards at the Medical School at Stanford, the University of Michigan Medical Center, and the Charles R. Drew Postgraduate Medical School in Los Angeles. This recognition from academic institutions, the CMA, and the AMA was especially gratifying to those who had endured the legal actions, harassments, and quiet ostracisms of the late 1940s and the attempts within the AMA in the 1950s to declare prepaid group medical practice unethical.

Not only was Cutting invited by the CMA, the AMA, and other organizations to speak or to write for various publications, but the program itself also began to receive a steady stream of visiting academics, medical economists, government officials, and other affiliates of organized medicine. A team from Johns Hopkins Medical School, led by the dean and associate dean, visited the program in 1966. Johns Hopkins later sponsored a group-practice prepayment health plan in Columbia, Maryland. During this same period, visiting teams from Mt. Sinai Medical School and Temple University Medical School also visited the program. The Surgeon General of the United States, William H. Stewart, inspected the program in 1966, as did Mrs. Marie Henderson, an official of the Federal Civil Service Commission, with which Kaiser-Permanente had a contract. The next year, 1967, The Permanente Medical Group was visited on February 20 by Charles M. Hudson, president of the AMA. Here indeed was a highly historical *tableau vivant:* the leader of organized medicine in America courteously visiting a medical group which the AMA, 10 years earlier, had speculated might be unethical.

Perhaps the most important of these mid-1960s recognitions and contacts came as a result of the 1966 visit of the Subcommittee on Technology of the National Advisory Commission on Health Manpower. "The quality of care provided by Kaiser," the commission reported in November 1967, "is equivalent, if not superior to, that available in most communities. Permanente physicians use standard medical practices and procedures. Patient satisfaction is indicated by the overall flow of patients into Kaiser from competing health plans under the dual choice available to all Kaiser subscribers." In its report the commission had cited the fact that Kaiser subscribers were found to have hospital use rates 30 percent below the state average. "The staff study group concluded that the majority of savings achieved by Kaiser result primarily from effective control over the nature of medical care that is provided and over the place where care is given."[1]

Five of the eight final recommendations of the commission, in fact, seemed to be directly inspired by Kaiser-Permanente. These were (1) the development of outpatient services, (2) the adjustment of Medicare and Medicaid payments to permit prepaid comprehensive care programs to share in the savings they effected through effective utilization of resources, (3) the reduction of hospital utilization, (4) the encouragement of health insurance organizations to share savings with health-care purveyors with less costly hospital utilization, and finally, (5) peer review as a technique for the control of hospitalization.

It soon became apparent that the Kaiser-Permanente Medical Care Program, with its long experience of comprehensive health care within a rigidly controlled cost structure, provided a wealth of insights and techniques applicable to Medicare, Medicaid, and a growing number of medical insurance programs. Within 1 week in October 1967, Cecil Cutting received invitations to discuss Kaiser-Permanente before three important groups: the American Association of Medical Clinics, the AMA Congress on the Socio-Economics of Medical Care, and the White House Conference on Medical Care Costs being convened under the auspices of HEW Secretary John Gardner. Some participants in the White House Conference left the meeting favoring a national system of prepaid group practice. One of the formal recommendations of the conference advocated support for legislation that would provide incentives for group-practice prepayment programs throughout the United States.

Needless to say, The Permanente Medical Group physicians were flattered that the federal government should be turning to Kaiser-Permanente as an illustrative model. They remained puzzled, however, by what they perceived to be the schizoid behavior of the federal government, praising them at the White House Conference, while pursuing through the IRS what the physicians believed was an unjustified tax claim on their retirement program.

Nor was this chorus of praise universal. Fee-for-service physicians practicing in the same communities as Kaiser-Permanente remained unconvinced that savings being realized under prepaid group practice were due to the system. The fee-for-service physicians continued to believe that Health Plan members were actually using fee-for-service practitioners instead of Permanente doctors. At the annual meeting of the CMA in May 1967, delegates from the Alameda–Contra Costa Medical Society introduced a resolution requesting that the CMA study whether or not Kaiser Health Plan members were actually utilizing fee-for-service physicians on the side, and if so, in what numbers?

The Permanente Medical Group Executive Committee welcomed the study and agreed to cooperate with it in every way. The study revealed that Health Plan members utilized non-Permanente physicians in three recurring instances. First and most obvious was in the case of services not covered by the Kaiser-Permanente system—cosmetic surgery, for example. Second, there were instances in which victims of industrial accidents were specifically directed by the insurance carrier to specified physicians and hospitals. Third, a small number of Health Plan members had previously bonded with fee-for-service physicians and continued to consult with them even after they had enrolled in Kaiser-Permanente. Even these, however, continued to consult Permanente physicians with about the same frequency as members who used Kaiser-Permanente only. The CMA study thus proved that the success of the Kaiser-Permanente program did not depend upon a use of non-Permanente physicians, although such outside consultations did occur.

Through the auspices of Kaiser Foundation International, an organization legally distinct from the Health Plan but related to the interest of Kaiser Industries in health enterprises abroad, the Kaiser-Permanente philosophy began to work its influence on the international scene as well. Keene, Saward, and a number of other physicians from the various Permanente Medical Groups provided consultation on hospital construction and management in Ghana, Nigeria, Argentina, Brazil, and

Australia, where various Kaiser companies were active. Keene and Saward made several trips to Argentina, where Kaiser automobiles were being manufactured in Cordova. On matters not related to Kaiser Industries abroad, Cecil Cutting traveled to Okinawa, Wally Cook to Mexico, and John Smillie to Sierra Leone as consultants in 1968. Both Smillie and, later, Gerald Stewart, a regional medical center administrator, went to Sierra Leone under the auspices of a New York–based foundation called the American Health Education for African Development. Neither Okinawa nor Sierra Leone, however, had a middle-class population sufficient to support a private prepayment group-practice plan.

As interest in prepaid group medical practice continued to grow, Cecil Cutting was inundated with requests for information. "I am suggesting," Cutting reported to the partnership on October 13, 1969, "that they not put their foot in it unless they can put their heart in it also. That is, first to be convinced of the principles, philosophy, and desire to provide good medical care at reasonable cost—to take pride in being part of an organization that is making the medical dollar go a little bit farther."[2] That same year, the American Association of Medical Clinics, later (in 1974) to rename itself the American Group Practice Association, established a commission to accredit medical groups. Cecil Cutting served on the task force dealing with quality of care.

2

From this increased complexity of activity—the expanded lines of credit, the growing need to gather statistics and to do long-range planning, the increasing requests for information and consultation from outside organizations, the invitations to expand to other regions—emerged two new major modes of administration and policy formation, the Central Office, and the Kaiser-Permanente Committee. The Central Office was not planned. It just happened. But as in the case of the Kaiser-Permanente program itself, which happened just as spontaneously in the Mojave Desert in the mid-1930s, the Central Office, once it had happened, soon assumed an aura of inevitability. The Kaiser-Permanente Committee, by contrast, evolved logically out of the conflicts during the 1950s between Health Plan–Hospitals and the Medical Groups. From this perspective, the Kaiser-Permanente Committee constituted a maturation of a dialogue between physicians and nonphysicians as to the policy and governance of the program.

Within a short time after his arrival in 1954, Clifford Keene had his own office at 1924 Broadway, the international headquarters of Kaiser Industries, but this office brought with it neither specific responsibilities nor support staff. Caught in a twilight world as a shadow administrator to the still formidable Sidney Garfield, Keene began to take an interest in the assemblage of data and statistics regarding the various regions. Gradually, all such activities began to coalesce around Keene, despite the fact that no formal title was given to him until 1960. "The Central Office," Keene later recalled, "was not a nicely thought out preconceived plan. It was just the progressive development of activities that occurred around myself."[3]

Keene began these operations with two staff assistants, attorney Scott Fleming, who also doubled as assistant to William Marks, secretary to the Health Plan and Hospitals, and medical economist and statistician Arthur Weissman, whom Henry J. Kaiser had personally recruited in 1951 from the U.S. Public Health Service. Two Kaiser-Permanente veterans, Ned Dodds and William Price, also joined Keene's staff. Dodds worked on facility planning, and Price served as office administrator. This nucleus was then joined by the treasurer of the Kaiser Industries, Joaquin Felix dos Reis (better known as Joe Reis) who introduced into the Central Office such Kaiser financial experts as Karl Palmaer, Irving Bolton, Howard Spaulding, and Walter Palmer. In 1957 Gibson Kingren, a Health Plan representative in northern California, was sent to Sacramento as a lobbyist. As of yet, however, the term "Central Office" had not come into use.

During the Hawaii crisis of the summer of 1960, Clifford Keene had acted decisively. He had dissolved the recalcitrant Pacific Medical Associates and had gotten Saward to reorganize it as the Hawaii Permanente Medical Group. He had personally appointed Dr. Philip Chu to be its director. It was an unusually bold step for the general manager of the Health Plan, the title Keene now bore, to appoint the leader of an independently contracting medical group of an autonomous region. By taking charge, Keene asserted his own authority, so ambiguous through the 1950s. Shortly after the Hawaii crisis, Keene was named director, vice president, and general manager of Kaiser Foundation Hospitals, Inc., and Kaiser Foundation Health Plan. He was also elected a vice president of the Kaiser Industries Corporation, with responsibilities for industrial medical programs, and a vice president of the Kaiser Foundation.

In 6 years Keene had emerged from his basement desk in a corner of Sidney Garfield's office to administrative preeminence in the Health Plan and the Hospitals, backed by a growing and increasingly involved support staff. As general manager, Keene made decisions in concert with regional management on Health Plan rates and the allocation of resources for facilities. He spearheaded the formation of capital for construction projects and together with the regional medical directors appointed regional managers. He selected key personnel for what was now the de facto Central Office. It was Keene who recommended Robert Glaser, vice president of medical affairs at Stanford University, for appointment to the board of directors of the Health Plan and Hospitals in 1964. Keene had become friendly with Glaser while lecturing at Harvard, where Glaser was then responsible for amalgamating the various hospitals associated with the Harvard Medical School under one umbrella organization.

Initially, The Permanente Medical Group experienced a sense of distance from these burgeoning Central Office activities. "I would call up and say," Cecil Cutting later recalled," 'Why in the world are you adding any more people there? Look at your budget, it's bigger than ours is!'"[4] But Permanente physicians realized that a growing multimillion dollar organization, increasingly involved in a maze of government relations, financial, planning, construction, and other administrative complexities required sophisticated staff support and coordination. As Executive Director of The Permanente Medical Group, Cecil Cutting worked closely with the Central Office in general and such individual Kaiser-Permanente administrators as Karl Steil, especially, Frank Jones, and Felix Day. Cutting later gave credit to these administrators for helping to create the generally harmonious atmosphere of this time of expansion and transition.

Structurally, this power and decision sharing among the medical directors of the four Medical Groups, the Central Office, and the regional administrations took the form of the Kaiser Permanente Committee. The Advisory Council of the mid-1950s had been torn apart by adversarial feelings. With the signing of the Medical Service Agreements, it soon became apparent that some structured form of dialogue among the various entities of Kaiser-Permanente had to be resumed. On Mother's Day 1960 Clifford Keene convened the first and only interentity conference on the theme "Planning for the 1960s." Perhaps the mood of Mother's Day spilled over into the proceedings, for in contrast to the 1950s, the physicians and the administrators, despite an initial standoffishness, were at least agreeing to plan their future together. "It was almost like a gathering of strange bulldogs," Clifford Keene later recalled of this Mother's Day meeting. "Everybody, I think, wanted to be nice and to forget the fights of the past, but everybody was suspicious of everybody else, and everybody was suspicious of me. So we started out talking about the simplest of things, just began talking. What kind of an organization are we? What are our common goals? What makes us different? Why are we succeeding when no one else seems to be? These were pretty basic questions which wouldn't start an argument, but did start everyone talking. We had to establish ways of talking to each other."[5]

This necessity for a forum for future planning became even more obvious as major policy decisions regarding expansion and growth came to the fore. The Health Insurance Plan of Greater New York began to send out tentative feelers about a possible merger with Kaiser-Permanente, thus coalescing the two largest prepaid programs of their type in the nation. The United Mine Workers (UAW) approached Kaiser-Permanente about assuming responsibility for health-care programs in Appalachia. In the 1950s Edgar Kaiser had formed a close working relationship with Walter Reuther, the head of the UAW. Several times in the early and mid-1960s Reuther approached Edgar Kaiser about the possibility of Kaiser-Permanente assuming responsibility for the health-care program of his union in Detroit. Each of these tentative offers involved a major policy decision. Responsible for planning and coordinating growth in the existing regions, the Central Office had neither the time nor the authority to make such policy decisions. The board of trustees of the Kaiser Health Plan and Hospitals was likewise reluctant to proceed unilaterally without the concurrence of the physicians and exhaustive preliminary research. The Medical Groups, for their part, had specifically worked out in the various Medical Service Agreements that there would be no expansion without their approval. Clearly, some structured dialogue among the various Kaiser-Permanente entities was necessary.

Meanwhile, an increasing number of requests for information and direction were coming into the various Kaiser-Permanente entities, and these also involved policy consideration. Visitors—consumers, providers, medical schools, management consultants, union leaders, health-care officials from abroad—would come to the Central Office, Cecil Cutting later remembered, and get one perspective. Others would come to the Medical Group and get another. Still others would come to both the Central Office and the Medical Group and receive guidelines that were not in conformity. In May 1967 the medical directors and the regional managers from each of the four regions met with key personnel from the Central Office at the Del Monte Lodge in Monterey to formulate a unified response to this growing number of outside inquiries and requests for help. At that meeting it was decided that the Kaiser-Permanente program was not at that time prepared to assume responsibility for the UAW-sponsored Community Health Association in Detroit. The question of expansion, however, was recognized as a recurring issue, and so the group agreed to meet again to deal with this and similar issues.

In September 1967 the same group reconvened at the Del Monte Lodge to reconsider the decision not to become involved in Detroit. Walter Reuther was still pressing his case. The Community Health Foundation of Cleveland was also pressing for a Kaiser-Permanente affiliation. To deal with these requests more in depth, a formal committee was established at this second Del Monte meeting. This committee consisted of the four regional medical directors, the four regional managers, plus Clifford Keene, MD, Arthur Weissman, and Scott Fleming from the Central Office. A staff person, Gordon Shields, was also assigned to this planning committee. When the committee next convened in August 1968 at Santa Barbara, it formally adopted the name Kaiser-Permanente Committee.

At both the September 1967 meeting at Monterey and the August 1968 meeting at Santa Barbara, the specific proposals from Cleveland and Detroit, together with the general question of expansion, were discussed. In the meanwhile, Clifford Keene had been approached about an expansion of Kaiser-Permanente to Denver. Ray Kay, medical director of the Southern California Permanente Medical Group, was in favor of the Denver option—particularly if The Permanente Medical Group in northern California took responsibility for Cleveland. Over the years, an opinion had formed in the eastern medical establishment that the success of Kaiser-Permanente was a localized west-of-the-Rockies phenomenon. Only the population boom and social displacements of the war years and postwar expansion on the west coast, it was argued, had made such an innovative program a success. Kaiser-Permanente was working on the Pacific coast because millions of Americans had migrated there in a short period of time, were in need of medical care, and did not have the more established connections and procedures of the American regions east of the Rockies. Proponents of this position thus considered Kaiser-Permanente a west coast aberration rather than a model for health-care delivery throughout the United States.

This argument was directly contradicted by the increased attention being paid to Kaiser-Permanente by the national medical establishment, beginning in the late 1950s, together with the specific requests for mergers that were coming in from New York, Detroit, and Cleveland. Needless to say, those within the Kaiser-Permanente organization remained unconvinced by the west-of-the-Rockies argument. This did not mean, however, that they favored imprudent expansion.

At the Santa Barbara meeting, the Kaiser-Permanente Committee, as it was now called, drew up seven specific criteria, not as absolutes, but as indicators of success for any possible expansions. They were legality, population, physicians, hospitals, impact, competition, and capital.

Prepaid comprehensive health care and group medical practice, first of all, must be legal in the state where expansion might occur. Since Kaiser-Permanente had just emerged from a period of hostility from local and state medical societies in the Pacific region, no one wanted a recurrence of such conflict elsewhere in the nation. Second, there was the question of population. In Hawaii, the program had faltered because there initially were not enough enrollees. At the Santa Barbara meeting it was determined that 50,000 enrollees constituted the minimum population necessary for a balanced multispecialty medical group and efficient medical center, including a hospital. Fifty thousand enrollees were necessary to guarantee financial self-sufficiency. Since between 10 and 20 percent of a community population could be expected to enroll in the Health Plan, a community population in excess of 250,000 would be necessary. The committee also expressed reluctance to go into a region whose economy was based upon a single industry. Other demographic indicators such as the median age and growth rate of the population would also have to be taken into consideration.

Then there was the question of physicians. There had to be a nucleus of competent physicians in the area willing to organize a medical group. While some seasoned Permanente physicians could be sent out to a new region, the basic staffing had to come from community physicians. The overall professional environment of a proposed region was also a critical factor. The region had to be a good place to practice medicine. Thus, beds and hospital services had to be available to the program from the outset. It also had to be determined whether existing hospitals could be purchased. Since new construction might be necessary, an effort should be made to ascertain the attitude of planning and governmental agencies toward hospital growth. Adequate capital had to be available without impairing the financial integrity of existing regions.

Finally, there remained the more subtle questions of competition and impact, together with the abiding requirement of available capital. Each new region, it was decided, should provide some national impact for Kaiser-Permanente. A program should not go into remote or obscure areas. A region under consideration should also serve as a springboard for expansion into nearby areas. In the matter of competition, the Kaiser Foundation Health Plan would have to make a significant contribution to the choices available in a region. It would make no sense whatsoever to go into an area where a program similar to Kaiser-Permanente was already flourishing.

On January 7, 1969, the Kaiser-Permanente Committee held a special meeting to reconsider Detroit and to examine more closely the Denver and Cleveland options. Some members of the Kaiser-Permanente Committee, concerned about the potential drain of finances and personnel from existing regions, were reluctant to expand at all, anywhere. Five years earlier, in fact, on October 9, 1964, Edgar Kaiser had sent a memorandum to Clifford Keene discouraging even thinking about expansion, "How are you going to do it, Keene? Where are you going to get the bucks?"[6] This reluctance on the part of Edgar Kaiser gradually softened. Keene, meanwhile, had tactfully agreed to apportion the Denver possibility to Ray Kay and the Southern California Permanente Medical Group, and the Cleveland option to Cecil Cutting and The Permanente Medical group. That way, responsibility for expansion, together with its possible financial and career benefits, would be equally shared by the two largest Permanente Medical Groups. Thus the Medical Groups did not per se oppose expansion.

At the January meeting, there were more possible long-range benefits from expansion that emerged in discussion and helped carry the day. Those favoring expansion argued that Kaiser-Permanente had to expand if it wanted to be in a position to be included in a national health insurance plan, should such a plan ever be adopted. After much discussion, it was decided to move ahead with the Denver and Cleveland expansion programs. Financial resources for these expansions were secured from a grant and a non-interest-bearing loan from the Henry J. Kaiser Family Foundation. Approximately $1.5 million was raised from the liquidation of Kaiser Industries stock donated by members of the Kaiser family and other Kaiser executives to Kaiser Foundation Hospitals. The trustees of the Family Foundation insisted that Kaiser-Permanente also make a financial commitment. As Kaiser-Permanente's contribution, a small per member per month contribution, rising gradually to a maximum of 5 cents per member per month by 1973, was approved for recommendation to the board of directors of the Kaiser Foundation Health Plan.

------------------------ **3** ------------------------

Ironically, the existing, if embattled, Community Health Foundation of Cleveland already sustained a significant Kaiser-Permanente connection. In 1961 the Group Health Institute met in Portland for its annual convention hosted by The Permanente Clinic. Avram Yedidia of the Kaiser Foundation Health Plan introduced Ernest Saward to a group of various union leaders from the Cleveland area, including Samuel Pollock of the Meat Cutters' Union. Saward took them on a tour of The Permanente Clinic and the new Bess Kaiser Hospital. The union leaders were impressed, especially Sam Pollock, a trade unionist–intellectual of the most unusual sort. Self-educated and widely read, Pollock maintained a large library at his office in Cleveland and another personal collection in his home. He also monitored European news on his shortwave radio and kept current with labor developments in a number of countries. Fascinated by social policy questions, Pollock was a dynamic visionary as well as a skilled pragmatic union leader and negotiator. After his retirement from the Meat Cutters' Union, Pollock lectured frequently at colleges and universities on labor and social policy questions.

Not surprisingly, once Pollock had seen the Permanente program in Oregon, and envisioned it happening in Cleveland, matters began to develop rapidly. Then and there, Pollock and other Cleveland leaders retained Yedidia as a consultant to help them organize a comprehensive prepaid program in their area. Interest in such a program had been percolating in Cleveland since the early 1950s but had been stifled by a 20-year-old statute that effectively blocked the formation of prepaid group-practice programs. In 1959 a labor-based coalition succeeded in getting this statute repealed. Several of the labor leaders who were spearheading the movement toward prepaid group practice in Ohio served as trustees of the Union Eye Care Center in Cleveland. A number of these trustees had been in Portland with Sam Pollock and, enthusiastically joining him in the drive for a prepaid program, persuaded the Union Eye Care Center to become involved as a sponsoring institution with a $25,000 enabling grant. This money allowed Yedidia to be hired as a consultant, together with healthcare manager Glenn Wilson and Dr. E. Richard Weinerman of Yale University. Later, Ernest Saward of The Permanente Clinic in Portland was also brought in as a consultant. Saward went out to Cleveland and organized several physicians on the faculty of Case Western Reserve into a medical group and served as temporary medical director and sole proprietor of the group until replaced by Dr. Gene Vayda when the group changed from a sole proprietorship to a partnership, following the pattern of the Permanente Medical Groups in California and Oregon.

Opening in July 1964, the Community Health Foundation (CHF) of Cleveland got off to a fairly good start, thanks to strong union support. One important component of the prepaid genetic code, however—the integration of facilities—had been ignored. The CHF program was dependent upon community hospital facilities. This inhibited smooth and efficient operations. The sole facility the CHF owned, moreover, was on the wrong side of the Cuyahoga River. Most of the potential enrollees of the CHF—blue-collar union members, that is—lived on the west side of the Cuyahoga River and were reluctant for reasons of ethnic and class identity to cross over to the east side of the river for hospital care. On the other hand, it was extremely difficult for the CHF to acquire hospital privileges on the west side of the Cuyahoga. The price for such hospital privileges in Cleveland was high. CHF doctors found themselves forced to donate several sessions per week of free service to hospital outpatient clinics so as to maintain their privileges in west-side hospitals. Obstetrical and pediatric services, moreover, could not be located in the same facility. By 1966 it had become clear that for the CHF to work, it had to have its own hospital.

Using labor union funds, in 1967 the CHF acquired a site in Independence, a suburban community west of Cleveland, for the construction of a new facility. As is often the case, the proposed hospital project involved zoning changes, which had to be put to a popular vote. The labor unions waged an intensive and very expensive campaign. They anticipated a successful outcome, for 80 percent of the working population in the Independence voting district were union members. The proposed zoning changes were voted down, however, by a narrow margin, presumably because blacks from the east side of the Cuyahoga River would be coming to the west-side hospital as patients and as employees. Racial conflict in Cleveland had left the CHF with a site, a $400,000 mortgage, obligations for $100,000 in legal and architectural fees, but no cash and no permission to build a hospital.

At this point, Ernest Saward, who had helped get the program going in 1964, reentered the situation, suggesting that CHF and Kaiser-Permanente initiate exploratory talks. Conversations continued when Sam Pollock and other Cleveland area labor leaders attended the annual meeting of the American Public Health Association held in San Francisco in 1967. A committed unionist, Pollock did not completely trust the Kaiser industrialists on the board of the Kaiser Foundation Health Plan, nor did his other labor colleagues. The distrust seemed mutual. In an effort to smooth matters out, Saward made reservations for the Cellar Room of the Blue Fox restaurant in San Francisco for the evening of October 31, 1967, and invited both the trustees and the labor union leaders together for a festive dinner. Over cocktails, tensions softened. Over dinner and generous servings of fine California vintages, geniality replaced the earlier standoffishness, and discussions regarding a possible merger continued in an atmosphere of cordiality.

Clifford Keene favored the Cleveland venture. Whatever problems the CHF was experiencing in the matter of its hospital, Cleveland stood at the geographical center of nearly half the population of the United States. Highly industrialized, this region also sustained a strong union movement, as evidenced in the very formation of the CHF 5 years earlier, and these unions in turn offered the potential for a strong membership. With its capital resources, Kaiser-Permanente could buy a hospital in the Cleveland area rather than repeat the expensive and problematic process of acquiring a new site and securing the necessary zoning approvals. Along with Karl Steil, northern California regional manager, Keene visited the struggling health plan in Cleveland and returned even more in favor of the merger.

In April and August 1968 Cecil Cutting made long visits to the medical group at the Cleveland CHF on behalf of The Permanente Medical Group. Upon his return, the Executive Committee questioned Cutting at length as to the costs of the proposed expansion. Cutting convinced the committee that the money required to acquire a hospital or to construct outpatient facilities in Cleveland would not adversely affect the facilities development program already capitalized and under way in northern California. Even then, the matter was not closed for discussion. One partner asked the Executive Director pointedly at a partnership meeting, "Why are we expanding to Cleveland when we have problems at home requiring attention?"

There was a dramatic pause as Cutting formulated his response, "We have been asked. We know of unsuccessful plans that did not follow our format. Failures may follow with plans in which lay persons take over responsibilities we think properly belong in the hands of progressive physicians. The medical group in Cleveland is a good group. They only lack a hospital."[7] With this argument—that the Cleveland physicians were strongly committed to prepaid group medical practice—Cutting helped create a climate of opinion in favor of the expansion. A few days after the partnership meeting, the Executive Committee approved Cutting's becoming a voting member of the executive committee of the medical group in Cleveland, later to be called the Ohio Permanente Medical Group.

On January 1, 1969, the board of directors of the Kaiser Foundation Health Plan approved the earlier recommendation of the Kaiser-Permanente Committee favoring the merger with the CHF of Cleveland. The northern California region of the Kaiser-Permanente program was assigned the responsibility for assisting with operations in Cleveland. The CHF now became the Kaiser Community Health Foundation. Its executive director Glenn Wilson was promoted to trustee, along with labor leader Sam Pollock and businessperson Lee C. Howley, general counsel of the Cleveland Illuminating Company and a leader in the politically powerful Catholic community. Howley later became a director of the Kaiser Foundations Hospitals and Health Plan.

In searching for ways to administer the new region, the Kaiser-Permanente committee devised a sponsor plan, with the northern California region acting as sponsor. Karl Steil, who also remained regional manager in northern California during the start-up period, assumed responsibility for the Health Plan and Hospitals, while Cecil Cutting assumed an advisory role with the Cleveland physicians. Shortly thereafter Dr. Sam Packer was elected medical director of the Ohio Permanente Medical Group.

4

In contrast to the Cleveland situation, in which Kaiser-Permanente reclaimed an organization it had helped get started, the Denver program started from scratch. Even here, however, there was a Permanente connection. In 1952 Dr. William Dorsey, regional medical director for the United Mine Workers' Welfare and Retirement Fund, based in Denver, and his assistant Ada Kruger had developed a positive working relationship with the northern California Permanente physicians working in Dragerton, Utah. During this time, Permanente physicians were operating the Utah Permanente Hospital, which served mine workers employed by Kaiser Steel and U.S. Steel companies. Both Dorsey and Kruger wanted the program to be made permanent and to be expanded, but in 1952 when they were replaced by non-Permanente physicians, The Permanente Medical Group physicians returned to their positions in the Bay Area. The seed planted at Dragerton, Utah, however, would eventually grow into a tree in Colorado.

Between 1952 and 1967 Dorsey made several overtures to Kaiser-Permanente to reconsider coming back to the Rocky Mountain region to inaugurate a health-care program for the United Mine Workers. In late 1967 interest in having Kaiser-Permanente come to Colorado was revived after a favorable study was issued by the faculty of the University of Colorado at Boulder. This study, in turn, quickened interest among labor leaders in the Denver area. Once again, William Dorsey contacted Clifford Keene about Kaiser-Permanente's expansion into the

Denver area. When he received a reply indicating interest in exploring the idea, Dorsey flew to California to make a personal presentation to the Kaiser-Permanente Committee. Dorsey brought with him the University of Colorado study indicating that there was a strong market for prepaid group practice in Denver. The Mine Workers in the Colorado region, Dorsey argued, were not getting the quality or quantity of medical care commensurate with the amount of money they were paying for insurance coverage. A consensus had emerged in the region that some sort of prepaid group medical practice program would be a better arrangement. UMW members who had been satisfactorily treated at the rehabilitation center in Vallejo in the 1950s helped to reinforce this opinion.

Several months after Dorsey's presentation, in February 1968, Clifford Keene and Karl Steil stopped over in Denver on their return from Cleveland to the San Francisco Bay Area. Both Keene and Steil were encouraged by the attractiveness of the Mile High City and its potential for growth. The following month, a number of Kaiser-Permanente representatives attended a 2-day seminar in Denver, entitled "Establishing Prepaid Group Health Plans in Colorado," sponsored by the Center for Labor Education and Research of the University of Colorado. Attended by an impressive cross section of local physicians, educators, labor representatives, government officials, and other community leaders, this conference heightened even further the growing interest in bringing Kaiser-Permanente to Denver.

As a follow-up to the conference, Karl Steil assigned Warren "Boots" Ogden, a marketing representative from the Health Plan, and Felix Day, who had worked closely with Dorsey at Dragerton, to do a feasibility study of the Denver area. Day and Ogden made a favorable report, which further encouraged the Kaiser-Permanente Committee. During the balance of 1968 the investigation continued into capital requirements, the availability of physicians and hospital beds, population statistics, and other critical questions. Since Ray Kay had committed the Southern California Permanente Medical Group to back the Denver expansion, Clifford Keene asked Kay and Jim Vohs, regional manager in southern California, to go to Denver and assess the situation. Kay and Vohs made several visits during the latter half of 1968. While in Denver, Kay talked to Wilbur L. Reimers, a respected surgeon with an ongoing interest in the socioeconomics of medicine. Years earlier, Reimers had applied to The Permanente Medical Group to be chief of surgery but had withdrawn his application after he had become discouraged by the hostility at the time of the San Francisco Medical Society. Encouraged by the positive attitude he was encountering in Colorado, Reimers volunteered to help form a new Permanente medical group.

Early in 1969 the Colorado expansion received a positive assessment from the Kaiser-Permanente Committee and approval from the Kaiser Foundation Health Plan and Hospitals Board of Trustees. The Henry J. Kaiser Family Foundation made a tentative grant of $2 million to help finance expansion into the region. Both the permission and the $2 million were conditional. If any major barriers were encountered, the project had to be halted. Operating out of a motel room in east Denver, newly appointed regional manager John Boardman led the search for suitable clinic space and saw to the other arrangements. "I knew we had our work cut out for us," Boardman stated at the time, "the day the telephone company asked for a credit reference."[8]

Boardman discovered available hospital beds at St. Joseph's Hospital, where the director, Sister Mary Andrew, was supportive of the proposed Kaiser-Permanente expansion to Denver. Office space was available next door in the Franklin Medical Building. St. Joseph's extended hospital privileges to the proposed cadre of the about-to-be-formed Colorado Permanente Medical Group. Boardman and the other planners did not foresee the need for a Kaiser Foundation hospital during the first 3 years of operation. Given this positive response, the tentative approvals and the tentative grant of $2 million were made permanent. On July 1, 1969, the Colorado Permanente Medical Group commenced medical treatment in Denver. Despite the encouragement of the labor unions, the Health Plan opened in Colorado with only 712 enrollees and no hospital. After 20 months of operation, enrollment had risen to 15,000, a figure still far short of the 50,000 minimum established by the Kaiser-Permanente Committee at the Santa Barbara meeting. The fact that Denver was overbuilt in hospitals, moreover, was a mixed blessing. On the one hand, this meant that beds were available to Kaiser-Permanente. On the other hand, this very availability delayed the integration of a Kaiser Hospital into the program, a component of the genetic code.

5

Considered from the perspective of the code, the move to Colorado was problematic. From the perspective of the rising tide of growth and acceptability that characterized Kaiser-Permanente in the late 1960s, the expansion to such a desirable city as Denver and such a desirable region as Colorado had to it an element of inevitability. The 1960s had opened with the medical world knocking at Kaiser-Permanente's door. The decade closed with Kaiser-Permanente taking its program to the nation.

As further evidence for this new national role, the Kaiser Foundation Health Plan joined the Group Health Association of America (GHAA) in 1969, after a long debate. Initially, the Executive Committee of The Permanente Medical Group in northern California had resisted joining the GHAA because a number of labor movement people in the association had made highly critical comments against physicians in general. The Permanente physicians resented this rhetoric. Thus, the Permanente physicians who were themselves criticized by organized medicine in the early stages of the program now found themselves defending their fellow physicians against the attacks of the GHAA. In the end, however, the Kaiser-Permanente Committee became convinced that it was not in the best interest of the program for the largest prepayment plan in the country to have no relationship with, or influence over, the national association which purported to speak for group practice prepayment plans. Before it joined the GHAA, however, the Kaiser Foundation Health Plan insisted that the GHAA amend its statement in the bylaws that the purpose of the Association was "consumer control" to read that the purpose was "in the interest of the consumer." Not surprisingly, the Kaiser Foundation Health Plan soon became the major force in the GHAA. Kaiser-Permanente paid dues to GHAA, which more than doubled its annual revenues. Two Health Plan vice presidents, Robert Erickson of the Central Office and Dan Wagster, assistant regional manager in southern California, were elected to the GHAA board of directors. As Clifford Keene later told the Group Health Institute meeting in Hawaii, "When the elephant comes into the tent, the tent assumes the shape of the elephant."

In March 1971, this outward movement of Kaiser-Permanente to the nation expressed itself in the Kaiser-Permanente Medical Care Program Symposium, a 3-day inquiry sponsored jointly by the Association of American Medical Colleges, the Commonwealth Fund, and Kaiser-Permanente. Two hundred and fifty attendees convened in Oakland, most of them medical academicians, including 31 deans of medical schools. Representatives also came from the Cleveland, Lahey, Lovelace, Mayo, and Ochsner Clinics, together with representatives from the Carnegie Corporation and the Rockefeller Foundation. Just a month previously, the Nixon administration had introduced proposed legislation to encourage health maintenance organizations (HMOs). "We suspect," Clifford Keene told the symposium, "that the similarity of the HMO concept and Kaiser-Permanente is more than coincidence. We ourselves don't see Kaiser-Permanente as a panacea. We do see it as one valid solution to some long-standing problems. We see it as an evolving method of organizing and delivering medical care which is intended to be responsive to the changing needs of the people it serves."[9]

This realistic note, of Kaiser-Permanente being one solution but not the only solution, characterized many of the talks delivered at the symposium by the 19 Permanente physicians who were featured speakers. Ably edited by Anne R. Somers, the proceedings of the symposium were published by the Commonwealth Fund later that year as *The Kaiser-Permanente Medical Care Program: One Valid Solution to the Problem of Health Care Delivery in the United States.* Valid, but making no claims to exclusivity, the program had at long last arrived to the point that Sidney Garfield, Henry J. Kaiser, and the Permanente physicians pioneers had envisioned for it since World War II when the possibility of providing quality health care to large groups on a prepayment basis had most boldly presented itself. A year after the proceedings of the Kaiser-Permanente Medical Care Symposium were published, more than 2.5 million Americans were receiving comprehensive medical care under the auspices of Kaiser-Permanente.

The sheer power of these numbers, the very vastness of the success of the Kaiser-Permanente concept, would have delighted Henry J. Kaiser, had he been around to review the enrollment statistics. Kaiser, after all, had always envisioned his projects on a large scale. Kaiser had glimpsed the possibility of millions of people in the United States and abroad enjoying the comprehensive medical care that he considered essential to human happiness and dignity. And now this dream had been actualized and Henry J. Kaiser had lived to see it. He died in 1967. His powerful body had taken 85 years of energetic use. Had he taken care of himself, his personal physician and brother-in-law Sidney Garfield later remarked, he would have lived to be 100.

"He visualized all of this," Eugene Trefethen later said of Henry J. Kaiser. "He thought it could be a plan that would take over the United States' health needs. He would go a lot further than any of us by saying that this is the one thing that will keep us from getting into socialized medicine, and it's the way to set up medicine so you get better quality care. You can spend the money on research, and you can get the best doctors, and you can get the best talents and the best facilities. It will be, as Henry Kaiser said, the one accomplishment he'll be remembered for."[13]

12

Into the Modern Era—Growth and Challenges

———————— 1 ————————

Changes in health care since 1960 have been called a revolution, involving an unprecedented role for government, rapid inflation in health-care costs, a technology explosion, a new emphasis on quality assurance, and the advent of competition among large managed-care organizations.[1]

Kaiser-Permanente was profoundly affected by these developments, but not surprised. Its history demonstrates its ability to cope with adverse conditions. Kaiser-Permanente did not always adapt by making internal changes. Indeed, it modified its environment in order to stay healthy. During the postwar years, Permanente Hospitals were established because physicians could not practice in community hospitals.

As growth continued, the program found its basic principles to be its guide to survival. Its structure remained intact, as Health Plan managers and Permanente physicians made necessary accommodations to demands of regulators, employers, and consumer groups. By the end of the 1980s, 3000 physicians of The Permanente Medical Group were caring for 2,300,000 members in the northern California region, utilizing 15 medical centers and 20 satellite medical offices. New regions had been established in Texas, the middle atlantic states, North Carolina,

Georgia, the northeastern states, and Kansas. Total nationwide membership exceeded 6 million.

Enacted in 1965, Medicare did not fit well with Kaiser-Permanente. Initially, a Part C with capitation payments to HMOs was proposed to augment Part A (hospitals) and Part B (mainly physicians). Part C would have reimbursed HMOs for both hospital and physician care by capitation, Kaiser-Permanente's mode of operation. Part C was dropped in the legislative process, a clear signal that Kaiser-Permanente had not yet matured enough to affect national health policy.[2] Forced to work under Part A, Kaiser Hospitals had to install a cost accounting system. Under Part B, the Medical Group was compensated on a complicated quasicapitation formula.[3] From the early 1960s until 1982, Kaiser-Permanente tried to get Congress to permit prepayment for managed-care systems. It was not until 1982, with the Tax Equity and Fiscal Responsibility Act (TEFRA) that remedial legislation approved a prepayment method that shifted the risk of unexpected utilization from Medicare Trust Funds to HMOs. Regulations were not approved until 1985. Kaiser-Permanente regions other than northern California accepted these "risk" contracts. The northern California region decided to wait until it became clearer that payment by the government would not be reduced over time to less than the usual, cost-based reimbursement.

Wage and price controls, imposed by President Nixon in 1971, created a problem until Kaiser-Permanente negotiated a satisfactory outcome by obtaining an agreement that the Health Plan was not considered as an "insurer," nor were doctors considered as "providers." Both were combined as "an institutional provider."[4]

Kaiser-Permanente's contribution to national health policy reached a peak with the enactment of the Health Maintenance Organization Act of 1973. Kaiser-Permanente was the model for this legislation. The law, however, contained provisions unfavorable to the program, especially a too comprehensive benefits package and open enrollment combined with community rating which allowed for adverse selection against the plan, a certain guarantee to make a health plan sick. A coalition of the Group Health Association of America, Kaiser-Permanente, the American Group Practice Association, the American Association of Foundations of Medical Care, the Health Insurance Association of America, and Blue Cross, calling itself the "Consensus Group" and amiably chaired by Jim Doherty of GHAA, was able to get corrective amendments enacted over the objections of an unlikely alliance of the American Medical Association and Senator Edward Kennedy.[5]

All regions of the Kaiser Foundation Health Plan finally became federally qualified HMOs in 1977, confirming the program's leadership role. The Department of Health, Education, and Welfare saluted the program in a ceremony in New York City, presided over by Secretary Joseph Califano. Dr. Bruce Sams, for The Permanente Medical Group, and the medical directors of all other regions of the program were present. Edgar Kaiser and Sidney Garfield were honored guests. At the same ceremony, Lady Bird Johnson presented Dr. Garfield with the Lyndon Baines Johnson Award for Humanitarian Service.[6]

The Health Planning and Resources Development Act was passed in 1973. This created Health Systems Agencies (HSAs) to curb overbuilding of hospitals and oversupply of expensive hospital technology. Kaiser-Permanente was not at first exempted, even though its ratio of hospital beds to members was well below the target set by HSAs and was frequently cited as an example of prudent allocation of resources. Congress eventually determined that HMOs were part of the solution, not part of the problem. HMOs were exempted from certificate-of-need requirements.[7]

The state of California entered the field of governmental scrutiny when it encouraged the formation of Prepaid Health Plans (PHPs) to contract with its Department of Health Services to provide medical care for MediCal (Medicaid) beneficiaries on a prepaid, capitation basis, following the Kaiser-Permanente model. A myriad of organizations sprang up like mushrooms. Some were fraudulent, owned and managed by persons with political influence in Sacramento. Their medical providers were frequently unavailable, and quality of care was ignored. Other PHPs had inept management; bankruptcies followed. To counter this disaster, the state enacted the Knox-Keene law, which addressed, by regulation, standards for accessibility, quality, marketing, and fiscal responsibility.[8]

2

Between 1965 and the late 1980s, the ability of providers of medical care to diagnose and treat disease exploded in a proliferation of new technology and skills. Kaiser-Permanente adopted an ever-enlarging standard of medical care with all deliberate speed. Special services—renal dialysis; coronary bypass grafting; CAT scanning, ultrasound, and nuclear imaging; numerous laboratory chemistry tests; genetic testing, bone marrow and heart and liver transplants—were established in regional medical centers or referred to community specialists. Kaiser-Permanente pioneered in offering hospice care. It also offered members a rich selection of health education courses. A regional office for preventive care and patient education was established under Dr. David Sobel. The medical care program saw its expenses increase alarmingly but was not alone. Costs for all providers and insurers of health care soared, and Kaiser-Permanente's dues increases were less, on the average, than its competitors' rates.[9]

The northern California region of Kaiser-Permanente used its own conservative policies, established during the Garfield pencil stub days, trying to blunt the impact of new technology on medical cost inflation. The Permanente Medical Group established a high technology committee to evaluate new services or purchases of new equipment. This committee analyzed effectiveness in diagnosis or treatment of patients, costs of new equipment and personnel, impact on facility space, and predictable obsolescence, as some of the factors to evaluate new technology. The Executive Committee also created "centers of excellence" to provide tertiary-care referral services such as neurosurgery, cardiac surgery, and genetics services at certain medical centers. The program had its own internal health planning and resource development activities in existence before Congress passed the 1973 Health Planning law.

Inflation in medical care costs were attributed to many factors, but among the most important were the Medicare Act and new technology. Medicare created a cost-plus system for hospitals and doctors. Fee-for-service providers were rewarded when they increased the costs of doing business, fueling the inflation flame. Medical care costs escalated rapidly after the enactment of Medicare. Medicare beneficiaries who retained their Kaiser-Permanente membership after 1966 proved less costly to Medicare Trust funds than those who received their care from fee-for-service providers.[10]

Kaiser-Permanente could do nothing to influence other causes of medical cost inflation: general inflation; costs of borrowing money; costs of construction; redefinition of social problems, such as alcoholism and self-inflicted injuries, as health problems; and accelerated increases in compensation for nurses, technicians, and other personnel. The program's efforts to moderate the escalation of its labor costs led to strikes in 1968, 1973, and 1974 that threatened to shut down its medical facilities. Physicians showed their loyalty to the program and to patients by performing tasks ranging from filing charts to cleaning floors. One physician, working in the outpatient pharmacy, commented that he had never been in a better position to perform peer review on his colleagues!

The strikes had a beneficial effect on management in The Permanente Medical Group. Chiefs of service had always been regarded as key managers in the organization. The Medical Group decided to train them for their management roles. In the early 1970s physicians were included in management training courses developed for all managers. In the 1980s a highly successful program was instituted for physician managers alone, in recognition of the finding that excellent physicians, lacking management skills, cannot lead the efforts of their peers in a busy group practice and that management of professional personalities is a special challenge!

3

Despite favorable recognition by government, employers, organized medicine, satisfied enrolled members, and the general public, some thought that Kaiser-Permanente did not measure up to what it should be. Unions, the foundation stones on which the program had been built, formed the California Council on Health Plan Alternatives in 1969. The council's intent was to develop its own statewide health plan for union members. Union leaders came to Kaiser-Permanente for advice. Arthur Weissman told them to proceed only if they could create a program that was superior to Kaiser-Permanente. Lack of capital and the failure of community physicians to support the venture convinced the council not to proceed. The proposal, however, sent its own message.[11,12,13]

This message was mild compared to an article in *Ramparts* magazine, November 10, 1970. The cover depicted a Permanente physician threatening to cut a patient's intravenous tubing. The caption: "Your Money or Your Life, Kaiser and the Health Business." The article described Henry J. Kaiser creating a health-care monopoly in order to block the development of federalized national health care—"socialized medicine." Kaiser executives on the Health Plan Board of Directors were accused of diverting funds from the Health Plan to swell the profits of Kaiser industries. Permanente physicians were especially enraged by stories of gruesome medical errors alleged by disgruntled, anonymous employees. The program was accused of racism and discrimination against urban black patients by making them wait for hours before receiving treatment.

"If Kaiser Health Plan is inefficient and alienating its members, why is it being boomed as an answer to America's critical medical problem?"

Writer Judith Carnoy answered her own question. Fee-for-service medicine was even worse. She argued that "Kaiser's aura of automated be-
nevolence and social planning allows it to occupy a vanguard
position.... With the cost of private 'vendor' physicians all but prohibi-
tive, Kaiser is fast moving into a monopoly position in supermarket
medical care."[14]

Dr. Cecil Cutting counseled the partnership, "Although the image
that we have achieved on a national level continues to mount, we do occasionally receive some criticism. In case we get too complacent, we can
refer to the *Ramparts* magazine for some areas in which to improve.
Sometimes, trumpery of that sort can be helpful if we can keep our cool
through the heat of inaccuracies and poor taste."[15]

The Executive Committee chose not to dispute the article point by
point, but to consider the source of the attack and to accept it as an
ideologically motivated pseudo-exposé. "It is clear that the [Kaiser-
Permanente] medical care organizations have evolved from a small,
unique, and highly controversial method of providing medical and hospital care into a nationally recognized institution. We should expect to
be the target of distorted and inaccurate representation in the media.
To the extent that there may be areas in which criticism has an element
of truth, there should be increasing vigilance to improve correctable situations and improve the quality of our service."[16]

On September 13, 1971, the *American Medical News,* the weekly newspaper of the AMA, published a feature headlined, "Kaiser-Permanente
Has Become a National Showcase."[17] The article admitted that Kaiser-
Permanente had become the most talked about phenomenon in American
medicine, especially after the President's Advisory Commission on Health
Manpower spent a week with Kaiser-Permanente in 1967 and reported
that it was delivering medical care at 30 percent less expense than other
systems. "Ever since and with increasing frequency," the AMA article reported, "Kaiser-Permanente has been criticized for delivering inferior, or
at best, ordinary medical care; scolded for being impersonal and even
rude; and chastised for lowering costs at the expense of the patient's welfare." The AMA writer did not ask the question: if service were so bad,
why were so many new members enrolling or retaining membership for
years?

Only one month later, October 18, 1971, the *New York Times* published a description of Kaiser-Permanente written by reporter Harry
Schwartz, who, for a variety of reasons, doubted that "it points the way
to a low-cost medical utopia for the nation." But despite these and other
criticisms, Schwartz concluded, "all available evidence suggests that

Kaiser-Permanente-type organizations are likely to increase. It is essentially that the Nixon Administration has this in mind in its espousal of 'health maintenance organizations.'"[18]

This prescient comment antedated the HMO Act of 1973. Originally criticized because prepaid health care was "unethical" and "socialistic," the program was now coming under attack because it was likely to become the creature of conservative cost-conscious payers for health care!

Twelve years later, the *New York Times* printed a feature article headlined, "The King of the HMO Mountain, Kaiser's prepaid health care plan has won converts coast-to-coast. But some skeptics see a darker side."[19]

The *Times* followed with a business feature in July 1989 headlined, "Why Kaiser Is Still the King—As the nation's health bill soars, companies and employees are flocking to the low-cost H.M.O."[20]

Health-care consumers were making their own choices and casting their own votes. For example, 35 percent of Kaiser-Permanente's largest group, federal employees, were subscribers. From 50 to 88 percent of other large employee groups were subscribers. Kaiser-Permanente's own employees were offered the choice of another carrier, but 98 percent enrolled in the Kaiser Health Plan. Physicians of the Medical Group chose to receive care for themselves and their families from fellow Permanente doctors. If the definition of quality care is the "kind of care I want for my family and myself," this attests to the level of confidence among persons with a unique advantage in evaluating quality of care.[21] A membership satisfaction survey conducted by an independent outside opinion survey, Field Research, showed that 90 percent of families would renew membership. Ninety-four percent found it to be a good value. Reasonable cost and complete coverage were principal reasons for this response. Only 2 percent of members polled had not used Permanente physicians. More than half of the families surveyed had used the plan within the last month. As Dr. Cutting advised the partners, "We must be doing something right!"[22]

4

Doing something right caused difficulties for Permanente physicians during the late 1980s. Rapid growth in membership had its pains. Physicians responded conscientiously with hard work and tolerance for

crowded offices and hospital space. Growth prediction, always a difficult art, produced figures that, as the 1980s ended, were too low.

As the program entered the modern era, challenges were many, and
they were met successfully. The most important feature of the previous
two decades was Kaiser-Permanente's steady adherence to its basic philosophy and mode of operation including constructive teamwork
among Permanente physician managers and Health Plan managers.

All around it were experiments in the organization of medical care
finance and delivery—so-called managed-care organizations. It was not
supposed to turn out this way. Sidney Garfield and Henry Kaiser envisioned a nation with one prepaid group-practice plan per community
with fee-for-service and indemnity insurance companies. Garfield expressed his concern in the late 1970s that the new managed-care plans
did not take into account the need for active physician participation in
the management of plans. Cecil Cutting, speaking indirectly to physicians who contract with managed-care plans, said, "they should not get
their feet wet unless their hearts are in it."

The post-World War II period began with ostracism of Permanente
physicians by county medical societies. The modern era saw the advice and
leadership of those physicians actively sought by these societies. In northern California, the program's share of the population in its service areas
rose to 29 percent. Other HMOs combined served 17 percent. Community
physicians were interested to learn what Kaiser-Permanente was all about.
Three county medical societies turned to Permanente physicians for a
president.[23]

Dr. Cutting's statement, "We must be doing something right" referred by inference to quality of care. Permanente physicians expressed
confidence in the quality of the group by choosing their colleagues as
physicians for themselves. They carefully evaluated each new physician
before hiring and by performance evaluations as time passed. One-
third of physicians who left the group in the first 2 years of association
were actively encouraged to resign as not "group suitable" and to enter
fee-for-service practice. More than 85 percent of Permanente physicians were eligible for certification or certified by specialty boards. Kaiser Hospitals continued to be considered physicians' workshops; the
medical staffs were zealous in maintaining the standards of the Joint
Commission for the Accreditation of Hospitals (JCAH).

Permanente physicians also employed a strong, informal and untitled
quality assurance system of daily peer review. Less than satisfactory
quality of care was more expensive to a medical group paid by capitation than optimum quality care, a fact of which all Permanent physi-

cians were reminded by their chiefs of service. Internal education programs and research also contributed significantly to the quality of care provided by Permanente physicians.

Initial attempts as early as 1964 by Permanente physicians to measure quality of care had not proved satisfactory. Dr. Leonard Rubin of the Department of Internal Medicine, Hayward, made a landmark contribution by developing the Comprehensive Quality Assurance System (CQAS) in 1969.[24] The steps in the CQAS system were: auditing outpatient medical records at random for instances of improvable care; developing standards; measuring performance against those standards; taking corrective action within a specified time through a responsible individual; and then remeasuring performance to determine improvement. CQAS was widely adopted in medical groups across the country in the 1970s.[25]

Employer groups soon joined the government in demanding to know what they were buying with their health-care dollars. They were no longer willing to accept on faith the quality of care provided by managed-care organizations. They asked whether all the care provided was necessary. As this employer emphasis shifted to appropriateness of care, organized systems were asked whether incentives arising from prepayment might motivate physicians to withhold care—going too far in the name of cost effectiveness. Kaiser-Permanente met this criticism by pointing out that underserved patients go elsewhere, sue for breach of contract, or return to the program with advanced illnesses that are more expensive to treat. In 1989, the Federal General Accounting Office carried out a detailed study of undesirable incentives for physicians working in prepaid practice and concluded that Kaiser-Permanente's incentives were appropriate.[26]

After 1970, competition became the greatest challenge to Kaiser-Permanente. Throughout the 30 years following World War II, population growth outstripped the supply of physicians, and there was work for all forms of medical practice. Then as a supposed "physician glut" and "patient shortages" developed, entities ranging from small entrepreneurs to huge insurance companies saw in the Kaiser-Permanente experience a model for attracting patients into managed-care, more efficient than fee-for-service practice supported by indemnity insurance. Kaiser-Permanente was suddenly beset with prepaid competition, its own creation. During the early 1980s, its growth slowed markedly. Its dues advantage over rates of competitors narrowed. Competitors were experimenting with prepayment in multiple forms, particularly Independent Practice Association (IPA) HMOs, through which individual physicians contracted with an HMO to serve its members in their own offices, on a fee schedule — sometimes discounted — without limitation on continuing their usual fee-for-service practice for non-HMO patients. This arrangement gave IPA HMOs multiple points of convenient service for their members, but lacked effective control of utilization or costs. As the decade dwindled, so did the fortunes for many IPA HMOs. Some were forced to withhold from contracting physicians larger and larger portions of their promised fees in order to cover unanticipated deficits. Bankruptcies occurred. By 1989, Kaiser-Permanente experienced record growth of membership in all regions, so much so that development of medical office and hospital space and personnel to meet the members' needs became the first priority of the program. Kaiser-Permanente's success in meeting the threat of competition had again created familiar problems for the organization.

13
The Old Guard Steps Down

———————————— 1 ————————————

Although the structure of Kaiser-Permanente's prepaid group practice in northern California did not change fundamentally in the years following the Tahoe agreement, adjustments were made in the medical group as new leadership replaced old. Physicians at the newer medical centers found themselves at a distance from the old guard Executive Committee, not understanding its processes. There was unrest even among the partners. A committee was assigned to study and make recommendations to correct this situation. After 1 year of intense investigation, the committee reported its findings and recommendations. The Executive Committee acted immediately. A more democratic representation on the Executive Committee of the partnership followed. Each medical center was granted two seats, one for the physician-in-chief, ex officio, for up to 6 years, and one for a representative elected by the physicians at his or her medical center to serve for 3 years.[1] The only other member was the Executive Director, Dr. Cutting.

Dr. Cutting's long service, begun in 1938 at Grand Coulee, was drawing to a close. His colleague from San Francisco General Hospital and Grand Coulee, Dr. Richard Moore, had retired in 1972. Dr. Moore's son, Stephen, born at Coulee, had become a physician and practiced pediatrics in The Permanente Medical Group in Santa Clara. Dr. Stephen

Moore was one among several two-generation physician families to work in the developing program.

In 1974 a search committee named Dr. Bernard Rhodes, chair of the Executive Committee and physician-in-chief at the Hayward medical center, and Dr. Bruce J. Sams, Jr., physician-in-chief at San Francisco, as nominees to succeed Dr. Cutting. The Executive Committee chose Dr. Sams in February 1975, and this choice was confirmed by a vote of all partners. Dr. Cutting stepped down in July of 1976.

Bruce Sams, a native of Savannah, Georgia, and a premedical graduate at Georgia Tech, received his medical degree from Harvard Medical School. His postgraduate training in internal medicine included a residency at the University of California at San Francisco (UCSF) and a senior residency and fellowship in hematology at the Massachusetts General Hospital in Boston. He practiced fee-for-service medicine in Savannah before accepting an academic appointment as instructor in medicine at UCSF. He joined The Permanente Medical Group in 1963, subsequently headed its medical residency program, and became chief of medicine in 1967. In 1971 he succeeded Dr. Smillie as physician-in-chief when Dr. Smillie became assistant to the executive director, Dr. Cutting. Reserved, with the charm of a southern gentleman, a first-rate mind, and a top medical education, Dr. Sams brought to the role of executive director firm leadership and an unrivaled capacity for work. To effect a smooth transition, he assumed the role of executive director-elect for the period between July 1975 and July 1976, when he became the second executive director of The Permanente Medical Group.

As the numbers of Permanente physicians passed 2000, Dr. Sams led his colleagues to consider the advantages of moving from a partnership to a professional corporation. This was a matter of some complexity. Incorporation would enhance the physicians' pension benefits and protect them from creditors of the Health Plan. Their personal assets would be immune from legal claims based on their partners' actions. But incorporation would change the group's tax year, accelerating the payment of income taxes in the process. Otherwise, the organization and its governance would be little changed. Expert legal advice was obtained. Incorporation committees studied the matter from 1977 to 1979, and the executive committee brought it to a vote of the partners in October 1980. Fifty-five percent were in favor. This was considered insufficient to proceed, and a second ballot was sent out in May 1981 after a loan program was secured to assist physicians with income tax payments. This time a 64.3 percent approval was obtained, and The Permanente Medical Group, Inc., became a reality on January 2, 1982. The physicians' future retirement contributions were no longer at risk of loss from financial reverses of the program as a whole.

2

Dr. Cutting, an articulate and energetic physician, devoted to the program he had founded and improved with Dr. Garfield, continued to be active in The Permanente Medical Group. After retirement from the position of executive director, he served in the role of elder statesperson and inspiring lecturer on the program's history to new physicians.

At Dr. Cutting's final Executive Committee meeting in June of 1976, Dr. Harry Kirby, who had been with Dr. Garfield on the desert in 1933, Dr. Wallace Neighbor, who had gone to Grand Coulee in 1938, and Dr. Sidney Garfield were guests. Dr. Cutting praised each of them and Karl Steil, northern California's regional manager for the Health Plan and Hospitals. Dr. Cutting said of Dr. Garfield and the program, "His advocacy of physician strength and physician control of the program earned him the loss of his management role but not the respect of all who know him....On the basis of our quality and our convictions, we stood and faced the opposition of those who felt we were wrong and those who were afraid we were right. We have gained stature in the nation and reputation around the world....We have the satisfaction of knowing we are doing something creative, with reasonable amenities, a freedom to practice and always the challenge that we can do better."[2]

Dr. Morris Collen retired from the Executive Committee in 1979 but continued as director of Medical Methods Research. His scholarly interests began with publications on the epidemics of pneumococcal pneumonia among Richmond shipyard workers in 1942 and continued through studies based on computer-organized data from multiphasic health examinations of health plan members. He had been an original Medical Group partner, a physician-in-chief in San Francisco, and for 25 years, chair of the Executive Committee. He was chief negotiator of the Tahoe Agreement. In 1971 he was elected to the Institute of Medicine of the National Academy of Science. A colleague remarked of him in 1973, "Our existence and our position today is in large part built on his strength and his genius."[3]

Gerald Stewart retired as the first Regional Medical Centers administrator in 1980 after the Clinics and Hospital Administration were combined in 1970. He was succeeded by Dr. Bernard Rhodes, Mr. Stewart had been clinic administrator at Oakland. Dr. Wallace Cook, the first physician-in-chief at the Walnut Creek Medical Center where he served from 1952 to 1977, retired in 1985 after additional service as regional director of medical-legal affairs for the medical group. He had been the first (and only) "permanent" member of the Executive Committee who was not a founding partner.

Dr. A. LaMonte Baritell died in 1980. "Monte" had first come to Permanente as a resident in surgery during World War II. He was a founding partner of the Medical Group, chief of surgery, and later physician-in-chief at Oakland, a permanent member of the Executive Committee, and an articulate spokesperson for all the Permanente Medical Groups at Tahoe.

Dr. John Mott also died in 1980. He started his career as a resident in surgery at the Permanente Hospital in Oakland. John started the semiautonomous Eden group in San Leandro which later joined Permanente. He became the first physician-in-chief at Hayward, moving on to Sacramento where he exerted strong leadership during the rapid growth of that medical center.

One of Dr. Garfield's earliest colleagues, starting during their residencies at Los Angeles County Hospital in the 1930s, Dr. Wallace Neighbor, died in 1984. "Wally" joined his friend at Grand Coulee, and selflessly became medical director of the troubled Permanente operation in Vancouver, Washington, during the shipyard days, later moving to the embryonic San Francisco expansion in 1948. He was a permanent member of the Executive Committee and after retirement from it at age 65 became the director of Kaiser-Permanente's medical-legal department in northern California.

With the retirement of so many physicians with long careers in The Permanente Medical Group, Dr. Irving Lomhoff was successful in founding a Retired Physicians Association in 1977.

32

Edgar Kaiser, Henry's son who had persuaded Dr. Sidney Garfield to come to Grand Coulee, had requested a Garfield prepaid health-care plan for shipyard workers in Vancouver, Washington, during World War II, and served as president of the Kaiser Foundation Health Plan and Hospitals, retired in 1980 and died in 1981. He shared his father's vision for health care, "I do not say that ours is the only approach," he remarked in 1973 upon the signing of the HMO Act, "but it would be in the country's best interest if a number of similar plans were undertaken. Not only would it be good for the country, it would stimulate competition which would be healthy for us."[4] Spoken like a true Kaiser! It was not easy being the son and heir of a father who exercised power well into his seventies, predeceasing his son by only 13 years. But Edgar managed it with grace, and like his father, he realized that the role he had played in establishing comprehensive prepaid medical care on a national basis had proved to be an accomplishment of startling dimensions.

James A. Vohs, regional manager of the southern California region, succeeded Edgar Kaiser as president of the Kaiser Health Plan and Hospitals. He appointed Dr. Bernard Rhodes, who had served as the first physician Regional Medical Centers administrator for both the Hospitals and the Medical Group, as executive vice president of the Health Plan and Hospitals and a member of the board of directors. Dr. Rhodes thus became the first Permanente physician, after Dr. Garfield, on that board. This increased interaction between the health plan and physicians indicated a need that grew as new regions were established. A nationwide program required coordination. Health Plan regions were interdependent, although each medical group was an autonomous entity. The Kaiser-Permanente Committee, including all regional medical directors and regional managers, formed to discuss programwide issues and to recommend policies to the regions, took on new importance. Increasing numbers of interregional committees were formed to address issues of common concern.

Every visionary movement has its prophets, and Kaiser-Permanente had several, beginning with Dr. Garfield and Henry J. Kaiser. As the program worked through the challenges of the 1970s, the partners heard a remarkable address by another prophet, Arthur Weissman, whom Mr. Kaiser had hired in the early 1950s as a medical economist and statistician. Prior to that, Weissman had directed special projects for the California Department of Public Health. In Kaiser-Permanente he developed in the central office a department of medical economics that guided the program through the early pragmatic years of financial planning without precedent. He served on state and national commissions and committees dealing with health care and public health and was a member of the National Advisory Health Manpower Council.

In June of 1978 he undertook to tell the northern California physicians the shape of the program's future so that long-range planning could succeed. No uniform national health policy or national health insurance plan would emerge in the 1980s, nor would any one entity emerge as dominant in the health-care community. Kaiser-Permanente should establish for the 1980s an advocacy on behalf of the whole group-practice prepayment movement in the United States. A strong Kaiser-Permanente and a strong prepaid group-practice movement could have great influence in shaping national health policy. The federal and state governments would continue to regulate HMOs; indeed, Weissman predicted, government would continue to expand its involvement in health care. Weissman urged Kaiser-Permanente to avoid the temptation to view everything the government was or would be doing in the health-care field with a hostile attitude.

In this prophetic position paper Weissman outlined a number of other trends that the experience of the following decade would corroborate. Cost containment would continue to be the key issue for both the government and the private sector. The number and size of HMOs would continue to grow. Within a short time, HMOs would become a major factor in national and state health-care economics and legislation. Kaiser-Permanente should maintain its leadership position.

On several fronts, Weissman continued, Kaiser-Permanente would be seriously affected by developing trends. The aging and growth of the population, the increased availability of physician and hospital services, the addition of new services based on technological advances, the increased expectations of consumers, and the increased availability of third-party payments would coalesce to create a spiraling demand for services and greater competition among providers of health care. The health aspects of broad social problems, such as alcoholism and drug addiction, malnutrition, and learning disabilities, were being redefined as problems to be treated by the health-care delivery sector. Although movements emphasizing responsibility for self-care and preventive health care had already emerged, Weissman cautioned against any appreciable reduction in demand or costs based on a revolution in personal behavior. "If any of you are tempted to relax in complacency," Weissman said, "please come to my anti-complacency clinic or call me at home."

Weissman, however, was optimistic about the program. Its principles and objectives were time-tested and strong. The program was flexible enough to adapt to the shifting situation of the 1980s. Not only was the plan better organized and stronger in the matter of administrative structure, but it had also moved beyond its first generation of leadership and now enjoyed a cadre of younger leaders capable of responding to new situations and taking the program in new directions.[5]

Arthur Weissman died in 1980 before he could see how correct his predictions had been or how far from solution many of the problems he identified remained. His optimism for the success of the Kaiser-Permanente program, however, was more than justified.

4

Unlike Henry J. Kaiser, who relished power to an advanced age, Dr. Sidney Garfield had stepped aside when it became evident that he had to leave the day-to-day management of the medical group and to assume the role of senior statesperson and visionary planner so congenial to his basic talents. In 1958 Garfield was appointed vice president for facility development for the Kaiser-Permanente program, continuing a role he had filled after Tahoe. In 1960 he joined the board of directors. He relinquished his vice presidency in 1969 and resigned from the board in 1971 but continued to be active in the program in the very same way he had begun, as a visionary physician seeking better ways to bring medicine to more people.

Before his death on December 29, 1984, Dr. Sidney Garfield had the satisfaction of knowing that his life's work had borne fruit and that he, after the divisions and misunderstandings of the 1950s, was truly appreciated as the founder of the Kaiser-Permanente program. The Group Health Association of America presented Garfield with its Distinguished Service Award in 1969. In October 1977 Garfield traveled to New York City to receive the Lyndon Baines Johnson Award for Humanitarian Service. At the time, Sidney Garfield was serving on the National Commission on the Cost of Medical Care of the American Medical Association—about 30 years after organized medicine had sought to discredit him.

Of greatest importance, appreciation came from the Permanente physicians themselves. Encounters with Permanente physicians meant much to Dr. Garfield. Following the lead of Garfield the entrepreneur, Permanente physicians had accepted responsibility for the economics, as well as for the quality, of medical care. Physicians of The Permanente Medical Group had struggled to retain equal participation with business professionals in controlling and directing the health care program they created together. When the medical establishment misunderstood what they were doing, Garfield and Permanente physicians had stood side by side before its criticisms. Eventually the medical establishment ceased its attack and turned to its pariah with respect and admiration.

On May 19, 1986, more than 50 years after Dr. Garfield had left the University of Southern California for the desert, USC held ceremonies dedicating the Sidney R. Garfield Chair in the Health Sciences, made possible by a million dollar grant from the Henry J. Kaiser Family Foundation. The holder of the Chair would be a medical scientist interested in preventive medicine and health policy studies. Dr. Garfield's work would continue, and his life would remain a source of inspiration to physicians concerned with the challenge of high-quality medical care at a reasonable cost.

"He captured the principles and significance of prepayment to a group of physicians as a more efficient and effective mechanism for health care," remarked his lifelong friend Dr. Cecil Cutting at the time of Sidney Garfield's death. "He developed the concept against opposition and obstructions that would have been overwhelming to many without his dedication and courage."[6]

Epilogue:
The Meaning
of It All

Cecil C. Cutting, MD

It has been said that history is the collision of chance and purpose. There could be no better example than in the evolution of the Kaiser-Permanente medical care program.

A visionary young Dr. Sidney Garfield, finding himself in an impossible economic situation, fortuitously discovered that prepayment for his medical services could be his salvation. Then, his reluctant decision to accept opportunities to develop prepaid group practice for a series of major construction projects which happened to present themselves, one after another, was critical to the flowering of his idea.

The clarity of his vision, recognizing the significance of prepaid group practice as a means of delivering high quality medical care at a reasonable cost, gave purpose to his zeal.

He became enamored of the potential in prepayment, when received directly by physicians, to reverse the economics of medicine. The well member became an asset; the sick patient a liability. Preventive health care became his lifelong obsession.

As the cost of medical care soared, the position of the physician within the medical care industry in this country changed. Blue Cross-Blue Shield, the indemnity insurance carriers, and especially governments became more involved in purchasing care, and were therefore compelled to control its costs. As they placed outside controls on the practices of fee-for-service physicians and hospitals, they became their adversaries. Patients, physicians, and payors suffered.

As the Kaiser-Permanente program evolved through difficult decades and struggles for control, it became evident that the role of the physician as partner with the health plan, rather than as adversary, was significant.

The group practice prepayment arrangement that is Kaiser-Permanente's tends to maintain the physician's responsibility, not only for the quality of the care, but also for its cost. This is more nearly as it was in a simpler time, before third-party involvement in the physician-patient relationship. This responsibility is surely an appropriate one for physicians. It seems unlikely that a satisfactory solution to the present, growing confusion in medicine can develop unless the physician is indeed a major, responsible participant in decisions which balance quality and cost.

This responsibility is difficult to establish in traditional fee-for-service practice when the purchaser of the medical care, a third party, feels obliged to control costs and quality by outside pressures on physicians and hospitals.

The prepaid group practice approach has proved a viable alternative to traditional practice, with a number of significant advantages. When properly organized, it employs physician motivation and participation to deliver cost-effective, high quality medical care.

I hope and believe that in the search for more satisfactory delivery of medical services in this country, and within the changes which must come, the principles developed over five decades in Kaiser-Permanente may be of some help and guidance.

Notes

Chapter One

1. Transcript of an interview by Daniella Thompson (20 September 1974), p. 1. The Permanente Archives. (Hereafter cited as Thompson interview.)
2. Ibid., p. 2.
3. Transcript of interviews by Daniella Thompson (4, 5, 6, 9, and 10 September 1974), p. 3 (4 September 1974). The Permanente Archives. (Hereafter cited as Thompson interview.)
4. Thompson interview (4 September 1974), p. 5.
5. Paul Starr, *The Social Transformation of American Medicine* (Basic Books, New York, 1982), pp. 209–210.
6. Thompson interview (4 September 1974), pp. 6–7.
7. Ibid., pp. 7–8.

Chapter Two

1. Sidney Garfield Oral History, transcript of an interview (no date), p. 2. The Permanente Archives. (Hereafter cited as Garfield Oral History.)
2. Garfield Oral History, p. 2; Thompson interview (4 September 1974), pp. 9–10.
3. Thompson interview (4 September 1974), p. 20.
4. Thompson interview (20 September 1974), p. 3.
5. Garfield Oral History, p. 1.
6. Transcript of an interview by Daniella Thompson, (16 October 1974), p. 2, The Permanente Archives (hereafter cited as Thompson interview); Oral

History, Cecil C. Cutting, MD (27 January 1982), p. 1. The Permanente Archives (hereafter cited as Cutting 1982 Oral History); Garfield, Thompson interview (4 September 1974), pp. 15–16.

7. Thompson interview (20 September 1974), p. 6.

8. Transcript of an interview by Daniella Thompson (16 October 1974), p. 3. The Permanente Archives. (Hereafter cited as Thompson interview.)

9. Cecil C. Cutting, MD, "The Early Years, From Grand Coulee through the Tahoe Conference," in Kaiser Foundation Hospitals, Kaiser Foundation Health Plan, "A Program for the Board of Directors," 16 April 1974, p. 2. The Permanente Archives.

10. Cutting 1982 Oral History, p. 2.

11. Thompson interview (4 September 1974), p. 13.

12. "The Early Years," p. 2.

13. Thompson interview (20 September 1974), p. 5.

14. Thompson interview (4 September 1974), p. 19.

15. "Cecil C. Cutting, MD: History of the Kaiser-Permanente Medical Care Program," an interview conducted by Malca Chall, 1985, the Regional Oral History Office of the Bancroft Library (1985), p. 11. (Hereafter cited as Cutting, Bancroft Oral History.)

16. Thompson interview (20 September 1974), p. 4.

17. Jerry Seavey, "Sidney Garfield, MD: Our Founder Remembered," *Reporter* (February 1985), p. 4.

18. Thompson interview (20 September 1974), p. 5.

19. Thompson interview (4 September 1974), p. 18.

20. Cutting, Bancroft Oral History, p. 10.

21. Thompson interview (4 September 1974), p. 21.

22. Thompson interview (5 September 1974), p. 1.

Chapter Three

1. Thompson interview (5 September 1974), pp. 3–4.

2. Cutting 1982 Oral History, p. 3.

3. Transcripts of interviews by Miriam Stein (17 February 1982 and 7 June 1984), pp. 3–4 (17 February 1982). The Permanente Archives. (Hereafter cited as Stein interview.)

4. Stein interview (17 February 1982, pp. 5–6; Thompson interview (5 September 1974), pp. 7–8; Garfield Oral History, p. 4.

5. Thompson interview (5 September 1974), p. 7.

6. "Morris Collen, MD: History of the Kaiser-Permanente Medical Care Program," an interview conducted by Sally Hughes, 28 February 1986, the Regional Oral History Office of the Bancroft Library (1989), p. 22. (Hereafter cited as Collen, Bancroft Oral History.) Kaiser biographer Mark S. Foster doubts this story, believing that Kaiser told it so many times that it became true in his mind. See Mark S. Foster, *Henry J. Kaiser, Builder in the Modern American West* (Austin, 1989), p. 13.

7. Garfield Oral History, p. 5; Thompson, Garfield interview (5 September 1974), pp. 9–10.

8. Thompson, Garfield interview (5 September 1974), p. 10.

9. Ibid.

10. Sidney R. Garfield, MD, "First Annual Report of the Permanente Foundation Hospital," *Permanente Foundation Medical Bulletin*, 2 (January 1944), 35.

11. Collen, Bancroft Oral History, p. 27.

12. "Editorial: Pneumonia in Shipbuilders," *New England Journal of Medicine*, 231 (21 September 1944), 433.

13. Sidney R. Garfield, MD, "Second Annual Report of the Permanente Foundation Hospital," *Permanente Foundation Medical Bulletin*, 3 (January 1945), 45.

14. "Editorial: Prepaid Medical Care à la Kaiser," *New England Journal of Medicine*, 231 (24 August 1944), 31.

15. Sidney R. Garfield, MD, "First Annual Report of the Permanent Foundation Hospital," *Permanente Foundation Medical Bulletin*, 2 (January 1944), 37–38.

16. Ibid., 3 (January 1945), 27.

17. Morris Collen, MD, "Sidney Garfield, MD: Our Founder Remembered," *Reporter* (February 1985), p. 4.

18. Thompson interview (16 October 1974), p. 4.

19. Thompson interview (5 September 1974), p. 13.

20. Ibid., p. 13.

21. Ibid., pp. 13–14.

22. Ibid., p. 16.

23. Sidney R. Garfield, MD, "First Annual Report of the Permanente Foundation Hospital," *Permanente Foundation Medical Bulletin*, 2 (January 1944), 35.

24. Ibid., p. 39.

25. Thompson interview (5 September 1974), p. 11.

Chapter Four

1. Cutting 1982 Oral History, p. 7.

2. "Eugene E. Trefethen, Jr.: History of the Kaiser-Permanente Medical Care Program," an interview conducted by Malca Chall, 1985, the Regional Oral History Office of the Bancroft Library (1986), p. 27. (Hereafter cited as Trefethen, Bancroft Oral History.)

3. Garfield Oral History, p. 9.

4. "Clifford H. Keene, MD: History of the Kaiser-Permanente Medical Care Program," an interview conducted by Sally Smith Hughes, 1985, the Regional Oral History Office of the Bancroft Library (1986), p. 30. (Hereafter cited as Keene, Bancroft Oral History.)

5. Cutting, Bancroft Oral History, p. 31.

6. *Life Among the Doctors* (Harcourt, Brace, New York, 1949), p. 417.

7. Thompson interview (5 September 1974), p. 18.

8. Thompson interview (20 September 1974), p. 12.

9. Garfield Oral History, p. 13.

10. Op. cit., p. 407.

11. Trefethen, Bancroft Oral History, p. 17.

12. Collen, Bancroft Oral History, pp. 41–42.

13. Thompson interview (6 September 1974), pp. 3–4.

14. "Historical Remarks Presented to the Executive Committee on 24 April 1974," p. 4. The Permanente Archives.

15. Thompson interview (6 September 1974), p. 12.

Chapter Five

1. Jun T. Ajari, "The Way We Were," *Reporter* (August 1982), p. 12.

2. Thompson interview (6 September 1974), p. 12.

3. Thompson interview (20 September 1974), p. 11.

4. Jun T. Ajari, "The Way We Were," *Reporter* (August 1982), p. 12.

5. Garfield Oral History, p. 12.

6. Ibid., p. 7.

7. Thompson interview (6 September 1974), p. 5.

8. "Address to Multnomah County Medical Association," 4 April 1945, typescript, p. 4. The Cutting Files, box 1, folder 1. The Permanente Archives.

9. Ibid.

Chapter Six

1. Sidney R. Garfield, MD, "A Report on Permanente's First Ten Years," *Permanente Foundation Medical Bulletin*, 10 (August 1952), p. 11.

2. Thompson interview (6 September 1974), p. 7.

3. "Lambreth Hancock: History of the Kaiser-Permanente Medical Care Program," an interview conducted by Sally Smith Hughes, 1986, the Regional Oral History Office of the Bancroft Library (1987), p. 111. (Hereafter cited as Hancock, Bancroft Oral History.)

4. Ibid., p. 37.

5. Stein interview (17 February 1982), p. 7.

6. Ibid., p. 8.

7. "Wallace H. Cook, MD: History of the Kaiser-Permanente Medical Care Program," an interview conducted by Sally Smith Hughes, 1986, the Regional Oral History Office of the Bancroft Library (1987), p. 48. (Hereafter cited as Cook, Bancroft Oral History.)

8. Cutting, Bancroft Oral History, p. 18.

9. Jack Chapman, interview by Daniella Thompson, 8 April 1975, two cassettes, the Permanente Archives.

10. Cook, Bancroft Oral History, p. 47.

11. Ibid., p. 55.

12. Hancock, Bancroft Oral History, p. 38.

13. Garfield Oral History, p. 11.

14. "Raymond M. Kay, MD: History of the Kaiser-Permanente Medical Care Program," an interview conducted by Ora Huth, 1985, the Regional Oral History Office of the Bancroft Library (1987), p. 76. (Hereafter cited as Kay, Bancroft Oral History.)

15. Collen, Bancroft Oral History, p. 72.

16. Ibid., p. 53.

17. Ibid., p. 53.

18. Garfield Oral History, p. 12.

19. Cook, Bancroft Oral History, pp. 27, 40.

20. Garfield Oral History, p. 15.

Chapter Seven

1. Cook, Bancroft Oral History, p. 21.

2. Keene, Bancroft Oral History, pp. 40–43, 47–48.

3. Ibid., p. 50.

4. "Abstract of Proceedings of the House of Delegates of the American Medical Association," *Journal of the American Medical Association*, 155 (31 July 1954), 1249. See also, "Medicine: What Is Free Choice?," *Time*, 64 (5 July 1954), 37.

5. Keene, Bancroft Oral History, p. 54.

6. Ibid., p. 62.

7. Thompson interview (20 September 1974), p. 9.

8. Quoted by Lester Velie in "Supermarket Medicine," *The Saturday Evening Post*, (20 June 1953), 49.

9. Statement included in the Hon. Charles A. Wolverton, "A Private Enterprise Solution to Medical Care by the Doctors of this Country," *The Congressional Record* (6 January 1954), 1.

10. Ibid., pp. 6–7.

11. Executive Committee, *Minutes*, 2 February 1954, 16 February 1954. The Permanente Archives.

12. Keene, Bancroft Oral History, p. 68.

13. Thompson interview (16 October 1974), p. 8.

14. Kay, Bancroft Oral History, p. 82.

15. Cutting, Bancroft Oral History, p. 49.

16. Ibid., p. 51.

17. Cook, Bancroft Oral History, p. 41.

18. Garfield Oral History, p. 8.

19. Bancroft Oral History, p. 54.

20. Thompson interview (6 September 1974), p. 4.

21. "Ernest W. Saward, MD: History of the Kaiser-Permanente Medical Care Program," an interview conducted by Sally Smith Hughes, 1985, the Regional Oral History Office of the Bancroft Library (1986), p. 86. (Hereafter cited as Saward, Bancroft Oral History.)

22. Hancock, Bancroft Oral History, p. 51.

23. Ibid., p. 52.

24. Keene, Bancroft Oral History, p. 50.

25. Saward, Bancroft Oral History, p. 87.

26. Ibid., pp. 83–84.

27. Cook, Bancroft Oral History, p. 73.

28. Keene, Bancroft Oral History, p. 89.

Chapter Eight

1. Executive Committee, *Minutes*, 1 June 1954. The Permanente Archives.

2. Cutting, Bancroft Oral History, p. 52.

3. Letter of 21 April 1955, attached to Working Council *Minutes* for 12–13 May 1955. The Permanente Archives.

4. George Link, "Memorandum to Working Council, 3 June 1955" and "Letter to the Board of Directors, Kaiser Foundation Hospitals, 3 June 1955." The Permanente Archives.

5. Statement attached to Working Council *Minutes* for 13 May 1955. The Permanente Archives.

6. Kay, Bancroft Oral History, p. 83.

7. Working Council *Minutes* for 21–22 June 1955. The Permanente Archives.

8. Ibid.

9. Cook, Bancroft Oral History, p. 52.

10. Kay, Bancroft Oral History, p. 84.

11. "George E. Link: History of the Kaiser-Permanente Medical Care Program," an interview conducted by Malca Chall, 1985, the Regional Oral History Office of the Bancroft Library (1986), p. 30. (Hereafter cited as Link, Bancroft Oral History.)

12. Hancock, Bancroft Oral History, p. 52.

13. Garfield Oral History, p. 10.

14. Link, Bancroft Oral History, pp. 32, 36.

15. Garfield Oral History, pp. 9–10.

16. Keene, Bancroft Oral History, p. 75.

17. Cutting, Bancroft Oral History, p. 59.

18. Scott Fleming, "Kaiser-Permanente Medical Care Program History," bound transcript (August 1982), pp. 2–3. The Permanente Archives.

19. Kay, Bancroft Oral History, p. 95.

20. Fleming, op. cit., pp. 27–30.

21. Cutting, Bancroft Oral History, p. 63.

22. Ibid., p. 59.

23. Trefethen, Bancroft Oral History, p. 45.

Chapter Nine

1. "Kaiser Foundation Hospitals of Northern California Fifteenth Anniversary Address by Sidney R. Garfield, MD," unpaged printed pamphlet of speech given 19 October 1957. The Permanente Archives.

2. Personal statement to John G. Smillie, 10 May 1982.

3. Hancock, Bancroft Oral History, pp. 112–113.

4. Ibid., pp. 61–62.

5. Ibid., pp. 56–57.

6. Stein interview (7 June 1982), pp. 14–15.

7. Keene, Bancroft Oral History, p. 82.

8. Ibid., p. 85.

9. Collen, Bancroft Oral History, p. 141.

10. Executive Committee *Minutes* for 1 June 1961. The Permanente Archives.

11. Cook, Bancroft Oral History, p. 79.

12. Quoted from typed transcription in the Cutting Files, box 1, folder 6. The Permanente Archives.

13. John G. Smillie, MD, "A History of the Permanente Medical Group and the Kaiser Foundation Health Plan," unpublished manuscript (1985), p. 106. The Bancroft Library and the Permanente Archives.

Chapter Ten

1. "Prepaid Medical Care: Nation's Biggest Private Plan," *Time*, (14 September 1962), 65.

2. Cutting, Bancroft Oral History, p. 78.

3. Ibid.

4. Saward, Bancroft Oral History, p. 99.

5. Cutting, Bancroft Oral History, p. 78.

Chapter Eleven

1. "The Kaiser Foundation Medical Care Program" in *Report of the National Advisory Commission on Health Manpower*, 2 vols. (November 1967), II, Appendix 4.

2. Partnership meeting *Minutes* for 13 October 1969. The Permanente Archives.

3. Keene, Bancroft Oral History, p. 127.

4. Cutting, Bancroft Oral History, p. 84.

5. Keene, Bancroft Oral History, p. 113.

6. Ibid., p. 105.

7. Partnership meeting *Minutes* for 7 October 1968. The Permanente Archives.

8. *Kaiser Foundation Medical Care Program 1969*, p. 19.

9. Somers, Anne R. (editor), "The Growing Demand for Information on Prepaid Group Practice," *The Kaiser-Permanente Medical Care Program, One Valid Solution to the Problem of Health Care Delivery in the United States* (New York, 1971) p. 4.

10. Trefethen, Bancroft Oral History, pp. 67–68.

Chapter Twelve

1. Fleming, Scott, "Evolution of the Kaiser-Permanente Medical Care Program, Historical Overview" (unpublished).

2. Falkson, Joseph L., "HMOs and the Politics of Health System Reform," American Hospital Association, 1980.

3. Minutes, Partnership meeting, February 25, 1965.

4. Minutes, Executive Committee meeting, May 4, 1972.

5. Smillie, John, "The Consensus Group: A History of Inter-Organizational Cooperation," Report to the Board of Directors (Kaiser Foundation Health Plan), March 13, 1975.

6. Annual Report, Kaiser Foundation Medical Care Program, 1977.

7. Brown, Lawrence, D., "Politics and Health Care Organization, HMOs as Federal Policy," The Brookings Institution, 1983.

8. California Health and Safety Code, Sec. 1340 et seq. (West, 1990).

9. Minutes, Executive Committee, March 18, 1976.

10. Corbin, Mildred, and Krute, Aaron, "Some Aspects of Medicare Experience with Group Practice Prepayment Plans," *Social Security Bulletin*, vol. 38, no. 3, March 1975.

11. Minutes, Executive Committee meeting, June 5, 1969.

12. Ibid., June 12, 1969.

13. Minutes, Partnership meeting, May 11, 1970.

14. Carnoy, Judith, "Kaiser: You Pay Your Money and You Take Your Chances," *Ramparts*, November 1970.

15. Minutes, Partnership meeting, October 26, 1970.

16. Minutes, Executive Committee meeting, November 12, 1970.

17. "Kaiser-Permanente Has Become a National Showcase," *American Medical News*, September 13, 1971.

18. Schwartz, Harry, "Health Plans: To Ease the Pain of the Doctor's Bill," *New York Times*, October 29, 1971.

19. Kleinfield, N. R., "The King of the HMO Mountain," *New York Times*, July 31, 1983.

20. Kamron, Glenn, "Why Kaiser is Still the King," *New York Times*, July 2, 1989.

21. Minutes, Executive Committee meeting, January 6, 1971.

22. Minutes, Partnership meeting, October 11, 1971.

23. Paul E. Stange, MD, Solano County, 1988; Anthony J. Nespole, MD, Santa Clara County, 1989; Donald Cheu, MD, San Mateo County, 1990.

24. Annual Report, Kaiser Foundation Medical Care Program, 1973.

25. Rubin, Leonard, "Comprehensive Quality Assurance System," American Group Practice Association, 1975.

26. "Medicare: Physician Incentive Payments by Prepaid Health Plans Could Lower Quality of Care," GAO/HRD-89-29, December 12, 1988, p. 15.

Chapter Thirteen

1. Minutes, Executive Committee meetings, May 13 and May 20, 1971.

2. Minutes, Partnership meeting, June 7, 1976.

3. Minutes, Partnership meeting, October 15, 1973.

4. Quoted in the Annual Report, Kaiser-Permanente Medical Care Program, 1981.

5. Minutes, Partnership meeting, October 12, 1980.

6. Annual Report, Kaiser-Permanente Medical Care Program, 1984, p. 39.

An Essay
on Sources

In 1985, "A History of the Permanente Medical Group and the Kaiser Foundation Health Plan" (by John Smillie, MD, a Permanente physician since 1949) was completed. This account constitutes the first and controlling draft of the present volume. Over the years, other long-time Kaiser-Permanente participants have also produced historical accounts, which are on deposit at the Archives of The Permanente Medical Group. Each of these accounts has been scrupulously cross-checked and utilized. They include Daniella Thompson, "Evolution of the Kaiser-Permanente Medical Care Program, An Historical Perspective," unpublished typescript, 25 pages (30 July 1975); Scott Fleming, "Evolution of the Kaiser Permanente Medical Care Program: Historical Overview," bound typescript, 89 pages, issued by the Kaiser Foundation Health Plan, Inc. (20 August 1982, reissued on 15 April 1988); and, Jack K. Chapman, "A Brief History of Kaiser-Permanente," unpublished typescript, 16 pages (1985). In 1979, Raymond M. Kay, MD, issued *Historical Review of the Southern California Permanente Medical Group, Its Role in the Development of the Kaiser-Permanente Medical Care Program in Southern California* (Southern California Permanente Medical Group, Los Angeles, California, 1979). See also Kay's "Kaiser-Permanente Medical Care Program: Its Origin, Development, and Their Effects on its Future," a paper presented to the Kaiser Permanente Regional Conference on January 28, 1985. For the personal recollections of another Permanente pioneer, see Ernest W.

Saward, MD, "Speech to Interregional Medical Directors," presented on October 16, 1988, at San Diego. Three historical surveys published in house organs are also relevant: "Kaiser Plan Is Twenty Years Old," *Kaiser-Permanente Reporter*, 5 (March 1962), 1–8; "Organized Health Care Delivery Systems: A Historical Perspective," *Kaiser Foundation Medical Care Program Annual Report 1978*, pp. 4–24; and Penny Anderson, "Caring and Growing Since 1942," *Kaiser-Permanente Reporter*, Special 40th Anniversary Issue (August 1982). For the larger social and historical context of medical practice patterns in the United States, see Paul Starr's authoritative *The Social Transformation of American Medicine, The Rise of a Sovereign Profession and the Making of a Vast Industry* (Basic Books, New York, 1982).

Founder Sidney R. Garfield, MD, wrote the "First Annual Report of the Permanente Foundation Hospital," for the *Permanente Foundation Medical Bulletin*, 2 (January 1944): 35–48, and the "Second Annual Report," Ibid., 3 (January 1945): 31–47. For the Tenth Anniversary Issue of the *Bulletin*, Garfield wrote, "A Report on Permanente's First Ten Years," Ibid., 10 (August 1952): 1–11. Other significant statements by Garfield include: "Address to Multnomah County Medical Association, April 4, 1945," typescript, 7 pages, the Permanente Archives; "Kaiser Foundation Health Plan," a speech to the Subcommittee on General Insurance of the Assembly Interim Committee on Finance and Insurance, meeting in San Francisco, November 3–4, 1955, typescript 12 pages, the Cutting Files, box 1, file 1; and "Kaiser Foundation Hospitals of Northern California, Fifteenth Anniversary Address," unbound pamphlet, the Cutting Files, box 1, file 1. See also Sidney Garfield, M. F. Collen, and C. C. Cutting, "Permanente Medical Group: 'Historical' Remarks," presented at a meeting of physicians-in-chief and medical directors of all six regions of the Kaiser-Permanente Medical Care Program, April 24, 1974, the Permanente Archives.

Daniella Thompson interviewed Garfield on September 5, 6, 9, and 10, 1974. Miriam Stein interviewed him on February 17, 1982, and June 7, 1984. The cassettes and transcripts of these interviews are in the Audio-Visual Department of the Kaiser Foundation Health Plan and in the Permanente Archives. Thompson also wrote "Chapter One of a Proposed Biography of Dr. Sidney Garfield," typescript, 25 pages (1976), the Permanente Archives. The Permanente Archives also has an "Oral History" by Garfield in question-and-answer format. The 15-page typescript has no date, nor is the interviewer known. The February 1985 issue of the *Reporter* contains "Sidney Garfield, MD: Our Founder Remembered," pp. 1–6. See also "An Ounce of Prevention: Kaiser Family Foundation Honors USC Alumnus," *USC Medicine*, 34 (Spring 1987): 24–32.

Cecil Cutting, MD, has deposited in the Permanente Archives two cartons of materials gathered over the course of his years as executive director of The Permanente Medical Group. Carton 1 contains file copies of numerous published articles by Cutting, transcripts of some 50 papers and speeches he delivered between 1954 and 1974, and numerous press and professional articles dealing with one or another aspect of the Kaiser-Permanente Medical Care Plan through the early 1970s. Carton 2 contains minutes, agreements, memoranda, and other administrative materials, largely from the 1950s and 1960s. Articles by Cutting that proved of value to this history include "Medical Care: Its Social and Organizational Aspects — Group Practice and Pre-Payment," *New England Journal of Medicine*, 269 (3 October 1963): 729–736; "Organization of Medical Services Under Group Practice with Pre-payment," *American Journal of Surgery*, 118 (October 1969): 546–549; "Pre-Paid Medical Care — A Panel Discussion," *Group Practice*, 18, no. 10 (October 1969): 11–16; 18, no. 11 (November 1969): 13–18, 23–29; "The What, Why and How of Group Practice Pre-payment for Medical Care," *Southern Medical Bulletin*, 58, no. 5 (October 1970): 23–28; "Group Practice Pre-payment in the National Setting," *Group Practice*, 20, no. 2 (February 1971): 16–17; and "A Comprehensive Medical Care Delivery System Born in Industry," *Journal of Occupational Medicine*, 13, no. 9 (September 1971): 411–414. Historical articles by Cutting include "Historical Development and Operating Concepts," in The Kaiser-Permanente Medical Care Program, edited by Anne R. Somers (1971), pp. 17–22, and "The Early Years: From Grand Coulee through the Tahoe Conference," included in "A Program for the Board of Directors, 16 April 1974," bound typescript, the Permanente Archives.

Cutting was interviewed on tape on October 16, 1974 (2 cassettes), January 27, 1982 (1 cassette), March 16, 1982 (1 cassette), and some time thereafter (2 cassettes). These cassettes are in the Permanente Archives. Also in the Permanente Archives is a recording of Cutting's historical reminiscences given on November 2, 1984 (1 cassette), which Dr. Richmond Prescott, assistant to the executive director, has described as "a classic speech, honed to perfection over thirty years of delivery." Also of importance is Cutting's "Transcription of Oral History Regarding the Early Years of the Permanente Group," typescript, 8 pages (January 27, 1982) in the Permanente Archives. Other taped interviews available at the Audio-Visual Department of the Kaiser Foundation Health Plan and/or the Permanente Archives include J. Wallace Neighbor, MD (2 cassettes, September 20, 1974); Harry Kirby, MD (1 cassette, September 24, 1974); Richard Moore, MD (1 cassette, October 2, 1974); James Cooke (1 cassette, October 4, 1974); Bill Davis (1 cassette, October 7, 1974); Ed Bell (2 cassettes, March 14, 1975); Jack Chapman (2 cassettes, April 8, 1975); Morris Collen, MD (2 cassettes, May 13, 1975); Scott Fleming (1 cassette, March 18, 1982); Ray Kay, MD (March 21, 1975, 2 cassettes; May 5, 1982, 1 cassette); and Ernest Saward, MD (May 20, 1982, 2 cassettes). Eugene E. Trefethen, Jr., was interviewed by Miriam Stein on February 16, 1982, and by Sheila O'Brien on February 19, 1982. Transcripts of these interviews are in the Audio-Visual Department of the Kaiser Foundation Health Plan.

Through its ambitious and comprehensive Kaiser-Permanente Medical Care Program Oral History Project, the Regional Oral History Office of the Bancroft Library is in the process of preparing 20 or more edited and bound oral interviews of Kaiser-Permanente pioneers. These fastidiously prepared volumes constitute a well of living testimony that will forever nurture any and all scholarly investigations into the early history of Kaiser-Permanente. Oral histories by the following pioneers have proved especially pertinent to this volume: Morris Collen, MD; Wallace Cook, MD; Cecil Cutting, MD; Lambreth Hancock; Frank Jones; Raymond Kay, MD; Clifford Keene, MD; George Link; Ernest Saward, MD; John Smillie, MD; and Eugene Trefethen, Jr.

Also at the Bancroft Library are the Papers of Henry J. Kaiser: 387 cartons and 208 volumes, for a total of 430 linear feet. Carton 147 contains materials of relevance to the 1941–1945 period, especially hospital construction and expansion. Carton 183 has two folders, "Permanente Health Plan, 1945," with drafts and position papers relating to the organization of the program after the war. Carton 183 also contains a five-page, single-spaced letter by Garfield to Secretary of Commerce Henry Wallace explaining the prepaid group-practice concept. Carton 43 contains an interesting report dated November 2, 1948, from a visiting team of the American College of Surgeons to the Permanente Hospital in Oakland, giving the hospital a total of 888 points out of 995, for an overall rating of 89.2 percent. Carton 43 also contains documents descriptive of the Permanente Health Plan in 1949, including the scope of program benefits. Carton 50 has a folder entitled "Organizational Planning to Extend Kaiser Permanente Work" showing the program taking stock of its resources and planning for the future in 1949 at a critical time of membership expansion. Another folder in Carton 50, "Highlight Points for Discussion with A.M.A.," notes the 38 major unions in the United States, with a total of 11 million members, as an important basis for growth. Cartons 92, 93, 105, 112, and 117 are replete with files expressive of the program's tumultuous relations with county, state, and national medical societies during the 1950s. Cartons 77 and 78 chronicle the often difficult relations with the Alameda County draft board during the Korean War. Carton 67 contains files of relevance to the expansion of the program to southern California. Material relating to hospital expansion in the 1950s can be found in cartons 67, 77, 78, 89, 90, and 104. Cartons 78, 89, 92, and 93 deal with the expansion to Walnut Creek. Files in these cartons thoroughly document Henry J. Kaiser's close personal involvement in every aspect of this venture, down to and including the selection of cabinets. Cartons 248, 249, 250, and 251 deal with the expansion to Hawaii. Kaiser's personal correspondence runs through cartons 293 to 300.

Mark S. Foster's *Henry J. Kaiser, Builder in the Modern American West*, foreword by William H. Goetzmann (Austin, Texas, 1989), answers a long-standing need for a critical biography of one of the most important industrialists of the twentieth century. Regarding Kaiser's wartime efforts, see, David Sudhalter, "How 'Hurry Up Henry' Helped Win the War," *Reporter*, April 1987, 4–6. For the atmosphere at the Richmond Shipyards, see the fictionalized sketches by Joseph Fabry gathered as *Swing Shift, Building the Liberty Ships* (Strawberry Hill Press, San Francisco, 1982). Paul De Kruif's *Kaiser Wakes the Doctors* (Harcourt, Brace, New York, 1943) is an early discussion of the Permanente program. See also De Kruif's *Life Among the Doctors* (Harcourt, Brace, New York, 1949), pp. 375–429, for a discussion of Garfield and the Permanente program in the postwar period as the medical establishment stepped up its resistance. Kaiser defended the Permanente program in Washington, DC, before the House Committee on Interstate and Foreign Commerce on January 11, 1954. A draft of Kaiser's statement, "A Private Enterprise Solution to Medical Care by the Doctors of this Country," can be found in the Cutting Files, carton 1. Regarding Edgar Kaiser, see the January 1982 memorial issue of the *Reporter*, especially Sidney Garfield's "The Coulee Dream, A Fond Remembrance of Edgar Kaiser," pp. 3–4. Defenses of Kaiser-Permanente in the *Congressional Record* include "The Kaiser-Permanente Medical Care Program" by Senator James E. Murray (July 6, 1949); "A Private Enterprise Solution to Medical Care by the Doctors of this Country" by Representative Charles A. Wolverton (January 6, 1954); and "Kaiser Foundation Medical Care Program—the Nation's Largest Prepaid Direct Service Medical and Hospital Plan" by Representative Chet Holifield (February 28, 1963).

The Minutes of the Executive Committee are in the Permanente Archives. The Cutting Files include a number of relevant documents. These include "Articles of Partnership" (February 22, 1948); the "Tahoe Agreement" (July 1955); the Minutes of the Regional Management Team of the Kaiser Foundation Hospitals in Northern California (1955–1957); the Minutes of the Board of Directors and the Minutes of the Regional Coordinating Committee of the Southern California Permanente Medical Group (1956–1962); and two versions of the "Policy Manual of the Permanente Medical Group," issued in July 1958 and updated in January 1964. There are also two volumes containing the "Contractual History" of the Permanente Medical Group through March 1958.

An early assessment of group practice was done by G. Halsey Hunt, MD, and Marcus S. Goldstein, PhD, *Medical Group Practice in the United States*, issued by the Federal Security Agency and the Public Health Service (1951). In March 1971 Kaiser-Permanente, the Commonwealth Fund, and the Association of American Medical Colleges sponsored a major symposium in Oakland. Anne R. Somers edited the proceedings as *The Kaiser-Permanente Medical Care Program: One Valid Solution to the Problem of Health Care Delivery in the United States* (1971). The Board of Directors of the Kaiser Foundation Hospitals and the Kaiser Foundation Health Plan reviewed its program on April 16, 1974. The briefing book for this meeting, "A Program for the Board of Directors," contains many useful assessments. See also Scott Fleming and Douglas Gentry's *A Perspective on Kaiser-Permanente Type Health Care Programs: The Performance Record, Criticisms and Responses* (January 1979); and Ernest W. Saward, MD, and Scott Fleming, "Health Maintenance Organizations," *Scientific American* 243 (1980): 47–53. In-house publications of varied usefulness to this history include the *Permanente Foundation Medical Bulletin* (1942–1952) and the *Annual Reports* of the Kaiser-Permanente Medical Care Program (1962–1984). See also Greer Williams, *Kaiser-Permanente Health Plan, Why It Works* (1971).

No complete listing of newspaper and periodical coverage of Kaiser-Permanente is possible in this space. Yet certain coverage has been of special importance to this study. These include Lester Velie, "Supermarket Medicine," *The Saturday Evening Post*, (20 June 1953): 22–23, 48–49; Hale Champion, "How New Kaiser Hospital Works," *San Francisco Chronicle*, 14, 15, and 16 February 1954; and, George Dusheck, "Henry Kaiser's 'Big Medicine'," *San Francisco News*, 29, 30, and 31 October, and 1 November 1957. Regarding the expansions to Denver and Cleveland, see "Giant Group Practice Heads East," *Medical World News*, 9, no. 44 (1 November 1968): 44–50. Important coverage in *Time* can be found in the issues for June 29, 1953, July 5, 1954, October 24, 1960, and September 14, 1962. See also Sheila K. Johnson's profile in the *New York Times* for April 28, 1974, "Kaiser Permanente Is a Good Legacy of the Great Depression."

Index

Throughout this index the name of Sidney Garfield has been abbreviated to SG.

About the Author

John G. Smillie, M.D. is a physician-manager now retired
from The Permanente Medical Group, Inc. Affiliating with
The Permanente Medical Group in San Francisco in 1949,
he served in a variety of capacities, including staff physician,
Chief of Pediatrics, Physician-in-Chief, Assistant to the
Executive Director, government relations representative, and
liaison from all of the Permanente medical groups to the
Central Office of the Kaiser Foundation Health Plan in
Oakland, California. He is a past trustee of the American
Group Practice Association, and former president and
chairman of the board of the Group Health Association of
America. Dr. Smillie is a graduate of the Harvard Business
School Program for Health Systems Management.